Bayesian Missing Data Problems

EM, Data Augmentation and Noniterative Computation

Chapman & Hall/CRC Biostatistics Series

Chapman & Hall/CRC Biostatistics Series

Published Titles

1. *Design and Analysis of Animal Studies in Pharmaceutical Development,* Shein-Chung Chow and Jen-pei Liu
2. *Basic Statistics and Pharmaceutical Statistical Applications,* James E. De Muth
3. *Design and Analysis of Bioavailability and Bioequivalence Studies, Second Edition, Revised and Expanded,* Shein-Chung Chow and Jen-pei Liu
4. *Meta-Analysis in Medicine and Health Policy,* Dalene K. Stangl and Donald A. Berry
5. *Generalized Linear Models: A Bayesian Perspective,* Dipak K. Dey, Sujit K. Ghosh, and Bani K. Mallick
6. *Difference Equations with Public Health Applications,* Lemuel A. Moyé and Asha Seth Kapadia
7. *Medical Biostatistics,* Abhaya Indrayan and Sanjeev B. Sarmukaddam
8. *Statistical Methods for Clinical Trials,* Mark X. Norleans
9. *Causal Analysis in Biomedicine and Epidemiology: Based on Minimal Sufficient Causation,* Mikel Aickin
10. *Statistics in Drug Research: Methodologies and Recent Developments,* Shein-Chung Chow and Jun Shao
11. *Sample Size Calculations in Clinical Research,* Shein-Chung Chow, Jun Shao, and Hansheng Wang
12. *Applied Statistical Design for the Researcher,* Daryl S. Paulson
13. *Advances in Clinical Trial Biostatistics,* Nancy L. Geller
14. *Statistics in the Pharmaceutical Industry, Third Edition,* Ralph Buncher and Jia-Yeong Tsay
15. *DNA Microarrays and Related Genomics Techniques: Design, Analysis, and Interpretation of Experiments,* David B. Allsion, Grier P. Page, T. Mark Beasley, and Jode W. Edwards
16. *Basic Statistics and Pharmaceutical Statistical Applications, Second Edition,* James E. De Muth
17. *Adaptive Design Methods in Clinical Trials,* Shein-Chung Chow and Mark Chang
18. *Handbook of Regression and Modeling: Applications for the Clinical and Pharmaceutical Industries,* Daryl S. Paulson
19. *Statistical Design and Analysis of Stability Studies,* Shein-Chung Chow
20. *Sample Size Calculations in Clinical Research, Second Edition,* Shein-Chung Chow, Jun Shao, and Hansheng Wang
21. *Elementary Bayesian Biostatistics,* Lemuel A. Moyé
22. *Adaptive Design Theory and Implementation Using SAS and R,* Mark Chang
23. *Computational Pharmacokinetics,* Anders Källén
24. *Computational Methods in Biomedical Research,* Ravindra Khattree and Dayanand N. Naik
25. *Medical Biostatistics, Second Edition,* A. Indrayan
26. *DNA Methylation Microarrays: Experimental Design and Statistical Analysis,* Sun-Chong Wang and Arturas Petronis
27. *Design and Analysis of Bioavailability and Bioequivalence Studies, Third Edition,* Shein-Chung Chow and Jen-pei Liu
28. *Translational Medicine: Strategies and Statistical Methods,* Dennis Cosmatos and Shein-Chung Chow
29. *Bayesian Methods for Measures of Agreement,* Lyle D. Broemeling
30. *Data and Safety Monitoring Committees in Clinical Trials,* Jay Herson
31. *Design and Analysis of Clinical Trials with Time-to-Event Endpoints,* Karl E. Peace
32. *Bayesian Missing Data Problems: EM, Data Augmentation and Noniterative Computation,* Ming T. Tan, Guo-Liang Tian, and Kai Wang Ng

Chapman & Hall/CRC Biostatistics Series

Bayesian Missing Data Problems

EM, Data Augmentation and Noniterative Computation

Ming T. Tan
University of Maryland School of Medicine
Baltimore, Maryland, U.S.A.

Guo-Liang Tian
The University of Hong Kong
Hong Kong, China

Kai Wang Ng
The University of Hong Kong
Hong Kong, China

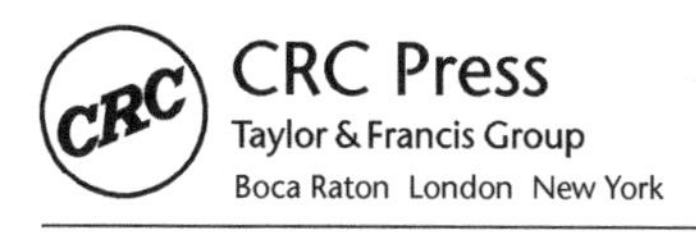

CRC Press is an imprint of the
Taylor & Francis Group, an **informa** business
A CHAPMAN & HALL BOOK

CRC Press
Taylor & Francis Group
6000 Broken Sound Parkway NW, Suite 300
Boca Raton, FL 33487-2742

First issued in paperback 2019

ISBN-13: 978-1-4200-7749-0 (hbk)
ISBN-13: 978-0-367-38530-9 (pbk)

Visit the Taylor & Francis Web site at
http://www.taylorandfrancis.com

and the CRC Press Web site at
http://www.crcpress.com

To Donna, Kenny, Calvin and Chloe

To Yanli, Margaret and Adam

To May, Jeanne and Jason

Contents

Preface

The *expectation-maximization* (EM) method, the *data augmentation* (DA) method, together with their improved versions are well-known techniques for handling *missing data problems* (MDPs). The **DA method** consists of two parts: (a) the **DA structure** of three constituents, namely a set of parameters, a set of observable data and a set of latent variables whose values are not available, and (b) the **DA algorithm(s)** for finding the observed posterior density of parameter or for sampling from observed posterior distribution. With regard to practical posterior computation in Bayesian analysis of MDPs, including the calculation of posterior densities or intervals, the last 20 years or so have seen the proliferation of methods based on iterative sampling until convergence, such as Gibbs and other *Markov chain Monte Carlo* (MCMC) sampling.

There are, however, two vital issues regarding such iterative samplers, which are all too easily overlooked by many users in applications. First, the values of the variate generated in the same iterative process are hardly ever independent. Second, although in theory an iterative sampler will generate the target variate in the limit, we still need to find a water-tight procedure that can check convincingly whether the stage of convergence has been reached upon termination of iteration. Otherwise, the generated variate may have a distribution other than the desired, which may be one that is unknown to the user. Obviously, formulating criteria for judging convergence of iterative sampling is hugely more difficult than is the case with iterative approximations of constants or functions in mathematics. So "in general, convergence can never be assessed," as pointed out by Gelfand (2002).

These issues have prompted some researchers to take the view that the MCMC methods are to be used only when there is no better alternative; see, e.g., discussions in Evans & Swartz (1995, 2000) and Hobert & Casella (1996). In fact, strenuous efforts have been expended to find alternatives, even though MCMC methods for posterior computation in Bayesian analysis have become overwhelmingly popular among methodologists and general users. For example, the so-called **perfect sampler** (Casella, Lavine & Robert, 2001) is an ideal alternative. However, it is unfortunately limited to rather simple statistical models.

It is natural to find other alternatives between the two extremes and this book aims to fill that void. We shall introduce noniterative methods in dealing with DA structures that allow us either to obtain the posterior density analytically, or to generate independent values of a variate following the posterior distribution through non-iterative sampling so that there is no issue with convergence, and to demonstrate their wide range of applications, especially in biostatistics. We shall also illustrate the roles of EM-type algorithms in such methods.

The non-iterative approach described in this book was discovered by one of us (KWN) in 1994. On re-examining the seminal paper of Tanner & Wong (1987), especially their process of solving an integral equation, which was the key to the "successive substitution" algorithm of the DA method proposed in the paper, Ng found a simple explicit solution (Ng, 1995a, 1995b). The solution had the interpretation of an inversion of the Bayes formula under the positivity condition, so he coined it the *Inverse Bayes Formula* (IBF).

The results were delivered in April 1996 and published in (Ng, 1997a). Non-iterative sampling and avenues for applications were discussed in a presentation (Ng, 1997b). With the intention of promoting joint research, Ng briefed Tian, a co-author of this book, the results and progress of IBF up to then and gave him reading materials during Tian's frequent visits to Hong Kong, initially from mainland China and later from the USA where he worked with Tan (the first author) in biostatistics and biomedical research.

While developing the MCMC solution for the hierarchical models of multi-level ordinal data (Tan *et al.*, 1999; Qiu *et al.*, 2002), Tan realized the advantages of having a non-iterative sampling procedure in Bayesian computation from a practical point of view, e.g., elimination of lengthy convergence diagnostics which do not necessarily ensure getting the stationary distribution when iteration is terminated and, equally importantly, the ease of presentation to nonstatisticians. Tian thus presented the results about IBF to Tan who then decided to replace the MCMC approach by the non-iterative sampling approach as facilitated by the function-wise formula. A solution was found next day by Tian in the normal linear model setting (Tan *et al.*, 2001).

That was a big boost to the first two authors' confidence in IBF methods. Since then, they persistently pursued applications of IBF methods to all kinds of problems wherever possible, and contributed many new ideas to facilitate IBF application and methodological developments, such as combining Rubin's *sampling/importance resampling* (SIR) procedure with IBF in cases where the envelope function in acceptance-rejection method is not easy to find, fine-tuning the noniterative sampling approach and developing methods for particular problems, etc. In recent years, the joint research of the three authors showed that the IBF-based methods, coupled with EM-type algorithms in certain situations, have a wide range of applications in *Bayesian analysis* of MDP such as the mixed-effects models and in *constrained parameter problems* for DA structures.

Our aim is to provide a systematic introduction to IBF-based methods, which combine the strengths of existing approaches via DA. We hope the systematic introduction may stimulate interest in the direct leading to solutions of both applied and theoretical problems. In particular, we anticipate that the more straightforward posterior computation would also be useful in Bayesian clinical trial design and analysis, where the final results have to be presented to a diverse audience including government agencies (such as the Food and Drug Administration), academia (e.g., scientific journals) and pharmaceutical companies.

The book is intended as a graduate text for a one- or two-semester course at the advanced Master or Ph.D. level, and as a reference book for researchers, teachers, applied statisticians and biostatisticians. The book is also useful to undergraduates in statistics and to practitioners (especially in drug development and biostatistics) who need a good understanding of Monte Carlo simulation and Bayesian approaches to MDPs. Knowledge of basic probability, statistics and Bayesian method is a prerequisite for this book, although reviews of these basic materials in Chapters 1 and 2, along with the Appendix on distributions and implementation, make the book quite self-contained. All R or S-plus codes for examples in this book are available at the following URLs:

http://medschool.umaryland.edu/facultyresearchprofile/
viewprofile.aspx?id=6775

http://www.hku.hk/statistics/staff/gltian/

http://www.hku.hk/statistics/staff/kaing/

A book such as this cannot be completed without substantial assistance from outside the team. Much of the original research findings presented is supported in part by U.S. National Cancer Institute grants CA119758 and CA106767. We gratefully acknowledge support by the Department of Mathematics, Hong Kong Baptist University, and Department of Probability and Statistics, Peking University, and especially the Department of Statistics & Actuarial Science of The University of Hong Kong where the final version was done. We are grateful to Prof. Z. Geng of Peking University, Dr. X.P. Xiong of St. Jude Children's Research Hospital, Dr. M.L. Tang of Hong Kong Baptist University, and Drs. H.B. Fang and Z.Q. Liu of University of Maryland Greenebaum Cancer Center, for the many constructive conversations. We thank Dr. C.X. Ma who helped a couple of LaTex novices get started on the long journey of writing this book.

Baltimore	Ming T. Tan
Hong Kong	Guo-Liang Tian
Hong Kong	Kai Wang Ng
December 2008	

CHAPTER 1

Introduction

1.1 Background

A *missing data problem* (MDP) refers to one where certain data are really missing, or where the problem itself has no data that are actually missing but can be reformulated as a problem of this type, say by augmenting latent variables whose values are not available. In fact, many statistical problems can be formulated as MDPs (Little & Rubin, 2002).

The *expectation-maximization* (EM) algorithm (Dempster *et al.*, 1977; Meng & van Dyk, 1997; McLachlan & Krishnan, 1997) is an iterative deterministic method for finding *maximum likelihood estimates* (MLEs) of the parameters of interest. The EM procedure is a powerful tool for likelihood-based inference, especially for missing (or incomplete) data problems. There are difficult challenges for likelihood-based inference, such as finding their standard errors in multiparameter problems (Meng & Rubin, 1991), dealing with nuisance parameters (see §1.4.2) and having samples of small to moderate size where the asymptotic theory of MLE may not apply. It is appealing therefore to use the Bayesian approach, especially when the sample size is small. In the latter case, the question is how to carry out the posterior computation.

As a Bayesian counterpart to the EM algorithm for incomplete data analysis, the *data augmentation* (DA) method was proposed in the seminal paper of Tanner & Wong (1987). To be specific, the **DA method** in the paper consisted of two parts: (a) the **DA structure** of three density functions, $\pi(\theta|y), f(z|y,\theta)$ and $p(\theta|y,z)$, where θ is the parameter (vector), y represents the observable data and z represents the augmented latent variables (whose values are not available); and (b) the **DA algorithm** to find the observed posterior density $\pi(\theta|y)$ given the other two density functions using the "successive substitution method" of functional analysis, to be implemented with Monte Carlo approximation in each substitution step.

The later trend of posterior computation in Bayesian analysis emphasizes sampling from the posterior distribution, like sampling from $\pi(\theta|y)$ instead of directly calculating $\pi(\theta|y)$ in the context of DA structure. The Gibbs sampler was first introduced by Geman & Geman (1984) as an application of *Markov chain Monte Carlo* (MCMC) sampling and made popular in the Bayesian computation literature by Gelfand & Smith (1990). Hence for the DA structure in this new trend, a two-block Gibbs sampling based on $f(z|y,\theta)$ and $p(\theta|y,z)$ became a new DA algorithm. Literature on Gibbs and MCMC methods prior to 1993 and interesting discussions on the subject in a Royal Statistical Society meeting can be found in JRSSB, vol.55, 3–102.

All iterative sampling methods face two issues: (i) the dependence nature of generated values in the same iterative process and (ii) the difficulty of certifying convergence. As pointed out by Gelfand (2002), "in general, convergence can never be assessed, as comparison can be made only between different iterations of one chain or between different observed chains, but never with the true stationary distribution." A nuanced opinion is that the MCMC methods are to be used only when there is no better alternative; see discussions in Evans & Swartz (1995, 2000) and Hobert & Casella (1996).

In 1994, a co-author of this book (KWN) was attracted to the paper of Tanner & Wong (1987), as Professor W. H. Wong was the new Head of Statistics in the Chinese University of Hong Kong around that time and the monograph (Tanner, 1993) expanding details of the paper in its third printing. Later the popular monograph was in its Third Edition (Tanner, 1996; Chapter 5). That paper was invited with discussions by prominent statisticians like A.P. Dempster, C.N. Morris, Donald B. Rubin, Shelby J. Haberman and A. O'Hagan. The successive substitution algorithm in the paper is to solve a key integral equation which, in the present notation, is as follows:

$$\pi(\theta|y) = \int p(\theta|y,z)\left\{\int f(z|y,\phi)\pi(\phi|y)d\phi\right\}dz. \qquad (*)$$

The authors provided sufficient conditions (see §1.5.3 for more details) for convergence of successive substitution, which was further studied by Schervish & Carlin (1992).

Since some of the sufficient conditions were not easy to check in practice, Ng intended to study the integral equation with his past experience in fixed-point theorems in functional analysis (Ng, 1969, 1970). But when he tried to formulate plainer sufficient conditions to ensure convergence, certain thoughts struck him. In the whole functional equation $(*)$ that connects $\pi(\theta|y)$, $f(z|y,\theta)$ and $p(\theta|y,z)$,

y was constant throughout. So dropping y, it was equivalent to finding $\pi(\theta)$ in terms of $f(z|\theta)$ and $p(\theta|z)$. That required going in the opposite direction to the Bayes formula: **from posterior to prior**! So he realized that the real question was finding the *Inverse Bayes Formula* (IBF) and thus he coined the solution as such.

In the basic version of Bayes formula concerning probabilities of non-void events, one has no obstacle at all in expressing the unconditional probability of an event in terms of conditional probabilities. The same is true for densities under the positivity condition as in the paper, replacing summation by integral. Thus the solution to the equation (*) has the following dual forms:

$$\pi(\theta|y) = \left\{ \int \frac{f(z|y,\theta)}{p(\theta|y,z)} \, dz \right\}^{-1} \tag{**}$$

$$= \left\{ \int \frac{p(\theta|y,z_0)}{f(z_0|y,\theta)} \, d\theta \right\}^{-1} \frac{p(\theta|y,z_0)}{f(z_0|y,\theta)}, \tag{***}$$

where in the second form (***), z_0 is arbitrary and the normalizing constant equals the predictive density $g(z|y)$ of Z given Y, by virtue of mathematical symmetry of z and θ in the first identity. When we substitute the second equality into (*), the inside integral gives $g(z|y)$ and hence the outside integral returns $\pi(\theta|y)$. The dual forms are respectively called the **point-wise formula** and the **function-wise formula**. The degree of simplicity of either form is on a par with the Bayes formula, which is good since simplicity is a virtue as argued in Lindley (1995).

Once said, it becomes obvious that we should have taught the IBF in any first course of probability and statistics in tandem with the Bayes formula as a two-way street. Given this simplicity, it is even possible that in areas other than statistics, the IBF has already appeared without our noticing it. For example, if there is a publication in medical research that can evaluate the prevalence of a certain disease in a population based on both the conditional probabilities of symptoms given the disease status and the conditional probabilities of disease status given the symptoms, then it is the IBF at work; and if, however, there is no such publication, this would be a very useful new application of IBF in medicine.

The basic results on IBF were summarized in a paper delivered in April 1996 to the editors of a volume in honor of Professor Samuel Kotz, which was published in (Ng, 1997a). For inversion of the Bayes formula without positivity condition, explicit or neat formulae may not be available. Algorithms instead of formulae to deal with such situations, for example in a projection-connected support space, were reported in the Sydney International Statistical Congress 1996, July 1996 (Ng, 1996). Avenues for application of IBF and noniterative sampling as alternative to MCMC methods were discussed in a conference presentation (Ng, 1997b).

With hindsight, Ng (1997a) has commented on the sudden emergence of IBF in unexpected circumstances:

> "However, the relative probability formula (2.2) of Besag (1974), the consistency condition (4.3) of Arnold and Press (1989), and the introductory discussion of Gelman and Speed (1993) were very close, but the authors did not turn the corner to get the Inverse Bayes formulae given here. Indeed, it is fair to say that all of us statisticians have been very close to the solution, since the identities (37.3) and (37.4) in Section 37.2 are well known."

Apparently without the opportunity of reading Ng's writings on IBF, Meng (1996) once raised an interesting enquiry in respect of the point-wise formula as follows [his equation (1) is equivalent to $(**)$ after dropping the y and his reference Ng (1995) is Ng (1995b) in this book]:

> "I learned the expression (1) from a presentation by Ng (1995). My immediate reaction was that it must be my ignorance that I had not seen (1) in this explicit form. However, Ng assured me that he had checked with several leading experts in this area (e.g., J. Besag, W. H. Wong), and it seemed that the identity (1) was 'mysteriously' missing from the general literature. An apparent explanation for this 'mystery' is that (1) is not useful in general for calculating $f_X(x)$ and thus $f_{(X,Y)}(x, y)$ since a main reason we use the Gibbs sampler is our inability to perform analytical integration, which is required by (1)."

Explanation for this "mystery" based on usefulness is not particularly convincing, however. It overlooks the duality that one form implies the other; indeed, we need the dual forms of the solution to satisfy the integral equation $(*)$. More importantly, it overlooks the fact that the point-wise formula $(**)$ reveals a **fundamental property** of the prior density in terms of the posterior density:

With respect to repeated sampling of data conditional on a fixed parameter value, the harmonic mean of the posterior density at that parameter value equals the prior density at the same parameter value.

Its **philosophical interpretation** is too dramatic to miss: *One can fix the prior distribution to get the desired posterior distribution.* With such an important implication for Bayesian inference, how could we statisticians have missed it for so many years simply because it was not useful, if any one of us had come across it?

In those continuous cases where the point-wise form $(**)$ is not useful for calculating the whole prior density, its dual form $(***)$ reduces that calculation to numerical approximation of a single constant corresponding to an arbitrary set of data, which we can choose for the purpose of easier approximation of the constant in question.

For the purpose of sampling, the function-wise formula $(***)$ can facilitate noniterative sampling, say through using acceptance-rejection method. In the case of DA structure, we shall choose a convenient z_0 to find an envelope function covering the target function $p(\theta|y, z_0)/f(z_0|y, \theta)$.

Around the year 2000, the first two authors joined research in this direction. Since then, application and development of the IBF-based methods to MDPs have progressed more quickly than before, including:

- Incomplete pre-post test problems (Tan *et al.*, 2001);
- Incomplete longitudinal data in tumor xenograft models (Tan *et al.*, 2002; Tan, Fang & Tian, 2005);
- Incomplete contingency tables (Tian *et al.*, 2003);
- Normal linear mixed-effects models (Tan, Tian & Ng, 2003);
- Multivariate normality test with incomplete data (Tan, Fang, Tian & Wei, 2005);
- Hierarchical models for repeated binary data (Tan, Tian & Ng, 2006);
- Discrete missing data problems (Tian, Tan & Ng, 2007);
- Generalized linear mixed models for correlated binary data (Tan, Tian & Fang, 2007);

- Changepoint problems (Tian, Ng, Li & Tan, 2009);
- Constrained parameter problems (Tan, Tian & Fang, 2003; Fang *et al.*, 2004, 2006; Tan, Fang, Tian & Houghton, 2005; Tan, Tian, Fang & Ng, 2007; Tian, Ng & Tan, 2008); and
- Checking compatibility and uniqueness for two given conditional distributions (Tian, Tan, Ng & Tang, 2009; Tian, Tang & Ng, 2009).

1.2 Scope, Aim and Outline

With the aforementioned background, we have restricted the scope of this book to

1° Bayesian MDPs,

2° constrained parameter problems, and

3° compatibility and uniqueness problems (arisen in distribution theory and the convergence diagnosis of the Gibbs sampler).

Although the models we present in this book can be used in many disciplines (e.g., medicine, public health, epidemiology, biology, engineering, reliability, economics and social science), the applications will focus on biomedical studies and health services research, especially, in cancer and HIV. There have been several textbooks (e.g., Gelman *et al.*, 1995; Gamerman, 1997; Robert & Casella, 1999; Carlin & Louis, 2000) and monographs (e.g., Tanner, 1996; Gilks *et al.*, 1996; Schafer, 1997; Chen *et al.*, 2000; Liu, 2001; Little & Rubin, 2002) that address to some extent MDPs and constrained parameter problems from a frequentist or Bayesian (say, MCMC) perspective. All these books have covered a broad range of topics and all use the MCMC method that produces dependent posterior samples. However, explicit (including closed-form) solutions to statistical problems and i.i.d. posterior samples are preferred in statistical theory and practice for obvious reasons. For example, they are theoretically simple, eliminating a harder convergence assessment problem, and can facilitate the communication of statistical analysis to a wider audience. One significant feature of the IBF-based methods presented in this book is their simplicity (e.g., explicit or exact solutions) and that the IBF sampling is *noniterative*, thus yielding i.i.d. posterior samples. All data analysis in this book is performed using R or S-plus on a personal computer.

Our aim is to provide a systematic introduction of the IBF-based methods for *missing data problems* (MDPs) which combine the strengths of the existing approaches via DA. Practically, the IBF sampler is a method to quickly generate i.i.d. samples approximately from the posterior once the posterior mode is identified. On the other hand, it combines the strengths of the SIR and EM-type algorithms. SIR generates i.i.d. samples but does not provide an efficient built-in importance sampling function directly from the model specification of a practical problem. It is easy to check if the EM has converged to the posterior mode or not, but it is difficult to find its standard error. The EM/DA and the sampling IBF share the structure of augmented posterior/conditional predictive distributions, thus no extra derivations are needed for the IBF sampler. This implies that the IBF sampler is applicable to problems where any EM-type algorithms apply.

In the remaining part of this chapter, we first introduce the dual forms of IBF and the derived versions, including Monte Carlo and the generalization to the case of three components. Next, we present the Bayesian methodology from a new perspective based on the IBF through a concise formulation of the posterior distribution, nuisance parameter problem, posterior predictive distribution, Bayes factor and estimation of marginal likelihood. We then address missing data problems by describing missing data mechanism, the notion of DA, the original DA algorithm of Tanner & Wong (1987), and its connections with both the Gibbs sampler and the IBF. Finally, we briefly introduce two useful concepts: Shannon entropy and Kullback–Leibler divergence, which have important applications in multivariate analysis and Bayesian statistics.

Chapter 2 covers basic statistical *optimization* techniques (e.g., the famous Newton–Raphson algorithm, Fisher scoring algorithm, EM-type and more general MM algorithms), useful *Monte Carlo simulation* tools (e.g., the inversion method, rejection, SIR, stochastic representation, conditional sampling and the vertical density representation method) and major *numerical integration* approaches including Laplace approximations, Riemannian simulation, importance sampling and the *cross-entropy* (CE) method. The CE method is usually not covered by standard statistics textbooks but is becoming increasingly important in modern Monte Carlo integration, especially in rare event simulation (Rubinstein & Kroese, 2004).

In Chapter 3, we first show that the IBF can be used to derive closed-form solutions to several Bayesian missing data problems including sample surveys with nonresponse, misclassified multinomial model, genetic linkage model, Weibull process, prediction problem, binormal model, 2×2 crossover trial with missing data and hierarchical models. Then we extend the IBF in product measurable space to nonproduct measurable space and focus on their applications in obtaining exact solutions.

Since many statistical problems can be formulated as discrete MDPs, Chapter 4 introduces an exact IBF sampling to obtain i.i.d. samples from posterior distribution in discrete MDPs. The algorithm is essentially a conditional sampling method, thus completely avoiding the issues with convergence in iterative algorithms such as Gibbs and MCMC. Examples such as genetic linkage model, contingency tables with one (or two) supplemental margin(s), hidden sensitivity model for surveys with two sensitive questions, zero-inflated Poisson model, changepoint problems and capture-recapture model are analyzed to illustrate the algorithm.

Chapter 5 provides a noniterative IBF sampling by combining the SIR with posterior mode estimates from EM-type algorithms to obtain an i.i.d. sample approximately from the posterior distribution for problems where the EM-type algorithms apply. First, incomplete pre-post test problems, right censored regression model, linear mixed models for longitudinal data, probit regression model for independent binary data, a probit-normal *generalized linear mixed model* (GLMM) for repeated binary data, hierarchical models for correlated binary data and several related real data sets are used to illustrate the method. Next, a hybrid algorithm by combining the IBF sampler with the Gibbs sampler is presented. Finally, three new monitoring approaches based on the IBF for assessing convergence of MCMC are introduced.

Chapter 6 illustrates how the EM, DA and IBF algorithms can be used for maximum likelihood and Bayesian estimation in normal distribution subject to linear inequality constraints, Poisson distribution and binomial distribution with a class of simplex constraints.

Checking compatibility for two given conditional distributions and identifying the corresponding unique compatible marginal distributions are important problems in mathematical statistics forming the theoretical underpinning of applications, especially in Bayesian statistical inferences. Chapter 7 gives a comprehensive review on the existing methods including the IBF for this topic. Product measurable space and nonproduct measurable space are distinguished and the continuous case and the finite discrete case are considered individually. Extension from two given conditionals to the case of given one marginal and another conditional are also presented.

In Appendix A, we outline some useful distributions including abbreviation, support, density, mean, variance, covariance, properties, relationship with other distributions and the random variable generation method or the existing S-plus function. In addition, we also provide a summary of the Poisson process and the nonhomogeneous Poisson process.

1.3 Inverse Bayes Formulae (IBF)

The Bayes formula, Bayes rule, or Bayes theorem, was published posthumously and named after Reverend Thomas Bayes (1763) and has been the foundation of Bayesian inference (Press, 1989). Historically, the Bayesian inference is the first default paradigm of statistical inference and was referred to the "classical procedure" by earlier European literature in contrast to the "modern formulation" of R.A. Fisher; see the later English translation of Gnedenko (1962, p.409 & p.419). Many modern writings seem to ignore this historical fact and call the latter approach "classical" while referring to the older one as "modern."

The Bayesian paradigm starts with a prior distribution of the parameter that reflects our information about, or subjective evaluation of, competing values of the parameter before collecting data and then revise the prior distribution to the posterior distribution with available data according to Bayes formula. It is therefore *unimaginable for people to even ponder the question of inverting the Bayes formula*, because that question would be equivalent to asking the following questions which might sound too sensitive:

> Can I find a prior distribution to get the posterior distribution I want? If yes, how?

That subconscious taboo might be the reason why the IBF has escaped the attention of so many statisticians for so long, until it arises unexpectedly in a problem (cf. §1.1) supposed to find a posterior distribution given available data. In the grand play of academic history, this act has both elements of drama and absurdity.

There have been some guesses on why Reverend Bayes did not send his finished fine essay to the Royal Society (e.g., see Stigler, 1983, p.295). One new guess now is that perhaps he realized the two-way nature/feature of the argument *from prior to posterior*, only after he had completed the essay and thus needed more time to revise it.

1.3.1 The point-wise, function-wise & sampling IBF

Since deriving the three IBF from the Bayes formula with rigor involving integration in the support of an r.v., we first need to distinguish two important notions: the product measurable space and the nonproduct measurable space. Let two random variables/vectors (X, Y) taking values in the space $(\mathcal{X}, \mathcal{Y})$ be absolutely continuous with respect to some measure μ on the joint support

$$\mathcal{S}_{(X,Y)} = \{(x, y) : f_{(X,Y)}(x, y) > 0,\ (x, y) \in (\mathcal{X}, \mathcal{Y})\},$$

where $f_{(X,Y)}(x, y)$ denotes the joint *probability density function* (pdf) of (X, Y). We denote the marginal and conditional pdfs of X and Y by $f_X(x)$, $f_Y(y)$, $f_{(X|Y)}(x|y)$ and $f_{(Y|X)}(y|x)$, respectively. Let $\mathcal{S}_X = \{x : f_X(x) > 0,\ x \in \mathcal{X}\}$ and $\mathcal{S}_Y = \{y : f_Y(y) > 0,\ y \in \mathcal{Y}\}$ denote the supports of X and Y, respectively. If $\mathcal{S}_{(X,Y)} = \mathcal{S}_X \times \mathcal{S}_Y$, then the measure μ is said to be *product measurable* and μ can be written as $\mu_X \times \mu_Y$; otherwise, it is said to be *nonproduct measurable*. The absolute continuous assumption allows discussion of a continuous variable (i.e., its density is Lebesgue measurable) with a discrete variable (i.e., its probability mass function gives rise to a counting measure). To fix the idea, we denote the conditional supports of $X|(Y{=}y)$ and $Y|(X{=}x)$ by

$$\begin{aligned} \mathcal{S}_{(X|Y)}(y) &= \{x : f_{(X|Y)}(x|y) > 0, x \in \mathcal{X}\} \quad \forall\, y \in \mathcal{S}_Y \ \text{ and} \\ \mathcal{S}_{(Y|X)}(x) &= \{y : f_{(Y|X)}(y|x) > 0, y \in \mathcal{Y}\} \quad \forall\, x \in \mathcal{S}_X. \end{aligned}$$

In practice, we usually have: $\mathcal{S}_{(Y|X)}(x) \subseteq \mathcal{S}_Y$ for all $x \in \mathcal{S}_X$, and $\mathcal{S}_{(X|Y)}(y) \subseteq \mathcal{S}_X$ for all $y \in \mathcal{S}_Y$. The joint pdf then is

$$f_{(X|Y)}(x|y) f_Y(y) = f_{(Y|X)}(y|x) f_X(x), \quad (x, y) \in \mathcal{S}_{(X,Y)}. \tag{1.1}$$

In product-measurable case, we have $\mathcal{S}_{(Y|X)}(x) = \mathcal{S}_Y$ for all $x \in \mathcal{S}_X$, and $\mathcal{S}_{(X|Y)}(y) = \mathcal{S}_X$ for all $y \in \mathcal{S}_Y$. Hence from (1.1) we get by division

$$f_Y(y) = \frac{f_{(Y|X)}(y|x)}{f_{(X|Y)}(x|y)} \cdot f_X(x), \qquad x \in \mathcal{S}_X,\ y \in \mathcal{S}_Y. \tag{1.2}$$

Integrating this identity with respect to y on support $\mathcal{S}_Y$, we immediately have the **point-wise formula** (1.3). Now substitute (1.3) into (1.2), we obtain the dual form of IBF for $f_Y(y)$ and hence by symmetry we obtain the **function-wise formula** of $f_X(y)$ as shown in (1.4), or the **sampling formula** in (1.5) when the normalizing constant is omitted.

$$\begin{aligned} f_X(x) &= \left\{ \int_{\mathcal{S}_Y} \frac{f_{(Y|X)}(y|x)}{f_{(X|Y)}(x|y)} dy \right\}^{-1}, \quad \text{for any } x \in \mathcal{S}_X. && (1.3) \\ f_X(x) &= \left\{ \int_{\mathcal{S}_X} \frac{f_{(X|Y)}(x|y_0)}{f_{(Y|X)}(y_0|x)} dx \right\}^{-1} \frac{f_{(X|Y)}(x|y_0)}{f_{(Y|X)}(y_0|x)} && (1.4) \\ &\propto \frac{f_{(X|Y)}(x|y_0)}{f_{(Y|X)}(y_0|x)}, && (1.5) \\ & \text{for all } x \in \mathcal{S}_X \text{ and an arbitrarily fixed } y_0 \in \mathcal{S}_Y. \end{aligned}$$

Often in practice, we know $f_{(X|Y)}(x|y)$ only up to a normalizing constant. In other words, $f_{(X|Y)}(x|y) = c(y) \cdot g(x|y)$, where $g(x|y)$ is completely known, then the function-wise IBF (1.4) and sampling IBF (1.5) still hold if we replace $f_{(X|Y)}(x|y_0)$ by $g(x|y_0)$.

The following three examples show that the IBF can be used to obtain exact joint distribution if two conditionals are given. It is worth noting that even in these simple examples, the Gibbs sampler does not reduce to such a simple form (Chen *et al.*, 2000, p.20–22).

Example 1.1 (*Bivariate normal distribution*). Assume that

$$\begin{aligned} X|(Y=y) &\sim N(\mu_1 + \rho(y-\mu_2), 1-\rho^2) \quad \text{and} \\ Y|(X=x) &\sim N(\mu_2 + \rho(x-\mu_1), 1-\rho^2). \end{aligned}$$

Since $\mathcal{S}_{(X,Y)} = \mathcal{S}_X \times \mathcal{S}_Y = \mathbb{R}^2$, from (1.3), we obtain

$$\{f_X(x)\}^{-1} = \sqrt{2\pi} \exp\{(x-\mu_1)^2/2\},$$

which means $X \sim N(\mu_1, 1)$. Therefore, the joint distribution of (X, Y) exists and is bivariate normal with means μ_1 and μ_2, unit variances and correlation coefficient ρ. When using (1.3), we need to evaluate an integral. In contrast, using (1.5), the integration can be avoided. In fact, let the arbitrary y_0 be μ_2, then

$$f_X(x) \propto \exp\{-(x-\mu_1)^2/2\}. \qquad \|$$

Example 1.2 (*Bivariate exponential distribution*). Let $\delta \geq 0$,

$$\begin{aligned} f_{(X|Y)}(x|y) &= (\alpha + \delta y)e^{-(\alpha+\delta y)x}, \quad x \in \mathbb{R}_+, \quad \alpha > 0, \quad \text{and} \\ f_{(Y|X)}(y|x) &= (\beta + \delta x)e^{-(\beta+\delta x)y}, \quad y \in \mathbb{R}_+, \quad \beta > 0. \end{aligned}$$

Note that $\mathcal{S}_{(X,Y)} = \mathcal{S}_X \times \mathcal{S}_Y = \mathbb{R}^2_+$. Setting $y_0 = 0$ in the sampling IBF (1.5), we obtain $f_X(x) \propto (\beta + \delta x)^{-1} \exp(-\alpha x)$. This is a univariate distribution, from which it is easy to generate i.i.d. samples by using the rejection method (see, e.g., §2.2.2) since

$$(\beta + \delta x)^{-1} e^{-\alpha x} \le (\alpha\beta)^{-1} \cdot \alpha e^{-\alpha x}.$$

Then, (X, Y) follows a bivariate exponential distribution with

$$f_{(X,Y)}(x, y) \propto \exp\{-(\alpha x + \beta y + \delta xy)\}.$$

Arnold & Strauss (1988) give more details on this joint pdf. ||

Example 1.3 (*Dimension reduction*). By utilizing the structure of the low-dimensional conditional densities, both the point-wise and function-wise IBF can effectively reduce the dimensionality that restricts the applications of direct Monte Carlo sampling. For example, given a joint density $f_{(X,Y)}(x, y_1, \dots, y_n)$, where X is a random variable and $Y = (Y_1, \dots, Y_n)^\top$ an n-dimensional random vector. Suppose we are interested in obtaining the marginal density

$$f_X(x) = \int \cdots \int f_{(X,Y)}(x, y_1, \dots, y_n)\, dy_1 \cdots dy_n.$$

There are many cases where the above n-fold integration is extremely difficult to perform, either analytically or numerically. In such cases the function-wise IBF (1.4) provides an alternative method to obtain $f_X(x)$. Noting that both the conditional pdfs $f_{(X|Y)}(x|y)$ and $f_{(Y|X)}(y|x)$ are easy to obtain and are usually available, we only need to perform a one-dimension integration to calculate the normalizing constant with formula (1.4) in order to obtain $f_X(x)$. On the other hand, if Y is univariate while X an n-dimensional vector, then the point-wise IBF (1.3) can be used to obtain $f_X(x)$. Therefore, we can choose between the point-wise and function-wise IBF depending on the practical problem at hand. ||

1.3.2 Monte Carlo versions of the IBF

(a) Harmonic mean formula

In some applications, the integrals in the right-hand side of Eq.(1.4) and Eq.(1.3) may be difficult to evaluate analytically. However, since the IBF already reduces the dimensionality by the conditional pdfs, we may use Monte Carlo methods to numerically calculate the normalizing constant in (1.4) or to numerically evaluate the integral in (1.3). For any given $x \in \mathcal{S}_X$, we have

$$f_X(x) \doteq \hat{f}_{1,X}(x) = \left\{ \frac{1}{n} \sum_{i=1}^{n} \frac{1}{f_{(X|Y)}(x|y^{(i)})} \right\}^{-1}, \tag{1.6}$$

where $\{y^{(i)}\}_{i=1}^{n} \overset{\text{iid}}{\sim} f_{(Y|X)}(y|x)$.

(b) Weighted point-wise IBF

Similar to the importance function in importance sampling method (cf. §2.3.3), we first derive a weighted version of the point-wise IBF (1.3). Let the weight $w(y)$ be a density function with the same support as $f_Y(y)$. From the identity (1.2), we have

$$w(y) = \frac{f_{(Y|X)}(y|x)w(y)}{f_{(X|Y)}(x|y)f_Y(y)} \cdot f_X(x), \quad \forall\, x \in \mathcal{S}_X,\ y \in \mathcal{S}_Y. \tag{1.7}$$

Integrating (1.7) with respect to y on the support $\mathcal{S}_Y$ gives

$$f_X(x) = \left\{ \int_{\mathcal{S}_Y} \frac{f_{(Y|X)}(y|x)w(y)}{f_{(X|Y)}(x|y)f_Y(y)}\, dy \right\}^{-1}, \quad \text{for any given } x \in \mathcal{S}_X, \tag{1.8}$$

which is called weighted point-wise IBF.

The first Monte Carlo version of (1.8) is given by

$$f_X(x) \doteq \hat{f}_{2,X}(x) = \left\{ \frac{1}{n} \sum_{i=1}^{n} \frac{w(y^{(i)})}{f_{(X|Y)}(x|y^{(i)})f_Y(y^{(i)})} \right\}^{-1}, \tag{1.9}$$

where x is a given point in $\mathcal{S}_X$, $\{y^{(i)}\}_1^n \overset{\text{iid}}{\sim} f_{(Y|X)}(y|x)$, and $f_Y(\cdot)$ is calculated by the point-wise IBF (1.3) via interchanging x and y. In particular, (1.8) and (1.9) will be reduced to (1.3) and (1.6), respectively, if we let $w(y) = f_Y(y)$ for all $y \in \mathcal{S}_Y$.

If the simulation from $f_{(Y|X)}(y|x)$ is very difficult but the evaluations of both $f_{(X|Y)}(x|y)$ and $f_{(Y|X)}(y|x)$ is relatively simple, then we may use the following Monte Carlo version of (1.8),

$$f_X(x) \doteq \hat{f}_{3,X}(x) = \left\{ \frac{1}{m} \sum_{j=1}^{m} \frac{f_{(Y|X)}(y^{(j)}|x)}{f_{(X|Y)}(x|y^{(j)})f_Y(y^{(j)})} \right\}^{-1}, \tag{1.10}$$

where $x \in \mathcal{S}_X$ is fixed, $\{y^{(j)}\}_1^m \overset{\text{iid}}{\sim} w(y)$, and $f_Y(\cdot)$ is computed by the point-wise IBF (1.3) via interchanging x and y.

(c) Rao–Blackwellized formula

Starting with two low-dimensional conditional densities $f_{(X|Y)}(x|y)$ and $f_{(Y|X)}(y|x)$, we can obtain i.i.d. joint samples of (X, Y) through the following two steps: First to draw x from the marginal $f_X(x)$ based on the sampling IBF (1.5), then to draw y from the conditional $f_{(Y|X)}(y|x)$. Any procedures such as the grid method (e.g., Gelman *et al.*, 1995, p.302), the rejection method (von Neumann, 1951) and the adaptive rejection method (Gilks & Wild, 1992) can be employed to the key first step.

For instance, with the grid method (cf. Ex.2.13), we select an appropriate grid of values $\{x^{(i)}\}_{i=1}^n$ that cover the support $\mathcal{S}_X$, and compute $f_X(x)$ by (1.3) at each point on the grid. Then the density $f_X(x)$ can be approximated by the discrete density at $\{x^{(i)}\}_{i=1}^n$ with probabilities $f_X(x^{(i)})/\sum_{j=1}^n f_X(x^{(j)})$, $i = 1, \ldots, n$. A random draw from $f_X(x)$ is obtained by drawing a sample from the uniform distribution on $[0, 1]$, and then transformed by the inversion method (Ross, 1991) to obtain a sample from the discrete approximate. Obviously, this method will also work for an unnormalized density function.

Let the joint samples $\{x^{(i)}, y^{(i)}\}_{i=1}^n$ be available, then the Rao–Blackwellized estimator is given by (Arnold, 1993)

$$f_X(x) \doteq \hat{f}_{4,X}(x) = \frac{1}{n}\sum_{i=1}^n f_{(X|Y)}(x|y^{(i)}), \quad \forall\, x \in \mathcal{S}_X. \tag{1.11}$$

1.3.3 Generalization to the case of three vectors

We now extend the IBF from two vectors to the case of three vectors. Consider three random vectors X_1, X_2 and X_3 and let $\mathcal{S}_{(X_1,X_2,X_3)} = \mathcal{S}_{X_1} \times \mathcal{S}_{X_2} \times \mathcal{S}_{X_3}$. Assume that three conditionals $f_1(x_1|x_2, x_3)$, $f_2(x_2|x_1, x_3)$ and $f_3(x_3|x_1, x_2)$ are given and are positive. The goal is to find the joint density. As

$$f_{(X_1,X_2,X_3)}(x_1, x_2, x_3) = f_{X_1}(x_1) f_{(X_2|X_1)}(x_2|x_1) f_3(x_3|x_1, x_2),$$

we need only to derive $f_{X_1}(\cdot)$ and $f_{(X_2|X_1)}(\cdot|\cdot)$. By (1.3), we have

$$f_{(X_2|X_1)}(x_2|x_1) = \left\{\int \frac{f_3(x_3|x_1, x_2)}{f_2(x_2|x_1, x_3)}\, dx_3\right\}^{-1} \quad \text{and}$$

$$f_{(X_1|X_2)}(x_1|x_2) = \left\{\int \frac{f_3(x_3|x_1, x_2)}{f_1(x_1|x_2, x_3)}\, dx_3\right\}^{-1}.$$

Hence, by using (1.3) again, we obtain

$$f_{X_1}(x_1) = \left\{ \int \frac{f_{(X_2|X_1)}(x_2|x_1)}{f_{(X_1|X_2)}(x_1|x_2)}\, dx_2 \right\}^{-1}.$$

1.4 The Bayesian Methodology

Bayesian inference starts with a probability model to a set of data together with a prior distribution of the model parameters, centers at calculating posterior distributions of the parameters and predictive distributions for latent variables or new observations, and possibly ends with presentation and interpretation of the posterior. Obtaining marginal (posterior) distributions or their characteristics, such as mean, modes and quantiles, is key to Bayesian inference. The fundamentals of the Bayesian analysis are to combine the prior distribution and the observed-data likelihood to yield the posterior distribution.

Bayesian approach to data analysis consists of the following three main steps (see, e.g., Gelman *et al.*, 1995, p.3):

(i) Constructing a full probability model summarized by a joint distribution for all observable and unobservable quantities (e.g., observed data, missing data, unknown parameters);

(ii) Summarizing the findings (e.g., mean, median, mode(s), posterior quantiles and intervals) for the unobserved quantities of interest based on the derived conditional distributions of these quantities given the observed data;

(iii) Assessing model adequacy (i.e., model checking) and suggesting improvements (e.g., model selection).

In this section, we only consider the complete data problem. Let Y_{com} denote the completely observed data and θ be the parameter vector of interest. Instead of treating θ as an unknown constant as in the classical (or frequentist) approach, the Bayesian approach treats θ as a realized value of a random variable that has a prior distribution $\pi(\theta)$.

1.4.1 The posterior distribution

In order to carry out Step (i), we must provide the joint distribution of Y_{com} and θ:

$$f(Y_{\text{com}}, \theta) = f(Y_{\text{com}}|\theta)\pi(\theta),$$

where $f(Y_{\text{com}}|\theta)$ is the *sampling distribution.* When $f(Y_{\text{com}}|\theta)$ is regarded as a function of θ with fixed Y_{com}, it is the familiar *likelihood function*, denoted by $L(\theta|Y_{\text{com}})$.

Step (ii) is accomplished by the Bayes theorem (see, e.g., (1.1)) to obtain the *posterior distribution*:

$$f(\theta|Y_{\text{com}}) = \frac{f(Y_{\text{com}}|\theta)\pi(\theta)}{f(Y_{\text{com}})} \propto f(Y_{\text{com}}|\theta)\pi(\theta), \tag{1.12}$$

where

$$f(Y_{\text{com}}) = \int f(Y_{\text{com}}, \theta)\, d\theta = \int f(Y_{\text{com}}|\theta)\pi(\theta)\, d\theta \tag{1.13}$$

is the normalizing constant of $f(\theta|Y_{\text{com}})$.

Example 1.4 (*The multinomial model*). Let N items be classified into n categories/cells, $Y_{\text{com}} = y = (y_1, \dots, y_n)^{\top}$ denote the observed counts of the n cells, and $\theta = (\theta_1, \dots, \theta_n)^{\top}$ the cell probabilities. The multinomial sampling distribution (cf. Appendix A.1.5) is

$$f(y|\theta) = \text{Multinomial}_n(y|N, \theta) = \binom{N}{y_1, \dots, y_n} \prod_{i=1}^{n} \theta_i^{y_i},$$

where $y \in \mathbb{T}_n(N)$. If the prior of θ is a conjugate Dirichlet (cf. Appendix A.2.3)

$$\pi(\theta) = \text{Dirichlet}_n(\theta|a) = \frac{\prod_{i=1}^{n} \theta_i^{a_i - 1}}{B_n(a)}, \quad \theta \in \mathbb{T}_n \equiv \mathbb{T}_n(1),$$

then, the posterior of θ and its normalizing constant are given by

$$\begin{aligned} f(\theta|y) &= \text{Dirichlet}_n(\theta|y + a), & \theta \in \mathbb{T}_n, \quad \text{and} \\ f(y) &= \binom{N}{y_1, \dots, y_n} \frac{B_n(y + a)}{B_n(a)}, & y \in \mathbb{T}_n(N), \end{aligned} \tag{1.14}$$

respectively. The density (1.14) is called the *Dirichlet multinomial* density (cf. Appendix A.3.4):

$$y \sim \text{DMultinomial}_n(N, a), \qquad y \in \mathbb{T}_n(N).$$

From (1.13), it is easy to see that (1.14) is a *mixture* of multinomial distribution with rates, θ, and it follows a Dirichlet distribution. Therefore, the Dirichlet multinomial distribution is a robust alternative to the multinomial distribution. ||

1.4.2 Nuisance parameters

A major difficulty with the classical likelihood approach is with nuisance parameters. Let $\theta = (\theta_1, \theta_{-1})$, where θ_1 is the parameter of interest and θ_{-1} denotes all but the first component. Then θ_{-1} becomes a *nuisance parameter* vector. A common approach to deal with the nuisance parameter is by the *profile likelihood method*, in which θ_{-1} is treated as known and is fixed usually at its MLE. However, this method underestimates the uncertainty in the estimation of θ_{-1} and may lead to biased estimate of θ_1 and incorrect conclusion, especially, when the dimension of θ_{-1} is high (Liu, 2001, p.304).

In Bayesian framework, θ_{-1} can be removed by integration:

$$f(\theta_1|Y_{\text{com}}) = \frac{\int f(Y_{\text{com}}|\theta_1, \theta_{-1})\pi(\theta_1, \theta_{-1})\, d\theta_{-1}}{\int\int f(Y_{\text{com}}|\theta_1, \theta_{-1})\pi(\theta_1, \theta_{-1})\, d\theta_{-1} d\theta_1}. \tag{1.15}$$

If we could obtain both $f(\theta_1|Y_{\text{com}}, \theta_{-1})$ and $f(\theta_{-1}|Y_{\text{com}}, \theta_1)$ in closed form, according to the sampling IBF (1.5), we would have

$$f(\theta_1|Y_{\text{com}}) \propto \frac{f(\theta_1|Y_{\text{com}}, \theta_{-1}^*)}{f(\theta_{-1}^*|Y_{\text{com}}, \theta_1)}, \tag{1.16}$$

where θ_{-1}^* is some arbitrary value in $\mathcal{S}_{\theta_{-1}}$. Therefore, the IBF provides a way to obtain the marginal distribution of interest and it does not require integration. Otherwise, sampling-based methods such as MCMC (e.g., the Gibbs sampler) or the IBF sampler detailed in Chapters 4 and 5 of this book can be utilized to evaluate such integrals.

Example 1.5 (*The normal model*). Let $y_1, \ldots, y_n \stackrel{\text{iid}}{\sim} N(\mu, \sigma^2)$ and $Y_{\text{com}} = \{y_i\}_{i=1}^n$. The likelihood function is

$$f(Y_{\text{com}}|\mu, \sigma^2) \propto (\sigma^2)^{-n/2} \exp\left\{ -\frac{\sum_{i=1}^n (y_i - \mu)^2}{2\sigma^2} \right\}.$$

Consider a noninformative prior distribution $\pi(\mu, \sigma^2) \propto 1/\sigma^2$, then, the joint posterior density is

$$f(\mu, \sigma^2|Y_{\text{com}}) \propto \sigma^{-n-2} \exp\left\{ -\frac{(n-1)s^2 + n(\bar{y} - \mu)^2}{2\sigma^2} \right\}, \tag{1.17}$$

where

$$\bar{y} = \frac{1}{n}\sum_{i=1}^n y_i \quad \text{and} \quad s^2 = \frac{1}{n-1}\sum_{i=1}^n (y_i - \bar{y})^2$$

are sufficient statistics for (μ, σ^2). We often are interested in μ, so σ^2 may be considered as a nuisance parameter. From (1.17), we readily have (cf. Appendix A.2.8)

$$\begin{aligned} \sigma^2|(Y_{\text{com}}, \mu) &\sim \text{IGamma}\left(\frac{n}{2}, \frac{(n-1)s^2 + n(\bar{y} - \mu)^2}{2}\right), \\ \mu|(Y_{\text{com}}, \sigma^2) &\sim N(\bar{y}, \sigma^2/n). \end{aligned}$$

Using (1.16) and letting the arbitrary value of nuisance parameter $\sigma^2 = 1$, we have (cf. Appendix A.3.5) the posterior of interest:

$$\mu|Y_{\text{com}} \sim t(\bar{y}, s^2/n, n-1). \qquad \|$$

1.4.3 Posterior predictive distribution

Model checking is crucial to Bayesian data analysis and is a major aspect of implementing Step (iii) as outlined at the beginning of Section 1.4. A common technique for model checking is to draw samples from the *posterior predictive distribution* of replicated data and compare these samples to the observed data. Any systematic discrepancies between the simulated data and the observed data imply potential lack of fit of the model.

Let $\tilde{y}$ denote a future observation or an unknown observable quantity. Predictive inference is to make inference on $\tilde{y}$ or its function. Before Y_{com} is observed, the distribution of the unknown but observable Y_{com} is $f(Y_{\text{com}})$ specified by (1.13). It is sometimes called the *prior predictive distribution* .

After Y_{com} is observed, we can predict or forecast $\tilde{y}$. The posterior predictive distribution of $\tilde{y}$ given the data Y_{com} is defined as (see, e.g., Aitchison & Dunsmore, 1975, p.24)

$$\begin{aligned} f(\tilde{y}|Y_{\text{com}}) &= \int f(\tilde{y}, \theta|Y_{\text{com}})\, d\theta \\ &= \int f(\tilde{y}|Y_{\text{com}}, \theta) f(\theta|Y_{\text{com}})\, d\theta. \end{aligned}$$

Most frequently, the future observation $\tilde{y}$ and Y_{com} are conditionally independent given θ. In this case, we have

$$f(\tilde{y}|Y_{\text{com}}, \theta) = f(\tilde{y}|\theta). \tag{1.18}$$

On the other hand, the function-wise IBF (1.4) can be used to derive the following alternative formula:

$$f(\tilde{y}|Y_{\text{com}}) = f(\tilde{y}|Y_{\text{com}}, \theta_0) \times \frac{f(\theta_0|Y_{\text{com}})}{f(\theta_0|Y_{\text{com}}, \tilde{y})}, \tag{1.19}$$

where θ_0 is an arbitrary value of θ in its support $\mathcal{S}_\theta$ and $f(\theta|Y_{\text{com}}, \tilde{y})$ is the posterior density of θ, with Y_{com} augmented by an additional observation $\tilde{y}$. Note that (1.19) gives $f(\tilde{y}|Y_{\text{com}})$ directly without integration. Eq. (1.19) appeared without explanation in a Durham University undergraduate final examination script of 1984 and was reported by Besag (1989). However, the writings of Besag (1989) indicates that they seem to be unaware that Eq. (1.19) could come from an exact formula, i.e., the function-wise IBF.

Example 1.6 (*Bernoulli experiments*). Let $\{y_i\}_{i=1}^n$ be observations (0 or 1) of n i.i.d. Bernoulli trials with success probability p. Define $Y_{\text{com}} = \{y_i\}_{i=1}^n$ and $y = \sum_{i=1}^n y_i$. Since y is the sufficient statistic for p, we could write $Y_{\text{com}} = y$. The sampling distribution is

$$f(y|p) = \binom{n}{y} p^y (1-p)^{n-y}, \quad y = 0, 1, \ldots, n.$$

Suppose that the prior distribution of p is the beta distribution $\text{Beta}(a, b)$, then the posterior distribution of p is

$$f(p|y) = \text{Beta}(p|y + a, n - y + b), \quad 0 \le p \le 1.$$

From (1.13), it is easy to see that the prior predictive distribution is a beta-binomial distribution (cf. Appendix A.3.3):

$$f(Y_{\text{com}}) = \text{BBinomial}(y|n, a, b) = \binom{n}{y} \frac{B(y + a, n - y + b)}{B(a, b)}.$$

Let $\tilde{y}$ denote the result of a new trial, from (1.18), we obtain

$$\begin{aligned} f(\tilde{y}|Y_{\text{com}}, p) &= f(\tilde{y}|p) = p^{\tilde{y}}(1-p)^{1-\tilde{y}} \quad \text{and} \\ f(p|Y_{\text{com}}, \tilde{y}) &= \text{Beta}(p|y + \tilde{y} + a, n + 1 - y - \tilde{y} + b). \end{aligned}$$

In (1.19) letting $p_0 = 0.5$, then the posterior predictive density is

$$f(\tilde{y}|Y_{\text{com}}) = \text{BBinomial}(\tilde{y}|1, y + a, n - y + b),$$

which is also a beta-binomial density. In particular, we have

$$\Pr(\tilde{y} = 1|Y_{\text{com}}) = \frac{y + a}{n + a + b}, \quad \Pr(\tilde{y} = 0|Y_{\text{com}}) = \frac{n - y + b}{n + a + b}. \quad \|$$

The next example shows that sometimes the assumption of conditional independence (1.18) is not valid.

Example 1.7 (*Homogeneous Poisson process*). Let $\{Y_i, i \geq 1\} \sim \text{HPP}(\lambda)$ (cf. Appendix A.4.1) and $Y_{\text{com}} = \{Y_i\}_{i=1}^n$. According to Property 3 in Appendix A.4.1, the joint pdf of the successive event times $Y_1, \ldots, Y_n$ is

$$f(Y_{\text{com}}|\lambda) = \lambda^n e^{-\lambda y_n}, \quad 0 < y_1 < \cdots < y_n.$$

Let the prior distribution of the rate λ be $\text{Gamma}(a, b)$, the conjugate prior, then the posterior is

$$f(\lambda|Y_{\text{com}}) = \text{Gamma}(\lambda|n + a, y_n + b).$$

From (1.13), the prior predictive distribution is given by

$$f(Y_{\text{com}}) = \frac{b^a}{\Gamma(a)} \cdot \frac{\Gamma(n+a)}{(y_n + b)^{n+a}}, \quad 0 < y_1 < \cdots < y_n.$$

Let $\tilde{y} = Y_{n+1}$, we obtain

$$\begin{aligned} f(y_{n+1}|Y_{\text{com}}, \lambda) &= \lambda e^{-\lambda(y_{n+1} - y_n)}, \quad y_{n+1} > y_n, \\ f(\lambda|Y_{\text{com}}, y_{n+1}) &= \text{Gamma}(\lambda|n + 1 + a, y_{n+1} + b). \end{aligned} \tag{1.20}$$

In (1.19) letting $\lambda_0 = 1$, then the posterior predictive density is

$$f(y_{n+1}|Y_{\text{com}}) = f(y_{n+1}|y_n) = \frac{(n+a)(y_n + b)^{n+a}}{(y_{n+1} + b)^{n+a+1}}, \quad y_{n+1} > y_n. \ \|$$

1.4.4 Bayes factor

The normalizing constant $f(Y_{\text{com}})$ defined by (1.13) is sometimes called the *marginal likelihood* of the data and is often denoted by $m(Y_{\text{com}})$ in the statistical literature. The marginal likelihood is closely related to the *Bayes factor*, which can be used for model selection (Kass & Raftery, 1995).

The Bayes factor is defined as the ratio of posterior odds vs. prior odds, which is simply a ratio of two marginal likelihoods. To compare two models, say M_1 and M_2, the Bayes factor for model M_1 vs. model M_2 is

$$B_{12} = \frac{m(Y_{\text{com}}|M_1)}{m(Y_{\text{com}}|M_2)}. \tag{1.21}$$

Jeffreys (1961) suggested interpreting B_{12} in half-units on the $\log_{10}$ scale, i.e., when B_{12} falls in intervals $(1, 3.2)$, $(3.2, 10)$, $(10, 100)$ and $(100, +\infty)$, the evidence against M_2 is considered not worth more than a bare mention, substantial, strong and decisive, respectively.

1.4.5 Marginal likelihood

Estimating the marginal likelihood $m(Y_{\text{com}})$ is crucial to the calculation of Bayes factor. If we replace X and Y in (1.6) by Y_{com} and θ, respectively, then from (1.6) we immediately obtain the first estimator of $m(Y_{\text{com}})$:

$$\hat{m}_1(Y_{\text{com}}) = \left\{ \frac{1}{n} \sum_{i=1}^{n} \frac{1}{f(Y_{\text{com}}|\theta^{(i)})} \right\}^{-1}, \tag{1.22}$$

where Y_{com} is a given point in its support, and $\{\theta^{(i)}\}_1^n \stackrel{\text{iid}}{\sim} f(\theta|Y_{\text{com}})$. The Monte Carlo version of the point-wise IBF, (1.22), coincides with the simulated harmonic mean formula of Newton & Raftery (1994, p.21) which is derived empirically in choosing an appropriate importance function. As explained again in Kass & Raftery (1995, p.779) that this simulated harmonic mean formula was obtained using the idea of choosing importance sampling in approximating the integral for the "marginal likelihood" via a "well-suited" choice of the importance function, which is justified empirically. Newton & Raftery (1994) further showed that $\hat{m}_1(Y_{\text{com}})$ converges almost surely to the correct value $m(Y_{\text{com}})$ for a given point Y_{com} as $n \to \infty$. However, $\hat{m}_1(Y_{\text{com}})$ does not generally satisfy the Gaussian central limit theorem. This manifests itself by the occasional occurrence of a value of $\theta^{(i)}$ with a small $f(Y_{\text{com}}|\theta^{(i)})$ and hence a large effect on the final result (Chib, 1995).

Similarly, from (1.9), the second estimator of $m(Y_{\text{com}})$ is

$$\hat{m}_2(Y_{\text{com}}) = \left\{ \frac{1}{n} \sum_{i=1}^{n} \frac{w(\theta^{(i)})}{f(Y_{\text{com}}|\theta^{(i)})\pi(\theta^{(i)})} \right\}^{-1}, \tag{1.23}$$

where Y_{com} is a given point in its support, $\{\theta^{(i)}\}_1^n \stackrel{\text{iid}}{\sim} f(\theta|Y_{\text{com}})$. In particular, (1.23) will be reduced to (1.22) if we let $w(\theta) = \pi(\theta)$. Eq. (1.23) was mentioned by Gelfand & Dey (1994) in the context of importance sampling. Kass & Raftery (1995) showed that $\hat{m}_2(Y_{\text{com}})$ is an unbiased and consistent estimator of $m(Y_{\text{com}})$, and satisfies a Gaussian central limit theorem if the tails of $w(\cdot)$ are thin enough. Therefore, $\hat{m}_2(Y_{\text{com}})$ does not have the instability of $\hat{m}_1(Y_{\text{com}})$. Chib (1995) found that the somewhat obvious choices of $w(\cdot)$ — a normal density or t density if $\mathcal{S}_\theta = \mathbb{R}$ — do not necessarily satisfy the thinness requirement. Using the importance-weighted marginal density estimation method of Chen (1994), Chen & Shao (1997, p.1570) also obtained (1.23). Therefore we may use the empirical procedure provided by Chen (1994) to achieve a fairly good $w(\cdot)$.

Alternatively, if generating samples from $f(\theta|Y_{\text{com}})$ is very difficult but evaluating both $f(Y_{\text{com}}|\theta)$ and $f(\theta|Y_{\text{com}})$ is relatively simple, from (1.10), then we can obtain the third estimator of $m(Y_{\text{com}})$:

$$\hat{m}_3(Y_{\text{com}}) = \left\{ \frac{1}{m} \sum_{j=1}^{m} \frac{f(\theta^{(j)}|Y_{\text{com}})}{f(Y_{\text{com}}|\theta^{(j)})\pi(\theta^{(j)})} \right\}^{-1}, \tag{1.24}$$

where Y_{com} is fixed, and $\{\theta^{(j)}\}_1^m \stackrel{\text{iid}}{\sim} w(\theta)$.

Finally, let $\{\theta^{(i)}\}_1^n \stackrel{\text{iid}}{\sim} \pi(\theta)$, from (1.11), then the fourth estimator of $m(Y_{\text{com}})$ is the Rao–Blackwellized estimator given by

$$\hat{m}_4(Y_{\text{com}}) = \frac{1}{n} \sum_{i=1}^{n} f(Y_{\text{com}}|\theta^{(i)}). \tag{1.25}$$

As mentioned by Gelfand *et al.* (1992), $\hat{m}_4(Y_{\text{com}})$ is better than the kernel density estimator under a wide range of loss functions. The disadvantages of the Rao–Blackwellized estimator are that (i) the closed form of $f(Y_{\text{com}}|\theta)$ must be known, and (ii) $\hat{m}_4(Y_{\text{com}})$ is a mixture density, which is relatively difficult to treat when n is sufficiently large.

1.5 The Missing Data Problems

In the previous sections, we assumed that the data set is completely observed. However, incomplete observations arise in many applications. For example, a survey with multiple questions may include nonresponses to some personal questions. In an industrial experiment some results are missing because of mechanical breakdowns unrelated to the experimental process. Some patients in a clinical trial may miss a treatment for various reasons. In cancer drug development, a mouse may die before the end of study or may be sacrificed when its tumor volume quadruples and its tumor may be suppressed for some time and may regrow. The incompleteness or missingness may also be caused by drastic tumor shrinkage (e.g., <0.01 cm^3) or random truncation. In addition, many other problems can be treated as a missing data problem (e.g, latent-class model, mixture model, some constrained parameter models, etc.). The missing data formulation is an important tool for modeling to address a specific scientific question. In this section, let $Y_{\rm obs}$ denote the observed values, $Y_{\rm mis}$ the missing values, θ the parameter vector of interest, and write $Y = (Y_{\rm obs}, Y_{\rm mis})$.

1.5.1 Missing data mechanism

We define a *missing-data indicator* M whose element taking value 1 if the corresponding component of Y is observed and 0 if the corresponding component of Y is missing. The joint distribution of (Y, M) is

$$f(Y, M|\theta, \psi) = f(Y|\theta) \times f(M|Y, \psi).$$

The missing-data mechanism is characterized by the conditional distribution of M given Y, which is indexed by an unknown parameter ψ. The distribution of observed data is obtained by integrating over the distribution of $Y_{\rm mis}$:

$$f(Y_{\rm obs}, M|\theta, \psi) = \int f(Y_{\rm obs}, Y_{\rm mis}|\theta) \times f(M|Y_{\rm obs}, Y_{\rm mis}, \psi)\, dY_{\rm mis}.$$

Missing data are said to be *missing at random* (MAR) if

$$f(M|Y_{\rm obs}, Y_{\rm mis}, \psi) = f(M|Y_{\rm obs}, \psi), \tag{1.26}$$

i.e., the distribution of the missing-data mechanism does not depend on the missing values, but depend on the observed values (including fully observed covariates) and the parameter ψ. Under the assumption of MAR, we have

$$f(Y_{\rm obs}, M|\theta, \psi) = f(M|Y_{\rm obs}, \psi) \times f(Y_{\rm obs}|\theta).$$

If the joint prior distribution $\pi(\theta, \psi) = \pi(\theta)\pi(\psi)$, then Bayesian inferences on θ can be obtained by considering only the observed-data likelihood $f(Y_{\rm obs}|\theta)$. In this case, the missing-data mechanism is said to be *ignorable.* Missing data are said to be *missing completely at random* (MCAR) if the distribution of the missing-data mechanism is completely independent of Y:

$$f(M|Y_{\rm obs}, Y_{\rm mis}, \psi) = f(M|\psi). \tag{1.27}$$

1.5.2 Data augmentation (DA)

Let θ be the parameter we want to make statistical inference for based on the observed posterior distribution $f(\theta|Y_{\rm obs})$. The EM algorithm (Dempster *et al.*, 1977; cf. §2.1.2 for more detailed discussions) and the DA algorithm are designed for obtaining the mode of

$f(\theta|Y_{\text{obs}})$ and for simulating from $f(\theta|Y_{\text{obs}})$, respectively. The EM and the DA share a simple idea that rather than performing a complicated optimization or simulation, the observed data is augmented with latent data so that a series of simple optimizations or simulations can be performed.

As a stochastic version of the EM algorithm, the DA algorithm was originally proposed by Tanner & Wong (1987). The basic idea is to introduce latent data Z so that the complete-data posterior distribution $f_{(\theta|Y_{\text{obs}},Z)}(\theta|Y_{\text{obs}}, z)$ and the conditional predictive distribution $f_{(Z|Y_{\text{obs}},\theta)}(z|Y_{\text{obs}}, \theta)$ are available, where by available it means either the samples can be easily generated from both, or each can be easily evaluated at any given point.

1.5.3 The original DA algorithm

(a) The fixed point iteration

The DA algorithm is motivated by two simple integral identities:

$$\begin{aligned} f(\theta|Y_{\text{obs}}) &= \int_{\mathcal{S}_{(Z|Y_{\text{obs}})}} f_{(\theta|Y_{\text{obs}},Z)}(\theta|Y_{\text{obs}}, z) f(z|Y_{\text{obs}})\, dz, \\ f(z|Y_{\text{obs}}) &= \int_{\mathcal{S}_{(\theta|Y_{\text{obs}})}} f_{(Z|Y_{\text{obs}},\theta)}(z|Y_{\text{obs}}, \phi) f(\phi|Y_{\text{obs}})\, d\phi, \end{aligned}$$

where $\mathcal{S}_{(Z|Y_{\text{obs}})}$ and $\mathcal{S}_{(\theta|Y_{\text{obs}})}$ denote the corresponding supports of Z and θ conditional on Y_{obs}. By substitution, we have

$$f(\theta|Y_{\text{obs}}) = \int K(\theta, \phi) f(\phi|Y_{\text{obs}})\, d\phi,$$

where the kernel function is

$$K(\theta, \phi) = \int f_{(\theta|Y_{\text{obs}},Z)}(\theta|Y_{\text{obs}}, z) f_{(Z|Y_{\text{obs}},\theta)}(z|Y_{\text{obs}}, \phi)\, dz. \tag{1.28}$$

The fixed point iteration in functional analysis is thus

$$f_{k+1}(\theta|Y_{\text{obs}}) = \int K(\theta, \phi) f_k(\phi|Y_{\text{obs}})\, d\phi, \quad k \in \mathbb{N}. \tag{1.29}$$

(b) Sufficient conditions for convergence

Tanner & Wong (1987) established the following sufficient conditions for the convergence of f_{k+1} to f in ℓ_1-norm, i.e.,

$$\int |f_k(\theta|Y_{\text{obs}}) - f(\theta|Y_{\text{obs}})|\, d\theta \to 0$$

as $k \to \infty$:

1) $K(\theta, \phi)$ is uniformly bounded;

2) $K(\theta, \phi)$ is equicontinuous in θ;

3) For any $\theta_0 \in \mathcal{S}_{(\theta|Y_{\text{obs}})}$, there is an open neighborhood $\mathcal{N}$ of θ_0 such that $K(\theta, \phi) > 0$ for all θ and ϕ in $\mathcal{N}$;

4) The starting function f_0 is such that $\sup\limits_{\theta} \frac{f_0(\theta|Y_{\text{obs}})}{f(\theta|Y_{\text{obs}})} < \infty$.

Note that, in addition to the integral (1.28) for obtaining the kernel function, the integral (1.29) is to be evaluated for each update from f_k to f_{k+1}. Tanner & Wong (1987) adopt the Monte Carlo method to perform the integration in (1.28).

(c) The original DA algorithm

The DA algorithm consists of iterations between the *imputation step* (I-step) and the *posterior step* (P-step), which is summarized as follows.

I-step: Draw $\{\theta^{(j)}\}_{j=1}^m$ from the current $f_k(\theta|Y_{\text{obs}})$; for each $\theta^{(j)}$, draw $z^{(j)}$ from $f_{(Z|Y_{\text{obs}},\theta)}(z|Y_{\text{obs}}, \theta^{(j)})$;

P-step: Update the posterior as

$$f_{k+1}(\theta|Y_{\text{obs}}) = \frac{1}{m}\sum_{j=1}^{m} f_{(\theta|Y_{\text{obs}},Z)}(\theta|Y_{\text{obs}}, z^{(j)}). \qquad (1.30)$$

The $\{z^{(j)}\}_{j=1}^m$ so produced are often called *multiple imputation* (Rubin, 1987a). The convergence rate and other aspects of the augmentation scheme (1.30) were further considered by Schervish & Carlin (1992) and Liu *et al.* (1994, 1995). It was stated without substantiation by Gelfand & Smith (1990) that the fixed point iteration can be extended to conditionals for more than two components. Since conditions 1)–4) and the proof involve considerable mathematics, the extension is not that obvious.

1.5.4 Connection with the Gibbs sampler

The Gibbs sampler is one of the best-known MCMC sampling algorithms in the Bayesian computation literature. It was developed originally by Geman & Geman (1984) for simulating posterior distributions in image reconstruction. The seminal paper of Gelfand & Smith (1990) introduces the Gibbs sampler to the mainstream statistical literature and has had far-reaching impact on the application of Bayesian method. The enormous potential of Gibbs sampling in complex statistical modeling is now being realized although there are still issues regarding convergence and the speed of computation. Various aspects of Gibbs sampler and MCMC methods are summarized by Smith & Roberts (1993), Besag & Green (1993), Gilks *et al.* (1993) and the discussions on all these papers.

Casella & George (1992) and Arnold (1993) provide excellent tutorial on the Gibbs sampler. Suppose we want to simulate a random vector $X = (X_1, \dots, X_d)^\top$ with a joint cdf $F(\cdot)$. Suppose that $F(\cdot)$ is either unknown or very complicated, but that for each i, the full univariate conditional distribution $f(X_i|X_1, \dots, X_{i-1}, X_{i+1}, \dots, X_d)$ is known and relatively easy to simulate. Choose a starting point $X^{(0)} = (X_1^{(0)}, \dots, X_d^{(0)})^\top$ and set $t = 0$, the Gibbs sampling iterates the following loop:

- Draw $X_1^{(t+1)} \sim f(X_1|X_2^{(t)}, \dots, X_d^{(t)})$;
- Draw $X_2^{(t+1)} \sim f(X_2|X_1^{(t+1)}, X_3^{(t)}, \dots, X_d^{(t)})$;

  $\vdots$
- Draw $X_d^{(t+1)} \sim f(X_d|X_1^{(t+1)}, \dots, X_{d-1}^{(t+1)})$.

Gelfand & Smith (1990) show that under mild conditions, the vector sequence $\{X^{(t)}\}_{t=1}^{\infty}$ has a stationary distribution $F(\cdot)$. Schervish & Carlin (1992) provide a sufficient condition that guarantees geometric convergence. Roberts & Polson (1994) discuss other properties regarding geometric convergence.

Example 1.8 (*Sampling from Dirichlet distribution*). To simulate $(X_1, X_2, X_3, 1 - \sum_{i=1}^3 X_i)^\top \sim \text{Dirichlet}(5, 4, 3, 2)$ using the Gibbs sampler, we first derive the full conditional distributions:

$$\begin{aligned}
X_1|(X_2, X_3) &\stackrel{d}{=} (1 - X_2 - X_3)Y_1, \quad Y_1 \sim \text{Beta}(5, 2), \\
X_2|(X_1, X_3) &\stackrel{d}{=} (1 - X_1 - X_3)Y_2, \quad Y_2 \sim \text{Beta}(4, 2), \\
X_3|(X_1, X_2) &\stackrel{d}{=} (1 - X_1 - X_2)Y_3, \quad Y_3 \sim \text{Beta}(3, 2),
\end{aligned}$$

where Y_1 is independent of (X_2, X_3), Y_2 is independent of (X_1, X_3), and Y_3 is independent of (X_1, X_2). Hence, first we need to choose a starting vector $(X_1^{(0)}, X_2^{(0)}, X_3^{(0)})$ such that $X_i^{(0)} > 0$, $i = 1, 2, 3$, $\sum_{i=1}^3 X_i^{(0)} < 1$. Then we independently simulate $Y_1^{(1)} \sim \text{Beta}(5, 2)$, $Y_2^{(1)} \sim \text{Beta}(4, 2)$ and $Y_3^{(1)} \sim \text{Beta}(3, 2)$. Let

$$\begin{aligned} X_1^{(1)} &= (1 - X_2^{(0)} - X_3^{(0)}) Y_1^{(1)}, \\ X_2^{(1)} &= (1 - X_1^{(1)} - X_3^{(0)}) Y_2^{(1)}, \\ X_3^{(1)} &= (1 - X_1^{(1)} - X_2^{(1)}) Y_3^{(1)}, \end{aligned}$$

then $(X_1^{(1)}, X_2^{(1)}, X_3^{(1)})$ is the first iteration of the Gibbs sampler. We can compute the second, third and higher iterations in a similar fashion. As $t \to +\infty$, the distribution of $(X_1^{(t)}, X_2^{(t)}, X_3^{(t)}, 1 - \sum_{i=1}^3 X_i^{(t)})^\top$ converges to the desired Dirichlet distribution. $\|$

Since the rate of convergence of the Gibbs sampler is controlled by the maximal correlation between the states of two consecutive Gibbs iterations, Liu *et al.* (1994) and Liu (1994) argued that grouping (or blocking) highly correlated components together in the Gibbs sampler can greatly improve its efficiency. For example, we can split $(X_1, \ldots, X_d)^\top$ into two blocks: $Y_1 = (X_1, \ldots, X_{d'})^\top$ and $Y_2 = (X_{d'+1}, \ldots, X_d)^\top$, resulting in the following two-block Gibbs sampler:

- Draw $Y_1^{(t+1)} \sim f(Y_1 | Y_2^{(t)})$;
- Draw $Y_2^{(t+1)} \sim f(Y_2 | Y_1^{(t+1)})$.

Particularly, in the original DA algorithm letting $m = 1$ and treating Z as the first block and θ the second block, we obtain

THE DA ALGORITHM:

$$\begin{aligned} &\text{I-step:} \quad \text{Draw} \quad z^{(t+1)} \sim f_{(Z|Y_{\text{obs}},\theta)}(z|Y_{\text{obs}}, \theta^{(t)}); \\ &\text{P-step:} \quad \text{Draw} \quad \theta^{(t+1)} \sim f_{(\theta|Y_{\text{obs}},Z)}(\theta|Y_{\text{obs}}, z^{(t+1)}). \end{aligned} \tag{1.31}$$

Example 1.9 (*Two-parameter multinomial model*). To illustrate the performance of the Gibbs sampler, Gelfand & Smith (1990) extended the genetic-linkage model (Tanner & Wong, 1987) to a two-parameter multinomial model: $Y_{\text{obs}} = (Y_1, \ldots, Y_5)^\top$,

$$Y_{\text{obs}} \sim \text{Multinomial}(n; a_1\theta_1 + b_1, a_2\theta_1 + b_2, a_3\theta_2 + b_3, a_4\theta_2 + b_4, c\theta_3),$$

where $a_i, b_i \geq 0$ are known, $0 \leq c = 1 - \sum_{i=1}^4 b_i = a_1 + a_2 = a_3 + a_4 \leq 1$ and $\theta = (\theta_1, \theta_2, \theta_3)^\top \in \mathbb{T}_3$. To split the first four cells, we introduce latent variables $Z = (Z_1, \dots, Z_4)^\top$ so that the augmented sampling distribution is

$$(Y_{\text{obs}}, Z) \sim \text{Multinomial}(n; a_1\theta_1, b_1, a_2\theta_1, b_2, a_3\theta_2, b_3, a_4\theta_2, b_4, c\theta_3).$$

Equivalently, the complete-data likelihood is

$$L(\theta|Y_{\text{obs}}, Z) \propto \theta_1^{z_1+z_2}\theta_2^{z_3+z_4}\theta_3^{y_5}. \tag{1.32}$$

A natural prior on θ is the Dirichlet distribution Dirichlet$(\alpha_1, \alpha_2, \alpha_3)$ so that the augmented posterior is given by

$$f(\theta|Y_{\text{obs}}, Z) = \text{Dirichlet}(\theta|z_1 + z_2 + \alpha_1, z_3 + z_4 + \alpha_2, y_5 + \alpha_3). \tag{1.33}$$

In addition, the conditional predictive density is

$$f(Z|Y_{\text{obs}}, \theta) = \prod_{i=1}^{4} \text{Binomial}(z_i|y_i, p_i), \tag{1.34}$$

where

$$p_i \hat{=} \frac{a_i\theta_1 I_{(1\leq i\leq 2)}}{a_i\theta_1 + b_i} + \frac{a_i\theta_2 I_{(3\leq i\leq 4)}}{a_i\theta_2 + b_i}. \tag{1.35}$$

Hence, the DA algorithm specified by (1.31) can be applied to (1.33) and (1.34). ‖

1.5.5 Connection with the IBF

In the DA scheme, we assumed that the complete-data posterior distribution $f_{(\theta|Y_{\text{obs}},Z)}(\theta|Y_{\text{obs}}, z)$ and the conditional predictive distribution $f_{(Z|Y_{\text{obs}},\theta)}(z|Y_{\text{obs}}, \theta)$ are available. Typically, in practice, we have $\mathcal{S}_{(\theta,Z|Y_{\text{obs}})} = \mathcal{S}_{(\theta|Y_{\text{obs}})} \times \mathcal{S}_{(Z|Y_{\text{obs}})}$. Corresponding to the point-wise IBF (1.3), for any given $\theta \in \mathcal{S}_{(\theta|Y_{\text{obs}})}$, we obtain

$$f(\theta|Y_{\text{obs}}) = \left\{ \int_{\mathcal{S}_{(Z|Y_{\text{obs}})}} \frac{f_{(Z|Y_{\text{obs}},\theta)}(z|Y_{\text{obs}}, \theta)}{f_{(\theta|Y_{\text{obs}},Z)}(\theta|Y_{\text{obs}}, z)} \, dz \right\}^{-1}. \tag{1.36}$$

Similarly, corresponding to the sampling IBF (1.5) and the function-wise IBF (1.4), for some arbitrary $z_0 \in \mathcal{S}_{(Z|Y_{\text{obs}})}$ and all $\theta \in \mathcal{S}_{(\theta|Y_{\text{obs}})}$, we have

$$f(\theta|Y_{\text{obs}}) \propto \frac{f_{(\theta|Y_{\text{obs}},Z)}(\theta|Y_{\text{obs}}, z_0)}{f_{(Z|Y_{\text{obs}},\theta)}(z_0|Y_{\text{obs}}, \theta)} \quad \text{and} \tag{1.37}$$

$$f(\theta|Y_{\text{obs}}) = c(z_0) \times \frac{f_{(\theta|Y_{\text{obs}},Z)}(\theta|Y_{\text{obs}}, z_0)}{f_{(Z|Y_{\text{obs}},\theta)}(z_0|Y_{\text{obs}}, \theta)}, \tag{1.38}$$

where the normalizing constant of $f(\theta|Y_{\text{obs}})$ is given by

$$\begin{aligned} c(z_0) &= f_{(Z|Y_{\text{obs}})}(z_0|Y_{\text{obs}}) \\ &= \left\{ \int_{\mathcal{S}_{(\theta|Y_{\text{obs}})}} \frac{f_{(\theta|Y_{\text{obs}},Z)}(\theta|Y_{\text{obs}}, z_0)}{f_{(Z|Y_{\text{obs}},\theta)}(z_0|Y_{\text{obs}}, \theta)} \, d\theta \right\}^{-1}. \end{aligned}$$

Therefore, the IBF gives explicit solutions to the fixed point iteration of the original DA algorithm in §1.5.3.

1.6 Entropy

One of the most important concepts in information theory is *entropy* that measures the *uncertainty* of a random variable. It has many applications in multivariate analysis and Bayesian statistics. In coding and communication theory, *Shannon entropy* (SE) measures the average amount of bits needed to transmit a message over a binary communication channel. In statistics, the amount of information contained in a random experiment can be quantified via a "distance" notion including the famous *Kullback–Leibler* (KL) divergence (or cross-entropy). This will be used to derive the ascent property of the EM algorithm (see §2.1.2(b)), to find an optimal reference parameter in the cross-entropy method (see §2.3.4(b)), and to develop (in conjunction with IBF) new criterion for checking convergence of the Gibbs sampler (see §5.9.3).

1.6.1 Shannon entropy

(a) Discrete distribution

Entropy is easily understood for discrete distribution. Let X be a discrete random variable taking values in $\mathcal{X}$ with probability mass function $p(\cdot)$. The Shannon entropy of X is defined as

$$\text{SE}(X) = -E \log_2 p(X) = -\sum_{\mathcal{X}} p(x) \log_2 p(x),$$

where $0 \log_2 0 \hat{=} 0$ and X is interpreted as a random character from $\mathcal{X}$ such that $\Pr(X = x) = p(x)$. It has been shown that the most efficient way to transmit characters sampled from $p(\cdot)$ over a binary channel is to encode them such that the number of bits required to transmit x is equal to $\log_2(1/p(x))$ (Cover & Thomas, 1991).

Example 1.10 (*Maximum entropy distribution*). Let $\mathcal{X} = \{x_1, \ldots, x_d\}$ and $X \sim p(\cdot)$, where $p(x_k) = 1$ and $p(x_i) = 0$ for $i \neq k$. Then clearly the probability distribution $p(\cdot)$ describes exactly and the "uncertainty" of X is zero, i.e., $\text{SE}(X) = -\sum_{i=1}^{d} p(x_i) \log_2 p(x_i) = 0$. At the other extreme, let $U \sim q(\cdot)$, where $q(x_i) = 1/d$ for all i. Then the "uncertainty" of U is maximized, i.e., $\text{SE}(U) = \log_2 d$ because $\text{SE}(X) \leq \log_2 d$ for any discrete random variable X defined in $\mathcal{X}$ (cf. Problem 1.7). Therefore, the $q(\cdot)$ is called the "most uncertain" or *maximum entropy* probability distribution. Note that this maximum entropy distribution is the same as the noninformative prior distribution in Bayesian statistics (Berger, 1980, p.75). ||

(b) Continuous distribution

Let X be a random vector with pdf f (with respect to the Lebesgue measure). The Shannon entropy of X is defined as

$$\text{SE}(X) = -E \log f(X) = -\int_{\mathcal{X}} f(x) \log f(x)\, dx. \tag{1.39}$$

It can be shown that $\text{SE}(X)$ is maximal if and only if f is the uniform distribution on $\mathcal{X}$ (Rubinstein & Kroese, 2004; cf. Problem 1.8).

For two random vectors X and Y, the *conditional entropy* of Y given X is defined by

$$\text{SE}(Y|X) = \text{SE}(X, Y) - \text{SE}(X). \tag{1.40}$$

It follows that $\text{SE}(X, Y) = \text{SE}(Y) + \text{SE}(X|Y)$. The *mutual information* of X and Y is defined as

$$\text{M}(X, Y) = \text{SE}(X) + \text{SE}(Y) - \text{SE}(X, Y). \tag{1.41}$$

1.6.2 Kullback–Leibler divergence

Let g and h be two pdfs with the same support, i.e., $\{x : g(x) > 0\} = \{x : h(x) > 0\}$. The *Kullback–Leibler* (KL) divergence between g and h is defined as

$$\text{KL}(g, h) = E_g \log \frac{g(X)}{h(X)} = \int g(x) \log \frac{g(x)}{h(x)}\, dx. \tag{1.42}$$

$\text{KL}(g, h)$ is also called the KL cross-entropy or the cross-entropy or the relative entropy. Note that $\text{KL}(g, h)$ is not a "distance" between

g and f since $\text{KL}(g,h) \neq \text{KL}(h,g)$. From Jensen's inequality (cf. Problem 1.10), we have

$$\text{KL}(g,h) \geq 0 \quad \text{and} \quad \text{KL}(g,h) = 0 \ \text{ iff } \ g(x) = h(x) \tag{1.43}$$

almost surely. In fact,

$$\text{KL}(g,h) = E_g\left[-\log\frac{h(X)}{g(X)}\right] \geq -\log\left[E_g\frac{h(X)}{g(X)}\right] = -\log 1 = 0.$$

Example 1.11 (*Normal distribution*). Let $Z \sim N(\mu, \sigma^2)$, then

$$\begin{aligned} \text{SE}(Z) &= -\int N(z|\mu,\sigma^2)\left[\log\frac{1}{\sqrt{2\pi}\sigma} - \frac{(z-\mu)^2}{2\sigma^2}\right] dz \\ &= \log(\sqrt{2\pi}\sigma) + 0.5. \end{aligned}$$

Furthermore, define $\mathcal{R}(\mu,\sigma^2) = \{X : E(X) = \mu, \text{Var}(X) = \sigma^2\}$, then we can prove the following assertion:

$$\text{SE}(Z) = \max_{X \in \mathcal{R}(\mu,\sigma^2)} \text{SE}(X).$$

In fact, let g denote the pdf of X and set $h(\cdot) = N(\cdot|\mu,\sigma^2)$. From (1.43), we have

$$\int g(x)\log g(x)\, dx \geq \int g(x)\log N(x|\mu,\sigma^2)\, dx.$$

Hence, $\text{SE}(X) \leq \log(\sqrt{2\pi}\sigma) + 0.5 = \text{SE}(Z)$, where equality holds iff $g(\cdot) = N(\cdot|\mu,\sigma^2)$. ||

Problems

1.1 Truncated normal distribution. An n-dimensional random vector W is said to follow a multivariate normal distribution truncated to the rectangle $[a,b] = \prod_{i=1}^n [a_i, b_i]$ if its density is proportional to $\exp\{-(w-\mu)^\top \Sigma^{-1}(w-\mu)/2\} \cdot I_{(a \leq w \leq b)}$, where $\mu = (\mu_1, \ldots, \mu_n)^\top$ is location parameter vector, Σ is an $n \times n$ positive definite matrix, $I_{(\cdot)}$ denotes the indicator function, and $a \leq w \leq b$ means that $a_i \leq w_i \leq b_i$ for all $i = 1, \ldots, n$. We write $W \sim TN_n(\mu, \Sigma; a, b)$ or $W \sim TN_n(\mu, \Sigma; [a,b])$ (Robert, 1995). Let both the conditionals are truncated uninormal, i.e.,

$$\begin{aligned} X|(Y=y) &\sim TN(\mu_1 + \rho\sigma_1\sigma_2^{-1}(y-\mu_2),\ \sigma_1^2(1-\rho^2);\ a_1, b_1), \\ Y|(X=x) &\sim TN(\mu_2 + \rho\sigma_2\sigma_1^{-1}(x-\mu_1),\ \sigma_2^2(1-\rho^2);\ a_2, b_2). \end{aligned}$$

Verify the following facts:

(a) The marginal density of X is proportional to

$$e^{-(x-\mu_1)^2/(2\sigma_1^2)} \times \left\{ \Phi\left(\frac{b_2 - \mu_2 - \rho\sigma_2\sigma_1^{-1}(x-\mu_1)}{\sigma_2\sqrt{1-\rho^2}} \right) \right.$$

$$\left. - \Phi\left(\frac{a_2 - \mu_2 - \rho\sigma_2\sigma_1^{-1}(x-\mu_1)}{\sigma_2\sqrt{1-\rho^2}} \right) \right\} \cdot I_{(a_1 \le x \le b_1)}.$$

(b) $(X, Y) \sim TN_2(\mu, \Sigma; a, b)$, where $\mu = (\mu_1, \mu_2)^\top$, and

$$\Sigma = \begin{pmatrix} \sigma_1^2 & \rho\sigma_1\sigma_2 \\ \rho\sigma_1\sigma_2 & \sigma_2^2 \end{pmatrix}, \quad a = \begin{pmatrix} a_1 \\ a_2 \end{pmatrix}, \quad b = \begin{pmatrix} b_1 \\ b_2 \end{pmatrix}.$$

1.2 **Derivation of prior from likelihood and a specified posterior** (Ng, 1997b). Let Y follow a shifted standard exponential distribution with new origin at unknown $\theta > 0$. Suppose we wish the posterior distribution of θ given $Y = y$ to be a truncated standard exponential distribution in the interval $(0, y)$. That is, we want

$$\begin{aligned} f_{(Y|\theta)}(y|\theta) &= e^{-(y-\theta)}, & y > \theta, \quad \text{and} \\ f_{(\theta|Y)}(\theta|y) &= e^{-\theta}/(1-e^{-y}), & \theta < y. \end{aligned}$$

Prove that the prior $\pi(\theta)$ is an exponential distribution with mean 0.5.

1.3 (Ng, 1997b). Let the conditional pdf of Y given θ be

$$f_{(Y|\theta)}(y|\theta) = \frac{e^{|\theta|}}{\sqrt{2\pi y}} \exp\left\{ -\frac{1}{2}\left(\frac{\theta^2}{y} + y \right) \right\}, \quad y > 0, \ \theta \in \mathbb{R}.$$

If one wishes the posterior distribution of θ to be very simple, say $N(0, y)$, then the prior could be computed by using (1.3) as $\pi(\theta) = e^{-|\theta|}/2$, which is the standard Laplace distribution. Show that the marginal distribution of Y is an exponential distribution with mean 2. This also leads to an interesting result that a Laplace distribution is the mixture of normal distribution with the variance being exponentially distributed. It contrasts with the Student's t distribution where the inverse of variance is being mixed with a gamma distribution.

1.4 (Hammersley & Clifford, 1970). Denote the full conditional density for n random variables as

$$f_i = f(x_i | x_1, \ldots, x_{i-1}, x_{i+1}, \ldots, x_n).$$

(a) Under the positivity conditions, show that the joint pdf of $(x_2, \dots, x_n)$ is given by

$$h_{2\cdots n}(x_2, \dots, x_n) = \left\{ \mathrm{I}_1 \left\{ \frac{f_1}{f_2} \mathrm{I}_2 \left[\frac{f_2}{f_3} \cdots \mathrm{I}_{n-1} \left(\frac{f_{n-1}}{f_n} \right) \right] \right\} \right\}^{-1},$$

where I_j denotes integration with respect to x_j.

(b) Suppose $h_{2\cdots n}(x_2^*, \dots, x_n^*)$ has been calculated at a particular point x^*, prove that

$$h_{1\cdots n-1}(x_1, \dots, x_{n-1}) =$$

$$h_{2\cdots n}(x_2^*, \dots, x_n^*) \frac{\prod_{i=1}^{n-1} f_i(x_i | x_1, \dots, x_{i-1}, x_{i+1}^*, \dots, x_n^*)}{\prod_{i=2}^{n} f_i(x_i^* | x_1, \dots, x_{i-1}, x_{i+1}^*, \dots, x_n^*)}.$$

1.5 Multivariate normal model. Let $y_1, \dots, y_n \stackrel{\text{iid}}{\sim} N_d(\mu, \Sigma)$ and $Y_{\text{com}} = \{y_i\}_{i=1}^n$. If the joint prior for (μ, Σ) is specified by $\Sigma \sim \text{IWishart}_d(\Lambda_0^{-1}, \nu_0)$ and $\mu|\Sigma \sim N_d(\mu_0, \Sigma/\kappa_0)$, then, the joint posterior $f(\mu, \Sigma | Y_{\text{com}})$ is proportional to

$$|\Sigma|^{-(\frac{n+\nu_0+d}{2}+1)} \exp\left\{ -0.5 \, \mathrm{tr}\, (\Sigma^{-1}[S_0 + \Lambda_0 + T_0]) \right\},$$

where $S_0 \hat{=} \Sigma_{i=1}^n (y_i - \mu)(y_i - \mu)^\top$, $T_0 \hat{=} \kappa_0(\mu - \mu_0)(\mu - \mu_0)^\top$. Verify the following facts:

$$\begin{aligned} \Sigma|(Y_{\text{com}}, \mu) &\sim \text{IWishart}_d([S_0 + \Lambda_0 + T_0]^{-1}, \nu_n + 1), \\ \mu|(Y_{\text{com}}, \Sigma) &\sim N_n(\mu_n, \Sigma/\kappa_n), \\ \mu|Y_{\text{com}} &\sim t_d\Big(\mu_n, \Lambda_n/[\kappa_n(\nu_n - d + 1)], \nu_n - d + 1\Big), \end{aligned}$$

where $\bar{y} = (1/n)\sum_{i=1}^n y_i$, $\mu_n = (n\bar{y} + \kappa_0\mu_0)/\kappa_n$, $\kappa_n = n + \kappa_0$, $\nu_n = n + \nu_0$, and

$$\Lambda_n = \sum_{i=1}^n (y_i - \bar{y})(y_i - \bar{y})^\top + \Lambda_0 + \frac{n\kappa_0}{\kappa_n}(\bar{y} - \mu_0)(\bar{y} - \mu_0)^\top.$$

1.6 Prove (1.20).

1.7 Let $x_i > 0, p_i > 0$, $i = 1, \dots, d$, and $\sum_{i=1}^d p_i = 1$, then

(a) $\sum_{i=1}^d p_i \log_2 x_i \le \log_2(\sum_{i=1}^d p_i x_i)$;

(b) $\sum_{i=1}^d p_i \log_2 p_i^{-1} \le \log_2 d$.

(*Hint*: Let X be a discrete r.v. with $\Pr(X = x_i) = p_i$ and use Jensen's inequality.)

1.8 Let r.v. X defined on $\mathcal{X}$ have pdf $f(x)$, show that $\mathrm{SE}(X)$ is maximal iff f is the uniform distribution on $\mathcal{X}$.
(*Hint*: Use (1.43).)

1.9 Let X, Y and Z be r.v.'s. Prove the following statements:

(a) $\mathrm{SE}(X|Y) \leq \mathrm{SE}(X)$;

(b) $\mathrm{SE}(X, Y|Z) = \mathrm{SE}(X|Z) + \mathrm{SE}(Y|X, Z)$;

(c) The mutual information of X and Y satisfies

$$\mathrm{M}(X, Y) = \mathrm{SE}(X) - \mathrm{SE}(X|Y) = \mathrm{SE}(Y) - \mathrm{SE}(Y|X).$$

1.10 Convexity and Jensen's inequality. Let ψ be a twice differentiable function defined on a convex set $\mathbb{S}$ and ∇ denote the derivative operator. The following statements are equivalent:

(a) ψ is convex;

(b) $\nabla^2\psi(x) \geq 0$ for all $x \in \mathbb{S}$;

(c) $\psi(x) \geq \psi(y_0) + \nabla\psi(y_0)(x - y_0)$ for all $x, y_0 \in \mathbb{S}$;

(d) $\psi(\alpha x + (1-\alpha)y) \leq \alpha\psi(x) + (1-\alpha)\psi(y)$ for all $x, y \in \mathbb{S}$ and $\alpha \in [0, 1]$;

(e) $\psi(\sum_i \alpha_i x_i) \leq \sum_i \alpha_i \psi(x_i)$ for any convex combination of points from $\mathbb{S}$.

Let X be an r.v. and ψ be a convex function (e.g., $-\log$), then $\psi(EX) \leq E\psi(X)$, provided both expectations exist. In addition, for a strictly convex function ψ, equality holds in Jensen's inequality iff $X = E(X)$ almost surely.
(*Hint*: Set $v_0 = E(X)$. The convexity yields $\psi(u) \geq \psi(v_0) + \nabla\psi(v_0)(u - v_0)$. Substitute X for u and take expectations.)

1.11 Extend the conclusions in Ex.1.11 from uninormal to multinormal.

1.12 Let $f_{(X,Y)}$, f_X and f_Y denote the joint, marginal pdfs of X and Y. Prove that

$$\mathrm{M}(X, Y) = \mathrm{KL}(f_{(X,Y)}, f_X f_Y).$$

CHAPTER 2

Optimization, Monte Carlo Simulation and Numerical Integration

Again, let Y_{obs} denote the observed (or observable) data and θ the parameter vector of interest. A central subject of statistics is to make inference on θ based on Y_{obs}. Frequentist/classical method arrives its inferential statements by combining point estimators of parameters with their standard errors. In a **parametric** inference problem, the observed vector Y_{obs} is viewed as a realized value of a random vector whose distribution is $f(Y_{\text{obs}}|\theta)$, which is the **likelihood** (function), usually denoted by $L(\theta|Y_{\text{obs}})$. Among all the estimation approaches, the *maximum likelihood estimation* (MLE) is the most popular one, where θ is estimated by $\hat{\theta}$ that maximizes $f(Y_{\text{obs}}|\theta)$. When sample sizes are small to moderate, a useful alternative to MLE is to utilize prior knowledge on the parameter and thus incorporate a prior distribution for the parameter into the likelihood and then compute the observed posterior distribution $f(\theta|Y_{\text{obs}})$. The posterior mode is defined as an argument $\tilde{\theta}$ that maximizes $f(\theta|Y_{\text{obs}})$ or equivalently maximizes its logarithm $\log f(\theta|Y_{\text{obs}})$. Computationally, finding the MLE or the mode becomes an **optimization** problem.

In addition, Bayesian computation of posterior mean, quantiles and marginal likelihood involves **high-dimensional integration** that usually does not have a closed-form solution. The "curse of dimensionality" coupled with rapid advances of computer technology has led to an enormous literature of sampling-based Bayesian methods. A variety of MCMC methods have been proposed to sample from posterior distributions. Essentially, they extend the univariate **simulation** method to multivariate situations. In this chapter, we focus on the introduction of some important and useful tools for optimization, Monte Carlo simulation and numerical integration.

2.1 Optimization

2.1.1 The Newton–Raphson (NR) algorithm

When the log-likelihood function $\ell(\theta|Y_{\rm obs})$ is well-behaved, a natural candidate for finding the MLE is the *Newton–Raphson* (NR) algorithm or the **Fisher scoring** algorithm because they converge quadratically (Tanner, 1996, p.26–27; Little & Rubin, 2002, Ch.8). The main objective of this subsection is to find the MLE of the parameter vector:

$$\hat{\theta} = \arg\max_{\theta\in\Theta} \ell(\theta|Y_{\rm obs}). \tag{2.1}$$

Let ℓ be a twice continuously differentiable and concave function and ∇ the derivative operator. Mathematically, $\nabla\ell$ is called the gradient vector and $\nabla^2\ell$ the Hessian matrix. Statistically, $\nabla\ell$ is called the **score** vector,

$$I(\theta|Y_{\rm obs}) = -\nabla^2\ell(\theta|Y_{\rm obs}) \tag{2.2}$$

is called the **observed information** matrix and

$$\begin{aligned} J(\theta) &= E\{I(\theta|Y_{\rm obs})|\theta\} \\ &= -\int \frac{\partial^2\ell(\theta|Y_{\rm obs})}{\partial\theta\partial\theta^{\top}} f(Y_{\rm obs}|\theta)\, dY_{\rm obs} \end{aligned} \tag{2.3}$$

is called the **Fisher/expected information** matrix.

(a) The formulation of the NR algorithm

Consider a second-order Taylor expansion of ℓ about $\theta^{(t)}$:

$$\begin{aligned} \ell(\theta|Y_{\rm obs}) &\doteq \ell(\theta^{(t)}|Y_{\rm obs}) + (\theta-\theta^{(t)})^{\top}\nabla\ell(\theta^{(t)}|Y_{\rm obs}) \\ &\quad + \frac{1}{2}(\theta-\theta^{(t)})^{\top}\nabla^2\ell(\theta^{(t)}|Y_{\rm obs})(\theta-\theta^{(t)}). \end{aligned}$$

Any stationary points of ℓ will satisfy (cf. Problem 2.1)

$$\nabla\ell(\theta|Y_{\rm obs}) \doteq \nabla\ell(\theta^{(t)}|Y_{\rm obs}) + \nabla^2\ell(\theta^{(t)}|Y_{\rm obs})(\theta-\theta^{(t)}) = \mathbf{0}.$$

Let $\theta^{(0)}$ be an initial guess of $\hat{\theta}$ and $\theta^{(t)}$ the guess at the t-th iteration, the NR algorithm is defined by

$$\theta^{(t+1)} = \theta^{(t)} + I^{-1}(\theta^{(t)}|Y_{\rm obs})\nabla\ell(\theta^{(t)}|Y_{\rm obs}). \tag{2.4}$$

Let $\mathrm{Se}(\hat{\theta})$ and $\mathrm{Cov}(\hat{\theta})$ denote the standard error and the asymptotic covariance matrix of $\hat{\theta}$, respectively. Under certain regularity conditions (Rao, 1973, p.364; Little & Rubin, 2002, p.105–108), it can be shown by the Central Limit Theorem that

$$\hat{\theta} - \theta \,\dot{\sim}\, N(\mathbf{0}, J^{-1}(\theta)),$$

so that $\text{Cov}(\hat{\theta}) = J^{-1}(\theta)$. It is important to note that $J^{-1}(\theta)$ is the covariance of the asymptotic distribution, not the limit of the exact covariance. The standard errors are the square roots of the diagonal elements of the inverse Fisher information matrix. We estimate $\text{Cov}(\hat{\theta})$ by

$$\widehat{\text{Cov}}(\hat{\theta}) = J^{-1}(\hat{\theta}). \tag{2.5}$$

In addition, the **delta method** can be used to derive the asymptotic distribution of $h(\hat{\theta})$, where h is differentiable (cf. Problem 2.2).

There are three potential problems with the NR algorithm. First, for complicated incomplete data or when the dimension of θ is large, it requires tedious calculations of the Hessian matrix at each iteration. Second, when the observed information evaluated at $\theta^{(t)}$ is apparently singular owing to collinearities among covariates, the NR does not work (cf. Ex.2.2). Third, the ℓ does not necessarily increase at each iteration for the NR algorithm, which may sometimes be divergent (Cox & Oakes, 1984, p.172). Böhning & Lindsay (1988, p.645–646) provided an example of a concave function for which the NR algorithm does not converge if a poor initial value is chosen.

(b) The Fisher scoring algorithm

A variant of the NR algorithm is the (Fisher) scoring algorithm, where the observed information in (2.4) is replaced by the expected information:

$$\theta^{(t+1)} = \theta^{(t)} + J^{-1}(\theta^{(t)})\nabla\ell(\theta^{(t)}|Y_{\text{obs}}).$$

An extra benefit of the scoring algorithm is that $J^{-1}(\hat{\theta})$ provides an estimated asymptotic covariance of the $\hat{\theta}$ (Lange, 1999, Ch.11).

(c) Application to logistic regression

Let $Y_{\text{obs}} = \{y_i\}_{i=1}^m$ and consider the following logistic regression

$$\begin{aligned} y_i &\stackrel{\text{ind}}{\sim} \text{Binomial}(n_i, p_i), \\ \text{logit}(p_i) &\hat{=} \log\frac{p_i}{1-p_i} = x_{(i)}^{\top}\theta, \quad 1 \le i \le m, \end{aligned} \tag{2.6}$$

where y_i denotes the number of subjects with positive response in the i-th group with n_i trials, p_i the probability of a subject in the i-th group with positive response, $x_{(i)}$ covariates vector and $\theta_{q\times 1}$ unknown parameters. The log-likelihood of θ is

$$\ell(\theta|Y_{\text{obs}}) = \sum_{i=1}^{m} \Big\{ y_i(x_{(i)}^{\top}\theta) - n_i \log[1 + \exp(x_{(i)}^{\top}\theta)] \Big\}.$$

Hence, the score and the observed information are given by

$$\begin{aligned} \nabla\ell(\theta|Y_{\text{obs}}) &= \sum_{i=1}^{m}(y_i - n_i p_i)x_{(i)} = X^{\top}(y - Np) \quad \text{and} \\ -\nabla^2\ell(\theta|Y_{\text{obs}}) &= \sum_{i=1}^{m} n_i p_i(1-p_i)x_{(i)}x_{(i)}^{\top} = X^{\top}NPX, \end{aligned} \tag{2.7}$$

respectively, where

$$\begin{aligned} X &= (x_{(1)}, \ldots, x_{(m)})^{\top}, \qquad y = (y_1, \ldots, y_m)^{\top}, \\ N &= \text{diag}(n_1, \ldots, n_m), \\ p &= (p_1, \ldots, p_m)^{\top}, \quad p_i = \exp[x_{(i)}^{\top}\theta]/(1 + \exp[x_{(i)}^{\top}\theta]), \\ P &= \text{diag}\Big(p_1(1-p_1), \ldots, p_m(1-p_m)\Big). \end{aligned}$$

From (2.4), we obtain

$$\theta^{(t+1)} = \theta^{(t)} + [X^{\top}NP^{(t)}X]^{-1}X^{\top}(y - Np^{(t)}). \tag{2.8}$$

Note that the observed information does not depend on the observed data Y_{obs}, then $J(\theta) = I(\theta|Y_{\text{obs}})$. From (2.5), we have

$$\widehat{\text{Cov}}(\hat{\theta}) = [X^{\top}N\hat{P}X]^{-1}, \tag{2.9}$$

which is a by-product of the NR iteration (2.8).

Example 2.1 (*Mice exposure data*). For illustration, we consider the mice exposure data in Table 2.1 reported by Larsen *et al.* (1979) and previously analyzed by Hasselblad *et al.* (1980). Here $m = 17$, y_i denotes the number of dead mice among n_i mice in the i-th group, and p_i is the probability of death for any mouse exposed to nitrous dioxide (NO_2) in the i-th group. We wish to investigate whether or not the probability of death depends on two further variables d_i (degree of exposure to NO_2), t_i (exposure time) and their interaction. We first take logarithms, $x_{i1} = \log(d_i)$ and $x_{i2} = \log(t_i)$, and then

Table 2.1 *Mice exposure data*

i	d_i	t_i	y_i	n_i	i	d_i	t_i	y_i	n_i
1	1.5	96.0	44	120	10	3.5	7.0	152	280
2	1.5	168.0	37	80	11	3.5	14.0	55	80
3	1.5	336.0	43	80	12	3.5	24.0	98	140
4	1.5	504.0	35	60	13	3.5	48.0	121	160
5	3.5	0.5	29	100	14	7.0	0.5	52	120
6	3.5	1.0	53	200	15	7.0	1.0	62	120
7	3.5	2.0	13	40	16	7.0	1.5	61	120
8	3.5	3.0	75	200	17	7.0	2.0	86	120
9	3.5	5.0	23	40					

Source: Leonard (2000).

standardize x_{i1} and x_{i2} by subtracting the sample mean and then dividing by the sample standard deviation (Leonard, 2000, p.147). The considered model is as follows:

$$\text{logit}(p_i) = \theta_0 + \theta_1 x_{i1} + \theta_2 x_{i2} + \theta_3 x_{i1} \times x_{i2}.$$

Using $\theta^{(0)} = \mathbf{1}_4$ as the starting values, the NR algorithm defined by (2.8) converged in 4 iterations. The MLEs associated with the intercept and three slopes are given by

$$\hat{\theta} = (0.1852, 1.0384, 1.2374, 0.2287)^{\top}.$$

The estimated covariance matrix of $\hat{\theta}$ is

$$\widehat{\text{Cov}}(\hat{\theta}) = \begin{pmatrix} 0.00391 & 0.00017 & 0.00136 & 0.00249 \\ 0.00017 & 0.00827 & 0.00725 & 0.00047 \\ 0.00136 & 0.00725 & 0.00964 & 0.00175 \\ 0.00249 & 0.00047 & 0.00175 & 0.00356 \end{pmatrix},$$

and estimated standard errors are $0.0624, 0.0909, 0.0981$ and 0.0597, respectively. ‖

The next example shows that the NR algorithm does not work because of the problem of collinearity.

Example 2.2 (*Cancer remission data*). We consider the cancer remission data (Lee, 1974) listed in Table 2.2. The binary outcome $y_i = 1$ implies that the i-th patient's remission occurred and $y_i = 0$ otherwise. There are six explanatory variables, where x1 =

Table 2.2 *Cancer remission data*

i	x1	x2	x3	x4	x5	x6	y_i	i	x1	x2	x3	x4	x5	x6	y_i
1	0.80	0.88	0.70	0.8	0.176	0.982	0	15	1.00	0.33	0.33	0.4	0.176	1.010	0
2	1.00	0.87	0.87	0.7	1.053	0.986	0	16	0.90	0.93	0.84	0.6	1.591	1.020	0
3	1.00	0.65	0.65	0.6	0.519	0.982	0	17	0.95	0.32	0.30	1.6	0.886	0.988	0
4	0.95	0.87	0.83	1.9	1.354	1.020	0	18	1.00	0.73	0.73	0.7	0.398	0.986	0
5	1.00	0.45	0.45	0.8	0.322	0.999	0	19	0.80	0.83	0.66	1.9	1.100	0.996	1
6	0.95	0.36	0.34	0.5	0.000	1.038	0	20	0.90	0.36	0.32	1.4	0.740	0.992	1
7	0.85	0.39	0.33	0.7	0.279	0.988	0	21	0.90	0.75	0.68	1.3	0.519	0.980	1
8	0.70	0.76	0.53	1.2	0.146	0.982	0	22	0.95	0.97	0.92	1.0	1.230	0.992	1
9	0.80	0.46	0.37	0.4	0.380	1.006	0	23	1.00	0.84	0.84	1.9	2.064	1.020	1
10	0.20	0.39	0.08	0.8	0.114	0.990	0	24	1.00	0.63	0.63	1.1	1.072	0.986	1
11	1.00	0.90	0.90	1.1	1.037	0.990	0	25	1.00	0.58	0.58	1.0	0.531	1.002	1
12	0.65	0.42	0.27	0.5	0.114	1.014	0	26	1.00	0.60	0.60	1.7	0.964	0.990	1
13	1.00	0.75	0.75	1.0	1.322	1.004	0	27	1.00	0.69	0.69	0.9	0.398	0.986	1
14	0.50	0.44	0.22	0.6	0.114	0.990	0								

Source: Lee (1974).

CELL/100, x2 = SMEAR/100, x3 = ABS.INFIL/100, x4 = LI/20, x5 = log(ABS.BLAST + 1) and x6 = Temperature/100. The logistic regression model is

$$\text{logit}(p_i) = \theta_0 + x_{i1}\theta_1 + \cdots + x_{i6}\theta_6.$$

Using $\theta^{(0)} = \mathbf{1}_7$ as the initial values, the NR algorithm (2.8) does not work because the observed information matrix evaluated at $\theta^{(0)}$ is apparently singular. The problem persists with other initial values. In fact, this is not surprising since the correlation coefficients for (x1, x2), (x1, x3), (x2, x3) are 0.98, −0.97 and −0.998, respectively. ||

2.1.2 The expectation-maximization (EM) algorithm

For incomplete data problems, an alternative to the NR algorithm is the EM algorithm (Dempster *et al.*, 1977) which does not require second derivatives to be calculated. The EM algorithm is an iterative deterministic method for finding the MLE or the posterior mode, and is remarkably simple both conceptually and computationally in many important cases. The basic principle behind the EM is that instead of performing a complicated optimization, one augments the observed data with latent data to perform a series of simple optimizations.

(a) The formulation of the EM algorithm

Let $\ell(\theta|Y_{\text{obs}}) \hat{=} \log L(\theta|Y_{\text{obs}})$ denote the log-likelihood function. Usually, directly solving the MLE $\hat{\theta}$ defined by (2.1) is extremely difficult. We augment the observed data Y_{obs} with latent variables Z so that both the complete-data log-likelihood $\ell(\theta|Y_{\text{obs}}, Z)$ and the conditional predictive distribution $f(Z|Y_{\text{obs}}, \theta)$ are available. Each iteration of the EM algorithm consists of an *expectation step* (E-step) and a *maximization step* (M-step).

Specifically, let $\theta^{(t)}$ be the current best guess of the MLE $\hat{\theta}$. The E-step is to compute the Q function defined by

$$\begin{aligned} Q(\theta|\theta^{(t)}) &= E\Big\{\ell(\theta|Y_{\text{obs}}, Z)\Big|Y_{\text{obs}}, \theta^{(t)}\Big\} \\ &= \int_{\mathcal{Z}} \ell(\theta|Y_{\text{obs}}, z) \times f(z|Y_{\text{obs}}, \theta^{(t)})\, dz, \end{aligned} \tag{2.10}$$

and the M-step is to maximize Q with respect to θ to obtain

$$\theta^{(t+1)} = \arg\max_{\theta \in \Theta} Q(\theta|\theta^{(t)}). \tag{2.11}$$

The two-step process is repeated until convergence occurs.

Example 2.3 (*Two-parameter multinomial model revisited*). In Ex. 1.9, we worked out a DA algorithm to simulate posterior draws of θ for the two-parameter multinomial model. Now suppose we are interested in finding the MLE of θ. From (1.32), the complete-data MLEs are given by

$$\hat{\theta}_1 = \frac{z_1 + z_2}{\Delta}, \quad \hat{\theta}_2 = \frac{z_3 + z_4}{\Delta}, \quad \hat{\theta}_3 = \frac{y_5}{\Delta}, \tag{2.12}$$

where $\Delta = \sum_{i=1}^4 z_i + y_5$. Thus, the E-step of the EM algorithm computes

$$E(Z_i|Y_{\text{obs}}, \theta) = y_i p_i$$

with p_i being defined by (1.35), and the M-step updates (2.12) by replacing $\{z_i\}_{i=1}^4$ with $E(Z_i|Y_{\text{obs}}, \theta)$.

For illustrative purpose, we consider the same dataset used in Gelfand & Smith (1990):

$$\begin{aligned} (y_1, \dots, y_5)^{\top} &= (14, 1, 1, 1, 5)^{\top}, \quad a_1 = \cdots = a_4 = 0.25, \\ b_1 = 1/8, &\qquad b_2 = b_3 = 0, \qquad b_4 = 3/8. \end{aligned} \tag{2.13}$$

Using $\theta^{(0)} = \mathbf{1}_3/3$ as initial values, the EM algorithm converged in 8 iterations. The obtained MLE is

$$\hat{\theta} = (0.585900,\ 0.0716178,\ 0.342482)^{\top}. \qquad \|$$

Example 2.4 (*Right censored regression model*). Consider the linear regression model (Wei & Tanner, 1990; Chib, 1992):

$$y = X\beta + \sigma\,\varepsilon, \quad \varepsilon \sim N(\mathbf{0}, \mathbf{I}_m),$$

where $y = (y_1, \dots, y_m)^\top$ is the response vector, $X = (x_{(1)}, \dots, x_{(m)})^\top$ the covariate matrix, β and σ^2 the unknown parameters. Suppose that the first r components of y are uncensored and the remaining $m - r$ are right censored (c_i denotes a censored time). We augment the observed data $Y_{\text{obs}} = \{y_1, \dots, y_r; c_{r+1}, \dots, c_m\}$ with the unobserved failure times $Z = (Z_{r+1}, \dots, Z_m)^\top$. If we had observed the value of Z, say $z = (z_{r+1}, \dots, z_m)^\top \,\hat{=}\, (y_{r+1}, \dots, y_m)^\top$ with $z_i > c_i$ $(i = r+1, \dots, m)$, we could have the complete-data likelihood

$$L(\beta, \sigma^2 | Y_{\text{obs}}, Z) = N(y | X\beta, \sigma^2 \mathbf{I}_m). \tag{2.14}$$

The conditional predictive density is the product of $(m - r)$ independent truncated normal densities:

$$f(Z | Y_{\text{obs}}, \beta, \sigma^2) = \prod_{i=r+1}^{m} TN(z_i | x_{(i)}^\top \beta, \sigma^2;\ c_i, +\infty). \tag{2.15}$$

The E-step requires to calculate (cf. Problem 2.3)

$$\begin{aligned} E\{Z_i | Y_{\text{obs}}, \beta, \sigma^2\} &= x_{(i)}^\top \beta + \sigma \Psi\Big(\frac{c_i - x_{(i)}^\top \beta}{\sigma}\Big) \quad \text{and} \\ E\{Z_i^2 | Y_{\text{obs}}, \beta, \sigma^2\} &= (x_{(i)}^\top \beta)^2 + \sigma^2 + \sigma(c_i + x_{(i)}^\top \beta) \Psi\Big(\frac{c_i - x_{(i)}^\top \beta}{\sigma}\Big), \end{aligned}$$

for $i = r+1, \dots, m$, where

$$\Psi(x) \,\hat{=}\, \phi(x) / \{1 - \Phi(x)\} \tag{2.16}$$

and $\phi(x)$ and $\Phi(x)$ denote the pdf and cdf of $N(0, 1)$, respectively. The M-step is to find the complete-data MLEs:

$$\beta = (X^\top X)^{-1} X^\top y \quad \text{and} \quad \sigma^2 = \frac{(y - X\beta)^\top (y - X\beta)}{m},$$

where $y = (y_1, \dots, y_r; z_{r+1}, \dots, z_m)^\top$.

We consider the dataset of accelerated life tests on electrical insulation in 40 motorettes (Schmee & Hahn, 1979). Ten motorettes were tested at each of the four temperatures: 150°C, 170°C, 190°C

Table 2.3 *Insulation life data with censoring times*

i	y_i	T_i	i	y_i	T_i	i	c_i	T_i	i	c_i	T_i
1	3.2464	2.2563	13	2.6107	2.0276	18	3.9066	2.3629	30	3.7362	2.2563
2	3.4428	2.2563	14	2.6107	2.0276	19	3.9066	2.3629	31	3.2253	2.1589
3	3.5371	2.2563	15	2.7024	2.0276	20	3.9066	2.3629	32	3.2253	2.1589
4	3.5492	2.2563	16	2.7024	2.0276	21	3.9066	2.3629	33	3.2253	2.1589
5	3.5775	2.2563	17	2.7024	2.0276	22	3.9066	2.3629	34	3.2253	2.1589
6	3.6866	2.2563				23	3.9066	2.3629	35	3.2253	2.1589
7	3.7157	2.2563				24	3.9066	2.3629	36	2.7226	2.0276
8	2.6107	2.1589				25	3.9066	2.3629	37	2.7226	2.0276
9	2.6107	2.1589				26	3.9066	2.3629	38	2.7226	2.0276
10	3.1284	2.1589				27	3.9066	2.3629	39	2.7226	2.0276
11	3.1284	2.1589				28	3.7362	2.2563	40	2.7226	2.0276
12	3.1584	2.1589				29	3.7362	2.2563			

and 220°C. Testing was terminated at different times at each temperature level. The linear model is

$$y_i = \beta_0 + \beta_1 T_i + \sigma\varepsilon_i, \quad \varepsilon_i \sim N(0,1),$$

where $y_i = \log_{10}(\text{failure time})$ and $T_i = 1000/(\text{Temperature} + 273.2)$. With this transformation, we summarize the new data in Table 2.3, where the first $r = 17$ units are uncensored and the remaining $m - r = 40 - 17 = 23$ are censored. Using $(\beta_0^{(0)}, \beta_1^{(0)}, \sigma^{(0)})^\top = (1,1,1)^\top$ as initial values, the EM algorithm converged to

$$\hat{\beta}_0 = -6.019, \quad \hat{\beta}_1 = 4.311 \quad \text{and} \quad \hat{\sigma} = 0.2592$$

after 40 iterations with precision 10^{-5}. ||

(b) The ascent property of the EM algorithm

The Bayes theorem gives

$$\frac{f(Y_{\text{obs}}, Z|\theta)}{f(Y_{\text{obs}}|\theta)} = f(Z|Y_{\text{obs}}, \theta)$$

so that the log-likelihood satisfies the following identity

$$\ell(\theta|Y_{\text{obs}}) - \ell(\theta|Y_{\text{obs}}, Z) = -\log f(Z|Y_{\text{obs}}, \theta). \tag{2.17}$$

Integrating both sides of this equation with respect to $f(Z|Y_{\rm obs},\theta^{(t)})$, we obtain

$$\ell(\theta|Y_{\rm obs}) - Q(\theta|\theta^{(t)}) = -H(\theta|\theta^{(t)}), \tag{2.18}$$

where Q is defined by (2.10) and

$$H(\theta|\theta^{(t)}) = E\{\log f(Z|Y_{\rm obs},\theta)|Y_{\rm obs},\theta^{(t)}\}. \tag{2.19}$$

By using (1.42) and (1.43), it follows that

$$H(\theta^{(t)}|\theta^{(t)}) - H(\theta|\theta^{(t)}) = \mathrm{KL}\Big(f(Z|Y_{\rm obs},\theta^{(t)}), f(Z|Y_{\rm obs},\theta)\Big) \ge 0,$$

and the equality holds iff $\theta = \theta^{(t)}$. Thus, for all θ and $\theta^{(t)}$, we have

$$\begin{aligned}\ell(\theta|Y_{\rm obs}) - Q(\theta|\theta^{(t)}) &= -H(\theta|\theta^{(t)}) \\ &\ge -H(\theta^{(t)}|\theta^{(t)}) \\ &= \ell(\theta^{(t)}|Y_{\rm obs}) - Q(\theta^{(t)}|\theta^{(t)}). \end{aligned} \tag{2.20}$$

In other words, $\ell(\theta|Y_{\rm obs})-Q(\theta|\theta^{(t)})$ attains its minimum at $\theta = \theta^{(t)} \in \Theta$. Inequality (2.20) is the essence of the EM algorithm because if we choose $\theta^{(t+1)}$ to maximize $Q(\theta|\theta^{(t)})$, then it follows that

$$\begin{aligned}&\ell(\theta^{(t+1)}|Y_{\rm obs}) - \ell(\theta^{(t)}|Y_{\rm obs}) \\ &\qquad \ge Q(\theta^{(t+1)}|\theta^{(t)}) - Q(\theta^{(t)}|\theta^{(t)}) \ge 0. \end{aligned} \tag{2.21}$$

Namely, the EM algorithm holds the **ascent property** that increasing $Q(\theta|\theta^{(t)})$ causes an increase in $\ell(\theta|Y_{\rm obs})$.

Generally, a GEM (generalized EM) algorithm chooses $\theta^{(t+1)}$ so that

$$Q(\theta^{(t+1)}|\theta^{(t)}) \ge Q(\theta^{(t)}|\theta^{(t)}).$$

From (2.21), a GEM algorithm also has the ascent property.

(c) Missing information principle and standard errors

Integrating both sides of (2.17) with respect to $f(Z|Y_{\rm obs},\theta)$, similar to (2.18), we have

$$\ell(\theta|Y_{\rm obs}) = Q(\theta|\theta) - H(\theta|\theta), \tag{2.22}$$

where Q and H are defined by (2.10) and (2.19). Differentiating Eq.(2.22) twice with respect to the left argument θ yields

$$-\nabla^2\ell(\theta|Y_{\rm obs}) = -\nabla^{20}Q(\theta|\theta) + \nabla^{20}H(\theta|\theta), \tag{2.23}$$

where $\nabla^{ij}Q(x|y)$ means $\partial^{i+j}Q(x|y)/\partial x^i \partial y^j$. If we evaluate the functions in Eq.(2.23) at the converged value $\hat{\theta}$, and call

$$\begin{aligned} I_{\text{obs}} &= -\nabla^2 \ell(\hat{\theta}|Y_{\text{obs}}) = I(\theta|Y_{\text{obs}})|_{\theta=\hat{\theta}}, & (2.24) \\ I_{\text{com}} &= -\nabla^{20} Q(\hat{\theta}|\hat{\theta}) \\ &= E\{-\nabla^2 \ell(\theta|Y_{\text{obs}}, Z)|Y_{\text{obs}}, \theta\}|_{\theta=\hat{\theta}}, & (2.25) \\ I_{\text{mis}} &= -\nabla^{20} H(\hat{\theta}|\hat{\theta}) \\ &= E\{-\nabla^2 \log f(Z|Y_{\text{obs}}, \theta)|Y_{\text{obs}}, \theta\}|_{\theta=\hat{\theta}}, & (2.26) \end{aligned}$$

the **observed information**, the **complete information** and the **missing information**, then Eq.(2.23) becomes

$$I_{\text{obs}} = I_{\text{com}} - I_{\text{mis}}. \tag{2.27}$$

Namely, the observed information equals the complete information minus the missing information.

Louis (1982) shows that

$$-\nabla^{20} H(\theta|\theta) = E\{[\nabla \ell(\theta|Y_{\text{obs}}, Z)]^{\otimes 2}|Y_{\text{obs}}, \theta\} - [\nabla \ell(\theta|Y_{\text{obs}})]^{\otimes 2}, \tag{2.28}$$

where $a^{\otimes 2} \mathrel{\hat{=}} aa^\top$. Since $\nabla \ell(\hat{\theta}|Y_{\text{obs}}) = 0$, Eq.(2.27) becomes

$$I(\hat{\theta}|Y_{\text{obs}}) = -\nabla^{20} Q(\hat{\theta}|\hat{\theta}) - E\{[\nabla \ell(\theta|Y_{\text{obs}}, Z)]^{\otimes 2}|Y_{\text{obs}}, \theta\}|_{\theta=\hat{\theta}}. \tag{2.29}$$

The estimated standard errors are the square roots of the diagonal elements for the inverse information matrix, i.e., $I^{-1}(\hat{\theta}|Y_{\text{obs}})$.

Example 2.5 (*Two-parameter multinomial model revisited*). In Ex. 2.3, we derived the MLEs of $\theta = (\theta_1, \theta_2, \theta_3)^\top$ by using an EM algorithm. From (1.32), the complete-data log-likelihood is

$$\ell(\theta|Y_{\text{obs}}, Z) = (Z_1 + Z_2)\log\theta_1 + (Z_3 + Z_4)\log\theta_2 + y_5 \log\theta_3.$$

It is easy to obtain

$$\begin{aligned} \nabla \ell(\theta|Y_{\text{obs}}, Z) &= \begin{pmatrix} \dfrac{Z_1 + Z_2}{\theta_1} \\ \dfrac{Z_3 + Z_4}{\theta_2} \end{pmatrix} - \frac{y_5}{\theta_3}\mathbf{1}_2, \\ -\nabla^2 \ell(\theta|Y_{\text{obs}}, Z) &= \begin{pmatrix} \dfrac{Z_1 + Z_2}{\theta_1^2} & 0 \\ 0 & \dfrac{Z_3 + Z_4}{\theta_2^2} \end{pmatrix} + \frac{y_5}{\theta_3^2}\mathbf{1}_2\mathbf{1}_2^\top. \end{aligned}$$

From (2.25), we have

$$
\begin{aligned}
-\nabla^{20}Q(\theta|\theta) &= E\{-\nabla^2\ell(\theta|Y_{\text{obs}}, Z)|Y_{\text{obs}}, \theta\} \\
&= \begin{pmatrix} \dfrac{z_1^* + z_2^*}{\theta_1^2} & 0 \\ 0 & \dfrac{z_3^* + z_4^*}{\theta_2^2} \end{pmatrix} + \frac{y_5}{\theta_3^2}\mathbf{1}_2\mathbf{1}_2^\top,
\end{aligned}
$$

where $z_i^* = E(Z_i|Y_{\text{obs}}, \theta) = y_i p_i$ with p_i being defined by (1.35). Substituting the dataset given by (2.13) and

$$\hat{\theta} = (0.585900,\ 0.0716178,\ 0.342482)^\top$$

in these expressions yields

$$-\nabla^{20}Q(\hat{\theta}|\hat{\theta}) = \begin{pmatrix} 67.5457 & 42.628 \\ 42.6280 & 246.478 \end{pmatrix}.$$

Similarly, we have

$$
\begin{aligned}
E\{[\nabla\ell(\theta|Y_{\text{obs}}, Z)]^{\otimes 2}|Y_{\text{obs}}, \theta\} &= \frac{y_5^2}{\theta_3^2}\mathbf{1}_2\mathbf{1}_2^\top \\
&+ \begin{pmatrix} \frac{z_{12}^*}{\theta_1^2} - 2y_5\frac{z_1^*+z_2^*}{\theta_1\theta_3}, & \frac{(z_1^*+z_2^*)(z_3^*+z_4^*)}{\theta_1\theta_2} - \frac{y_5}{\theta_3}\left[\frac{z_1^*+z_2^*}{\theta_1} + \frac{z_3^*+z_4^*}{\theta_2}\right] \\ * & \frac{z_{34}^*}{\theta_2^2} - 2y_5\frac{z_3^*+z_4^*}{\theta_2\theta_3} \end{pmatrix},
\end{aligned}
$$

where $z_{12}^* \mathrel{\hat{=}} E\{(Z_1 + Z_2)^2|Y_{\text{obs}}, \theta\}$, $z_{34}^* \mathrel{\hat{=}} E\{(Z_3 + Z_4)^2|Y_{\text{obs}}, \theta\}$ and $E(Z_i^2|Y_{\text{obs}}, \theta) = y_i p_i(1 - p_i + y_i p_i)$. Numerically, we obtain

$$E\{[\nabla\ell(\theta|Y_{\text{obs}}, Z)]^{\otimes 2}|Y_{\text{obs}}, \theta\}|_{\theta=\hat{\theta}} = \begin{pmatrix} 10.1320 & 0 \\ 0 & 8.47962 \end{pmatrix}.$$

Hence, from (2.29), the observed information matrix is

$$I(\hat{\theta}|Y_{\text{obs}}) = \begin{pmatrix} 57.4137 & 42.628 \\ 42.6280 & 237.998 \end{pmatrix},$$

and the estimated standard errors are $\widehat{\text{Se}}(\hat{\theta}_1) = 0.1417$ and $\widehat{\text{Se}}(\hat{\theta}_2) = 0.0696$. Using the delta method (cf. Problem 2.2), we obtain $\widehat{\text{Se}}(\hat{\theta}_3) = 0.1332$.

‖

2.1.3 The ECM algorithm

One limitation of the EM algorithm is that the M-step may be difficult to achieve (e.g., has no closed form) in some problems. Meng & Rubin (1993) proposed an *expectation/conditional maximization* (ECM) algorithm to replace a complicated M-step with several computationally simpler conditional maximization steps. As a consequence, it typically converges more slowly than does the EM algorithm in terms of number of iterations, but possibly faster in total computer time. Importantly, the ECM algorithm preserves the monotone convergence property of the EM algorithm.

More precisely, the ECM replaces each M-step of the EM by a sequence of K conditional maximization steps, i.e., CM-steps, each of which maximizes the Q function defined in (2.10) over θ but with some vector function of θ, $g_k(\theta)$ $(k = 1, \ldots, K)$, fixed at its previous value. Ex.2.6 illustrates ECM in a simple but rather general model in which, partitioning the parameter into a location parameter and a scale parameter, leads to a simple ECM with two CM-steps, each involving closed-form solution while holding the other fixed.

Example 2.6 (*A multinormal regression model with missing data*). Suppose that we have n independent observations from the following m-variate normal model

$$\mathbf{y}_j \sim N_m(X_j\beta, \Sigma), \quad j = 1, \ldots, n, \tag{2.30}$$

and X_j is a known $m \times p$ design matrix for the j-th observation, β is a $p \times 1$ vector of unknown coefficients and Σ is an unknown $m \times m$ covariance matrix. Let $\theta = (\beta, \Sigma)$. If Σ were given, say $\Sigma = \Sigma^{(t)}$, the conditional MLE of β would be simply the weighted least-squares estimate:

$$\beta^{(t+1)} = \left\{\sum_{j=1}^{n} X_j^{\top}(\Sigma^{(t)})^{-1}X_j\right\}^{-1}\left\{\sum_{j=1}^{n} X_j^{\top}(\Sigma^{(t)})^{-1}\mathbf{y}_j\right\}. \tag{2.31}$$

On the other hand, given $\beta = \beta^{(t+1)}$, the conditional MLE of Σ is

$$\Sigma^{(t+1)} = \frac{1}{n}\sum_{j=1}^{n}(\mathbf{y}_j - X_j\beta^{(t+1)})(\mathbf{y}_j - X_j\beta^{(t+1)})^{\top}. \tag{2.32}$$

The E-step of the ECM algorithm computes

$$E(\mathbf{y}_j|Y_{\text{obs}}, \theta^{(t)}) \quad \text{and} \quad E(\mathbf{y}_j\mathbf{y}_j^{\top}|Y_{\text{obs}}, \theta^{(t)}), \quad j = 1, \ldots, n,$$

where $\theta^{(t)} = (\beta^{(t)}, \Sigma^{(t)})$. The first CM-step is to calculate $\beta^{(t+1)}$ using (2.31) with $\mathbf{y}_j$ being replaced by $E(\mathbf{y}_j|Y_{\text{obs}}, \theta^{(t)})$. The second CM-step calculates $\Sigma^{(t+1)}$ using (2.32) where $\mathbf{y}_j$ and $\mathbf{y}_j\mathbf{y}_j^{\top}$ being replaced by $E(\mathbf{y}_j|Y_{\text{obs}}, \theta^{(t)})$ and $E(\mathbf{y}_j\mathbf{y}_j^{\top}|Y_{\text{obs}}, \theta^{(t)})$, respectively. ||

Ex.2.7 illustrates that even if some CM-steps do not have analytical solutions, ECM may still be computationally simpler and more stable because it involves lower-dimensional maximizations than EM.

Example 2.7 (*A gamma model with incomplete data*). Let

$$y_1, \dots, y_m \stackrel{\text{iid}}{\sim} \text{Gamma}(\alpha, \beta)$$

(cf. Appendix A.2.7) and we are interested in finding the MLEs of α and β based on the observed data Y_{obs}, which, for example, are the results of censoring the complete data $Y = \{y_i\}_{i=1}^m$. The E-step of the ECM computes

$$E(y_i|Y_{\text{obs}}, \alpha^{(t)}, \beta^{(t)}) \quad \text{and} \quad E(\log y_i|Y_{\text{obs}}, \alpha^{(t)}, \beta^{(t)})$$

for some i. The complete-data log-likelihood is

$$\ell(\alpha, \beta|Y) = (\alpha - 1)\sum_{i=1}^m \log y_i - m\bar{y}\beta + m[\alpha \log \beta - \log \Gamma(\alpha)],$$

where $\bar{y} = \frac{1}{m}\sum_{i=1}^m y_i$. For given $\alpha = \alpha^{(t)}$, the first CM-step is to calculate the conditional MLE of β as

$$\beta^{(t+1)} = \alpha^{(t)}/\bar{y}.$$

On the other hand, for given $\beta = \beta^{(t+1)}$, the second CM-step is to find the conditional MLE of α, $\alpha^{(t+1)}$, which satisfies the following equation

$$\frac{\partial\Gamma(\alpha)/\partial\alpha}{\Gamma(\alpha)} = \frac{1}{m}\sum_{i=1}^m \log y_i + \log \beta^{(t+1)}. \tag{2.33}$$

Although (2.33) does not provide an analytic solution for $\alpha^{(t+1)}$, a value can be easily obtained by a one-dimensional Newton–Raphson algorithm. ||

2.1.4 Minorization-maximization (MM) algorithms

Although EM-type algorithms (Dempster *et al.*, 1977; Meng & Rubin, 1993) possess the ascent property that ensures monotone convergence, they may not apply to generalized linear models (e.g., logistic regression, log-linear models) and Cox proportional models due to the absence of a missing-data structure in these models. Therefore, for problems in which the missing-data structure does not exist or is not readily available, *minorization-maximization* (MM) algorithms (Lange *et al.*, 2000; Hunter & Lange, 2004) are often useful alternatives. In the sequel, MM refers to a class of algorithms.

(a) A brief review of MM algorithms

According to Hunter & Lange (2004), the general principle behind MM algorithms is first enunciated by numerical analysts Ortega & Rheinboldt (1970, p.253–255) in the context of linear search methods. De Leeuw & Heiser (1977) presented an MM algorithm for multidimensional scaling in parallel to the classic Dempster *et al.* (1977) article on EM algorithms. Although the work of de Leeuw & Heiser did not draw the same degree of attention from the statistical community as did the Dempster *et al.* (1977) article, development of MM algorithms has continued. The MM principle reappears, among other places, in robust regression (Huber, 1981), in correspondence analysis (Heiser, 1987), in the quadratic lower-bound principle of Böhning & Lindsay (1988), in the psychometrics literature on least squares (Bijleveld & de Leeuw, 1991; Kiers & Ten Berge, 1992), and in medical imaging (De Pierro, 1995; Lange & Fessler, 1995). The recent survey articles by De Leeuw (1994), Heiser (1995), Becker *et al.* (1997), and Lange *et al.* (2000) deal with the general principle, but it is not until the rejoinder of Hunter & Lange (2000) that the acronym MM first appears. This acronym pays homage to the earlier names "majorization" and "iterative majorization" of the MM principle, emphasizes its crucial link to the well-known EM principle, and diminishes the possibility of confusion with the distinct subject in mathematics known as majorization (Marshall & Olkin 1979).

(b) The MM idea

Let $\ell(\theta|Y_{\text{obs}})$ denote the log-likelihood function and we want to find the MLE $\hat{\theta}$ defined by (2.1). Let $\theta^{(t)}$ represent the current guess of $\hat{\theta}$ and $Q(\theta|\theta^{(t)})$ a real-valued function of θ whose form depends on

$\theta^{(t)}$. The function $Q(\theta|\theta^{(t)})$ is said to **minorize** $\ell(\theta|Y_{\text{obs}})$ at $\theta^{(t)}$ if

$$\begin{aligned} Q(\theta|\theta^{(t)}) &\le \ell(\theta|Y_{\text{obs}}) \quad \forall\, \theta \in \Theta, &(2.34)\\ Q(\theta^{(t)}|\theta^{(t)}) &= \ell(\theta^{(t)}|Y_{\text{obs}}). &(2.35)\end{aligned}$$

In an MM algorithm, we maximize the minorizing function $Q(\theta|\theta^{(t)})$ instead of the target function $\ell(\theta|Y_{\text{obs}})$. If $\theta^{(t+1)}$ is the maximizer of $Q(\theta|\theta^{(t)})$, i.e.,

$$\theta^{(t+1)} = \arg\max_{\theta \in \Theta} Q(\theta|\theta^{(t)}), \tag{2.36}$$

then from (2.34) and (2.35), we have

$$\ell(\theta^{(t+1)}|Y_{\text{obs}}) \ge Q(\theta^{(t+1)}|\theta^{(t)}) \ge Q(\theta^{(t)}|\theta^{(t)}) = \ell(\theta^{(t)}|Y_{\text{obs}}). \tag{2.37}$$

Consequently, an increase in $Q(\theta|\theta^{(t)})$ forces $\ell(\theta|Y_{\text{obs}})$ uphill. Under appropriate additional compactness and continuity conditions, the ascent property (2.37) guarantees convergence of the MM algorithm, and lends the algorithm monotone convergence. From (2.37) it is clear that it is not necessary to actually maximize the minorizing function, it suffices to find $\theta^{(t+1)}$ such that

$$Q(\theta^{(t+1)}|\theta^{(t)}) \ge Q(\theta^{(t)}|\theta^{(t)}).$$

(c) The quadratic lower-bound (QLB) algorithm

Let $\ell(\theta|Y_{\text{obs}})$ denote the log-likelihood function and we want to find the MLE $\hat{\theta}$ defined by (2.1). The *quadratic lower-bound* (QLB) algorithm developed by Böhning & Lindsay (1988) is a special MM algorithm. The key idea is to transfer the optimization from the intractable $\ell(\theta|Y_{\text{obs}})$ to a quadratic **surrogate** function $Q(\theta|\theta^{(t)})$. A key for the QLB is to find a positive definite matrix $B > 0$ such that

$$\nabla^2 \ell(\theta|Y_{\text{obs}}) + B \ge 0 \qquad \forall\, \theta \in \Theta. \tag{2.38}$$

Then, for a given $\theta^{(t)} \in \Theta$, we can construct a quadratic function

$$\begin{aligned} Q(\theta|\theta^{(t)}) \hat{=} {}& \ell(\theta^{(t)}|Y_{\text{obs}}) + (\theta - \theta^{(t)})^{\top} \nabla \ell(\theta^{(t)}|Y_{\text{obs}}) \\ & -\frac{1}{2}(\theta - \theta^{(t)})^{\top} B (\theta - \theta^{(t)}), \quad \theta \in \Theta. \end{aligned} \tag{2.39}$$

It is easy to see that this Q minorizes $\ell(\theta|Y_{\text{obs}})$ at $\theta^{(t)}$ (cf. Problem 2.4). The QLB algorithm is defined by (2.36), i.e.,

$$\theta^{(t+1)} = \theta^{(t)} + B^{-1} \nabla \ell(\theta^{(t)}|Y_{\text{obs}}). \tag{2.40}$$

Just like an EM algorithm, the QLB algorithm also holds the ascent property (2.37), leading to monotone convergence. The algorithm has the advantage of requiring a single matrix inversion instead of repeated matrix inversions.

Example 2.8 (*Logistic regression models*). In §2.1.1, we applied the NR algorithm to logistic regression. The key to the application of the QLB algorithm is to find a positive definite matrix B satisfying the condition (2.38). Since $p_i(1-p_i) \leq 1/4$, from (2.7), we have

$$B \hat{=} \frac{1}{4} X^{\top} N X \geq -\nabla^2 \ell(\theta | Y_{\text{obs}}). \tag{2.41}$$

From (2.40), we obtain

$$\theta^{(t+1)} = \theta^{(t)} + 4[X^{\top} N X]^{-1} X^{\top}(y - N p^{(t)}), \tag{2.42}$$

where

$$p_i^{(t)} = \frac{\exp\{x_{(i)}^{\top} \theta^{(t)}\}}{1 + \exp\{x_{(i)}^{\top} \theta^{(t)}\}}$$

is the i-th component of $p^{(t)}$. Applying the QLB algorithm (2.42) to the cancer remission data (cf. Ex.2.2), where the NR algorithm does not work, we arrived at

$$\hat{\theta} = (58.039, 24.661, 19.293, -19.601, 3.896, 0.151, -87.434)^{\top},$$

after 1500 iterations starting from $\theta^{(0)} = \mathbf{1}_7$. ||

Example 2.9 (*Cox's proportional hazards models*). Cox's regression (Cox, 1972) is a semi-parametric approach to survival analysis in which the hazard function

$$h(t) = h_0(t) \exp(x^{\top} \theta)$$

is modeled, where $h_0(t)$ is the baseline hazard function and can be viewed as nuisance parameters, x a vector of covariates and $\theta_{q \times 1}$ regression parameters. Suppose that among a total of N subjects there are m ordered **distinct** survival times $\{y_{(i)}\}_{i=1}^m$ (i.e., there are no ties in the data) and $N - m$ right censored survival times. We also assume that censoring is noninformative in the sense that inferences do not depend on the censoring process. Let $\mathbb{R}_i$ denote the risk set at $y_{(i)}$ so that $\mathbb{R}_i$ is the set of individuals who are event-free and uncensored at a time just prior to $y_{(i)}$. The parameters θ are estimated by maximizing the partial log-likelihood

$$\ell(\theta|Y_{\text{obs}}) = \sum_{i=1}^{m} \log\left\{\frac{\exp(x_{(i)}^{\top}\theta)}{\sum_{j\in I\!R_i}\exp(x_j^{\top}\theta)}\right\}, \tag{2.43}$$

where $x_{(i)}$ denotes the vector of covariates for an individual who has an event at $y_{(i)}$. The score and the observed information are given by

$$\begin{aligned}\nabla\ell(\theta|Y_{\text{obs}}) &= \sum_{i=1}^{m}\Big\{x_{(i)} - \sum_{j\in I\!R_i} x_j p_{ij}\Big\},\\ -\nabla^2\ell(\theta|Y_{\text{obs}}) &= \sum_{i=1}^{m}\Big\{\sum_{j\in I\!R_i} x_j x_j^{\top} p_{ij} - \Big(\sum_{j\in I\!R_i} x_j p_{ij}\Big)^{\otimes 2}\Big\},\end{aligned}$$

where

$$p_{ij} = \frac{\exp(x_j^{\top}\theta)}{\sum_{k\in I\!R_i}\exp(x_k^{\top}\theta)}, \qquad j \in I\!R_i. \tag{2.44}$$

Note that, for given i, $\{p_{ij}\}$ is a probability distribution with support points in the set $\{x_j : j \in I\!R_i\}$. Let U_i denote a random vector taking the value x_j with probability p_{ij}, then we have

$$\begin{aligned}E(U_i) &= \sum_{j\in I\!R_i} x_j p_{ij} \quad \text{and}\\ \text{Var}(U_i) &= \sum_{j\in I\!R_i} [x_j - E(U_i)][x_j - E(U_i)]^{\top} p_{ij}.\end{aligned}$$

Thus, $-\nabla^2\ell(\theta|Y_{\text{obs}}) = \sum_i \text{Var}(U_i)$ is positive definite for all θ, which implies the concavity of the log-likelihood $\ell(\theta|Y_{\text{obs}})$. Utilizing the result in Problem 2.5, we have

$$\begin{aligned}-\nabla^2\ell(\theta|Y_{\text{obs}}) &\le \sum_{i=1}^{m}\frac{1}{2}\Big\{\sum_{j\in I\!R_i} x_j x_j^{\top} - \frac{1}{n_i}\Big(\sum_{j\in I\!R_i} x_j\Big)^{\otimes 2}\Big\}\\ &\hat{=}\ B, \quad \text{for any } \theta \in \Theta,\end{aligned}$$

where n_i denotes the number of individuals in $I\!R_i$. Thus, the QLB algorithm can be applied to find the MLE of θ. ||

Another important application of the MM algorithm is in Problem 2.6.

(d) The De Pierro's algorithm

Although the QLB algorithm is elegant, its applicability depends on the existence of a positive definite B satisfying (2.38). In examples such as Poisson regression, this algorithm fails because of the absence of such a matrix B. The **De Pierro's** algorithm originally proposed by De Pierro (1995) is also a special member of the family of MM algorithms. The main idea is to transfer the optimization of a high dimensional function $\ell(\theta|Y_{\text{obs}})$ to the optimization of a low dimensional **surrogate** function $Q(\theta|\theta^{(t)})$ in the sense that $Q(\theta|\theta^{(t)})$ is a sum of convex combinations of a series of one-dimensional concave functions. Maximizing $Q(\theta|\theta^{(t)})$ can be implemented via the Newton–Raphson method.

Let the log-likelihood function be of the form

$$\ell(\theta|Y_{\text{obs}}) = \sum_{i=1}^{m} f_i(x_{(i)}^{\top}\theta), \tag{2.45}$$

where $X_{m\times q} = (x_{(1)}, \ldots, x_{(m)})^{\top}$ is the design matrix, $x_{(i)} = (x_{i1}, \ldots, x_{iq})^{\top}$ denotes the i-th row vector of X, θ the parameters of interest, $\{f_i\}_{i=1}^{m}$ are twice continuously differentiable and strictly concave functions defined in one-dimensional real space $\mathbb{R}$. From (2.45), the score and the observed information are given by

$$\begin{aligned}
\nabla\ell(\theta|Y_{\text{obs}}) &= \sum_{i=1}^{m} \nabla f_i(x_{(i)}^{\top}\theta)x_{(i)}, \quad \text{and} \\
-\nabla^2\ell(\theta|Y_{\text{obs}}) &= \sum_{i=1}^{m} \Big\{-\nabla^2 f_i(x_{(i)}^{\top}\theta)\Big\}x_{(i)}x_{(i)}^{\top}.
\end{aligned}$$

Thus, $\ell(\theta|Y_{\text{obs}})$ is strictly concave provided that each $\nabla^2 f_i < 0$.

To construct a surrogate function, we first define two index sets:

$$\mathbb{J}_i = \{j : x_{ij} \neq 0\}, \quad 1 \le i \le m, \tag{2.46}$$

$$\mathbb{I}_j = \{i : x_{ij} \neq 0\}, \quad 1 \le j \le q. \tag{2.47}$$

Furthermore, for a fixed $r \in \mathbb{R}_+ = \{r : r \ge 0\}$ and a fixed i, we define weights

$$\lambda_{ij} = \frac{|x_{ij}|^r}{\sum_{j'\in\mathbb{J}_i} |x_{ij'}|^r}, \quad j \in \mathbb{J}_i. \tag{2.48}$$

Obviously,

$$\lambda_{ij} > 0 \quad \text{and} \quad \sum_{j\in\mathbb{J}_i} \lambda_{ij} = 1.$$

It can be shown that when $r = 1$, the algorithm converges most quickly. Note that when $r = 0$, $\lambda_{ij} = 1/n_i$, where n_i denotes the number of elements in $\mathbb{J}_i$. Now, we can construct a surrogate function for a given $\theta^{(t)} \in \Theta$ as follows:

$$Q(\theta|\theta^{(t)}) = \sum_{i=1}^{m} \sum_{j \in \mathbb{J}_i} \lambda_{ij} f_i\Big(\lambda_{ij}^{-1} x_{ij}(\theta_j - \theta_j^{(t)}) + x_{(i)}^{\top}\theta^{(t)}\Big), \tag{2.49}$$

for $\theta \in \Theta$. It can be shown that this Q minorizes $\ell(\theta|Y_{\text{obs}})$ at $\theta^{(t)}$ (cf. Problem 2.7). The De Pierro's algorithm is defined by

$$\theta^{(t+1)} = \arg\max_{\theta \in \Theta} Q(\theta|\theta^{(t)}). \tag{2.50}$$

Note that Q defined in (2.49) is a sum of convex combinations of a series of one-dimensional concave functions since all parameters are separated. In this sense, Q is essentially a one-dimensional function, which is much easier to optimize. The $(t+1)$-th iterate $\theta^{(t+1)}$ can be obtained as the solution to the system of equations

$$\sum_{i \in \mathbb{I}_j} \nabla f_i\Big(\lambda_{ij}^{-1} x_{ij}(\theta_j - \theta_j^{(t)}) + x_{(i)}^{\top}\theta^{(t)}\Big)\, x_{ij} = 0, \tag{2.51}$$

for $1 \le j \le q$. When (2.51) cannot be solved explicitly, one step of the NR algorithm provides the approximate solution

$$\theta_j^{(t+1)} = \theta_j^{(t)} + \tau_j^2(\theta^{(t)}, r) \sum_{i \in \mathbb{I}_j} \nabla f_i(x_{(i)}^{\top}\theta^{(t)})\, x_{ij}, \tag{2.52}$$

where $1 \le j \le q$ and

$$\tau_j^2(\theta, r) = \left\{ \sum_{i \in \mathbb{I}_j} \{-\nabla^2 f_i(x_{(i)}^{\top}\theta)\}\, x_{ij}^2/\lambda_{ij} \right\}^{-1}. \tag{2.53}$$

Example 2.10 (*Generalized linear models*). Consider GLM with canonical link function. Let $\{y_i\}_{i=1}^m$ be m independent observations from an underlying exponential family (McCullagh & Nelder, 1989):

$$f_e(y|\psi) = \exp\{[y\psi - b(\psi)]/a(\gamma) + c(y, \gamma)\}, \tag{2.54}$$

where ψ denotes the canonical or natural parameter, $a(\cdot)$, $b(\cdot)$ and $c(\cdot, \cdot)$ are known real-valued functions, γ is the dispersion parameter and is assumed to be known. Let $Y_i \sim f_e(y_i|\psi_i)$, then

$$E(Y_i) = \nabla b(\psi_i) \quad \text{and} \quad \text{Var}(Y_i) = \nabla^2 b(\psi_i) a(\gamma),$$

respectively. For index i, let $\psi_i = x_{(i)}^{\top}\theta$, then the log-likelihood function for θ is given by (2.45) with $f_i(\psi) = y_i\psi - b(\psi)$. Noting that

$$\begin{aligned} \nabla f_i(\psi) &= y_i - \nabla b(\psi) \quad \text{and} \\ -\nabla^2 f_i(\psi) &= \nabla^2 b(\psi), \end{aligned}$$

from (2.52), we have

$$\theta_j^{(t+1)} = \theta_j^{(t)} + \frac{\sum_{i\in\mathbb{I}_j} [y_i - \nabla b(x_{(i)}^{\top}\theta^{(t)})]\, x_{ij}}{\sum_{i\in\mathbb{I}_j} \nabla^2 b(x_{(i)}^{\top}\theta^{(t)})\, x_{ij}^2/\lambda_{ij}} \tag{2.55}$$

for $1 \le j \le q$. ‖

Example 2.11 (*Log-linear models for lymphocyte data*). Let $Y_{\rm obs} = \{y_i\}_{i=1}^m$ and consider the following Poisson regression

$$\begin{aligned} y_i &\overset{\text{ind}}{\sim} \text{Poisson}(\mu_i), \\ \log(\mu_i) &= x_{(i)}^{\top}\theta, \qquad 1 \le i \le m, \end{aligned}$$

then the log-likelihood function for θ is

$$\ell(\theta|Y_{\rm obs}) = \sum_{i=1}^{m} \{y_i(x_{(i)}^{\top}\theta) - \exp(x_{(i)}^{\top}\theta)\}.$$

Setting $b(\psi) = e^{\psi}$ in (2.55), then the algorithm (2.55) reduces to

$$\theta_j^{(t+1)} = \theta_j^{(t)} + \frac{\sum_{i\in\mathbb{I}_j} [y_i - \exp(x_{(i)}^{\top}\theta^{(t)})]\, x_{ij}}{\sum_{i\in\mathbb{I}_j} \exp(x_{(i)}^{\top}\theta^{(t)})\, x_{ij}^2/\lambda_{ij}} \tag{2.56}$$

for $1 \le j \le q$. When $r = 1$, we can re-express the algorithm (2.56) in matrix form (cf. Problem 2.8). We consider the lymphocyte data as summarized in Table 2.4, whose medical background is given in Groer & Pereira (1987). Here $m = 7$, y_i denotes the number of dicentrics for individual i, c_i is the number of cells (in thousands), and d_i is the dose level. It is of interest to relate the expectation μ_i

Table 2.4 *Lymphocyte data*

i	1	2	3	4	5	6	7
c_i	269	78	115	90	84	59	37
d_i	0.50	0.75	1.00	1.50	2.00	2.50	3.00
y_i	109	47	94	114	138	125	97

with the explanatory variables c_i and d_i. The considered model is as follows:

$$\log(\mu_i) = \theta_0 + \theta_1 \log(c_i) + \theta_2 \log(d_i).$$

Applying the algorithm (2.56), we have

$$\hat{\theta} = (-0.125, 0.985, 1.022)^{\top}$$

after 12,000 iterations starting from $\theta^{(0)} = \mathbf{1}_3$. The estimated standard errors are 0.751, 0.156 and 0.148, respectively. ||

2.2 Monte Carlo Simulation

In this section, we describe basic Monte Carlo simulation techniques for generating random samples from univariate and multivariate distributions. These techniques also play a critical role in Monte Carlo integration. We assume that **random numbers** or r.v.'s uniformly distributed in $(0, 1)$ can be satisfactorily produced on the computer. Our focus here is on fast methods for generating non-uniform r.v.'s.

2.2.1 The inversion method

Let X be an r.v. with cdf F. Since F is a nondecreasing function, the inverse function F^{-1} may be defined by

$$F^{-1}(u) = \inf\{x : F(x) \geq u\}, \quad u \in (0, 1).$$

If $U \sim U(0, 1)$, then $F(X) \sim U(0, 1)$ or equivalently

$$X = F^{-1}(U)$$

has the cdf F. Hence, in order to generate one sample, say x, from r.v. $X \sim F$, we first draw u from $U \sim U(0, 1)$, then compute $F^{-1}(u)$ and set it equal to x. Figure 2.1 illustrates the inversion method. We summarize the algorithm as follows.

THE INVERSION METHOD:

Step 1. Draw U from $U(0, 1)$;

Step 2. Return $X = F^{-1}(U)$.

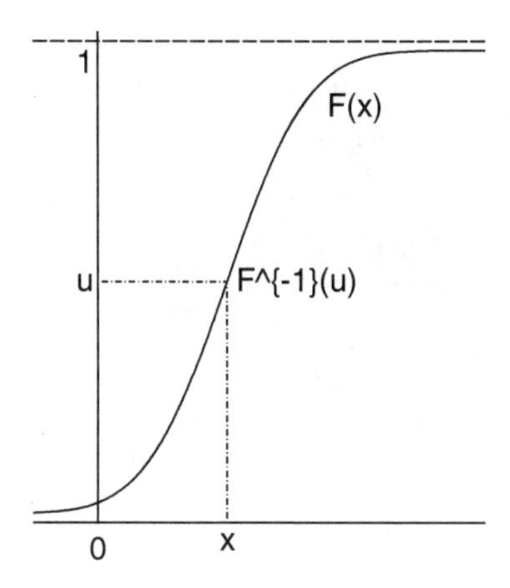

Figure 2.1 The inversion method.

Example 2.12 (*Generation of standard Laplace*). Let X follow the standard Laplace distribution, then its pdf and cdf are given by $f(x) = 0.5e^{-|x|}$, $x \in \mathbb{R}$, and $F(x) = 0.5e^x I_{(x<0)} + (1 - 0.5e^{-x})I_{(x \ge 0)}$, respectively. It is easy to obtain

$$F^{-1}(u) = \log[2u] \cdot I_{(0<u<0.5)} - \log[2(1-u)] \cdot I_{(0.5 \le u < 1)}.$$

An S-plus code for simulating N i.i.d. samples of X is given in the Appendix A.2.5. ||

Distributions that have analytical F^{-1} include the exponential, Weibull, logistic and Cauchy distributions (Johnson, 1987). If F^{-1} is not available analytically, the inversion method may not be efficient.

Example 2.13 (*Generation of marginal distribution of truncated binormal via the grid method*). Let $X \sim f_X(x)$ and $\mathcal{S}_X$ denote its support. To generate X, we first select an appropriate grid of values $\{x_i\}_{i=1}^d$, which cover the support $\mathcal{S}_X$, and then approximate the pdf $f_X(x)$ by a discrete density at $\{x_i\}_{i=1}^d$ with probabilities $p_i = f_X(x_i)/\sum_{j=1}^d f_X(x_j)$, $i = 1, \dots, d$. In other words, we have

$$X \dot{\sim} \text{FDiscrete}_d(\{x_i\}, \{p_i\}).$$

To generate this finite discrete distribution, we may use the built-in S-plus function "`sample`" (cf. Appendix A.1.1). Obviously, the grid method will also work for an unnormalized density function (Gelman *et al.*, 1995, p.302).

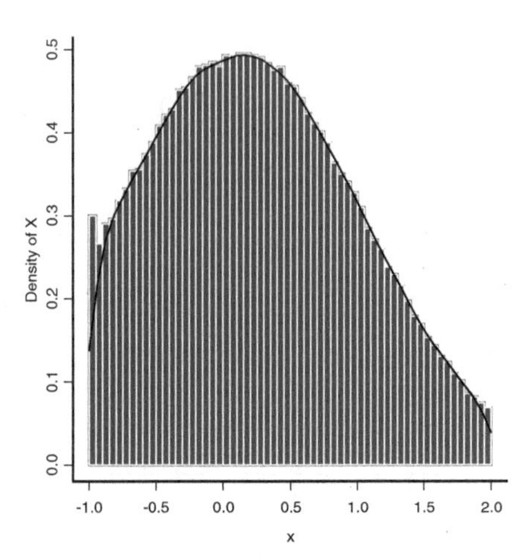

Figure 2.2 The histogram of the marginal density of X based on 200,000 i.i.d. samples generated via the grid method with `sample` (x, 200,000, prob $= p$, replace $=$ T), where $(X, Y) \sim TN_2(\mu, \Sigma; a, b)$, $\mu_1 = \mu_2 = 0$, $\rho = 0.5$, $\sigma_1 = \sigma_2 = 1$, $a = (-1, -1)^\top$ and $b = (2, 2)^\top$.

For illustration, let (X, Y) follow a **truncated binormal distribution** with known parameters $(\mu, \Sigma; a, b)$, then the marginal density of X is (cf. Problem 1.1)

$$\begin{aligned} f_X(x) \;\propto\; & e^{-(x-\mu_1)^2/(2\sigma_1^2)} \times \left\{ \Phi\left(\frac{b_2 - \mu_2 - \rho\sigma_2\sigma_1^{-1}(x - \mu_1)}{\sigma_2\sqrt{1-\rho^2}} \right) \right. \\ & \left. - \Phi\left(\frac{a_2 - \mu_2 - \rho\sigma_2\sigma_1^{-1}(x - \mu_1)}{\sigma_2\sqrt{1-\rho^2}} \right) \right\}, \end{aligned} \tag{2.57}$$

where $x \in \mathcal{S}_X = [a_1, b_1]$. When $-\infty < a_1 < b_1 < +\infty$, we may select $x_i = a_1 + (b_1 - a_1)i/d$ for $i = 1, \ldots, d$, and $d = 300$, say. Figure 2.2 shows the histogram based on 200,000 i.i.d. samples generated via the grid method with `sample` (x, 200,000, prob $= p$, replace $=$ T). $\|$

2.2.2 The rejection method

Suppose that we want to draw random samples from a **target** density $f(x)$, $x \in \mathcal{S}_X \subseteq \mathbb{R}^d$. If we can find some **envelope** constant $c\,(\geq 1)$ and an **envelope** density $g(x)$ having the same support $\mathcal{S}_X$ so that $f(x)$ minorizes $cg(x)$, i.e.,

$$f(x) \leq cg(x), \quad \forall x \in \mathcal{S}_X,$$

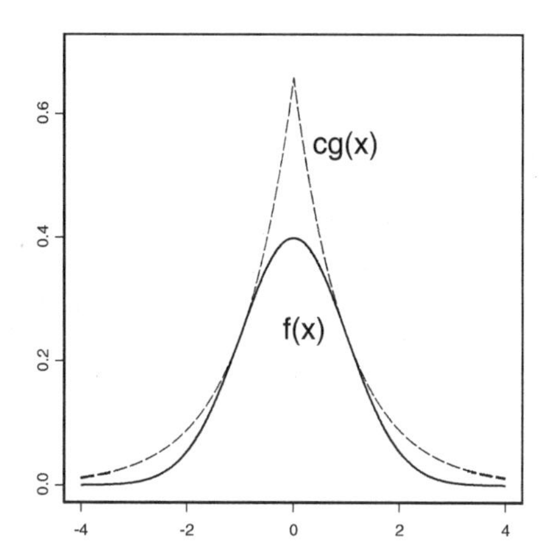

Figure 2.3 The rejection method.

see Figure 2.3, then we can apply the following procedure suggested by von Neumann (1951).

THE REJECTION METHOD:

Step 1. Draw $U \sim U(0,1)$ and independently draw $Y \sim g(\cdot)$;

Step 2. If $U \le \frac{f(Y)}{cg(Y)}$, return $X = Y$; otherwise, go to Step 1.

(a) Theoretical justification

Let $h(Y) = f(Y)/[cg(Y)]$. The theoretical justification of the rejection method follows from the Bayes theorem (Rubinstein & Kroese, 2004, p.23):

$$f_Y(x|U \le h(Y)) = \frac{\Pr\{U \le h(Y)|Y = x\}g(x)}{\Pr\{U \le h(Y)\}}. \tag{2.58}$$

Since Y is independent of U, we have

$$\Pr\{U \le h(Y)|Y = x\} = h(x)$$

and

$$\begin{aligned} \Pr\{U \le h(Y)\} &= \int_{\mathcal{S}_X} \Pr\{U \le h(Y)|Y = x\}g(x)\,dx \\ &= \int_{\mathcal{S}_X} h(x)g(x)\,dx = 1/c. \end{aligned} \tag{2.59}$$

Therefore, (2.58) becomes $f_Y(x|U \le h(Y)) = f(x)$. In other words, the generated r.v. (or random vector) X has density $f(x)$.

(b) The efficiency of the rejection method

From (2.59), the efficiency of the rejection method is determined by the acceptance probability $1/c$. Thus a smaller c will result in a better rejection method. We determine c via maximizing the ratio of f over g:

$$c = \max_{x \in \mathcal{S}_X} \frac{f(x)}{g(x)}. \tag{2.60}$$

In practice, we usually consider a family of densities indexed by θ, say $\{g_\theta(x) : \theta \in \Theta\}$, as the candidate envelopes. Define

$$c_\theta = \max_{x \in \mathcal{S}_X} \frac{f(x)}{g_\theta(x)}, \tag{2.61}$$

then, the optimal θ is that for which c_θ is minimal.

Example 2.14 (*Normal generation from Laplace*). To generate an $N(0,1)$, we consider the Laplace envelope family, $\text{Laplace}(x|0,\sigma^2) = \frac{1}{2\sigma} e^{-|x|/\sigma}$ indexed by $\sigma \in \mathbb{R}_+$. From (2.61), it is easy to obtain

$$\begin{aligned} c_\sigma &= \max_{x \in \mathcal{S}_X} \frac{N(x|0,1)}{\text{Laplace}(x|0,\sigma^2)} \\ &= \sqrt{\frac{2}{\pi}}\, \sigma \exp\left(\frac{1}{2\sigma^2}\right). \end{aligned}$$

The optimal $\sigma = 1$ so that the optimal envelope constant is

$$c_{\text{opt}} = \min_{\sigma \in \mathbb{R}_+} c_\sigma = \sqrt{2e/\pi} = 1.3155.$$

Thus, the acceptance probability is $1/c_{\text{opt}} = 0.76$. ||

The representation of (2.60) implies that the rejection method is also available if we replace the normalizing pdf f with its unnormalizing density f^*, that is, the normalizing constant of f need not be known (see Ex.2.15). This property is particularly important in Bayesian calculations.

Let N be the number of iterations in the algorithm, i.e., the number of pairs (U, Y) required before a successful pair (U, X) occurs, then N has a geometric distribution

$$\Pr\{N = n\} = p(1-p)^{n-1}, \quad n = 1, 2, \ldots,$$

where

$$p = \Pr\{U \le h(Y)\} = 1/c.$$

Thus, the expected number of iterations until one variable is accepted is $E(N) = 1/p = c$.

(c) Log-concave densities

We say a density function $f(x)$ is **log-concave** if its logarithm is **concave**, i.e., $\nabla^2 \log f(x) \le 0$. On a log scale, an exponential pdf is a straight line. If a pdf $f(x)$ is log-concave, then any line **tangent** to $\log f(x)$ will lie above $\log f(x)$. Thus, log-concave pdfs are ideally suited to the rejection method with piece-wise exponential envelopes (Lange, 1999, p.273). Table 2.5 gives some log-concave densities.

Table 2.5 *Some log-concave densities*

Distribution	Kernel of $f(x)$	$\nabla^2 \log f(x)$	Condition
Normal	$\exp\{-\frac{(x-\mu)^2}{2\sigma^2}\}$	$-\frac{1}{\sigma^2}$	$\sigma \in \mathbb{R}_+$
Gamma	$x^{\alpha-1}e^{-\beta x}$	$-\frac{\alpha-1}{x^2}$	$\alpha \ge 1,\ \beta > 0$
Beta	$x^{a-1}(1-x)^{b-1}$	$-\frac{\alpha-1}{x^2} - \frac{\beta-1}{(1-x)^2}$	$\alpha \ge 1,\ \beta \ge 1$
Logistic	$e^{-\frac{x-\mu}{\sigma}}/(1+e^{-\frac{x-\mu}{\sigma}})^2$	$\frac{-2}{\sigma^2}e^{-\frac{x-\mu}{\sigma}}/(1+e^{-\frac{x-\mu}{\sigma}})^2$	$\sigma \in \mathbb{R}_+$
Gumbel	$e^{-\frac{x-\mu}{\sigma}}\exp(-e^{-\frac{x-\mu}{\sigma}})$	$-\frac{1}{\sigma^2}e^{-\frac{x-\mu}{\sigma}}$	$\sigma \in \mathbb{R}_+$
Weibull	$x^{\alpha-1}e^{-\beta x^\alpha}$	$-(\alpha-1)[\frac{1}{x^2}+\beta\alpha x^{\alpha-2}]$	$\alpha \ge 1,\ \beta > 0$

A strictly log-concave pdf $f(x)$ defined on an interval is unimodal. The model $\tilde{x}$ of $f(x)$ may occur at either endpoint or on the interior of the interval. In the former case, we suggest using a truncated exponential envelope (see Ex.2.15 and Figure 2.4). In the latter case, we suggest using two truncated exponential envelopes oriented in opposite directions from the mode $\tilde{x}$ (see Figure 2.3).

Example 2.15 (*Generation of truncated uninormal*). Suppose we want to draw random samples from $X \sim TN(\mu, \sigma^2; a, \infty)$. The pdf of X is

$$f(x) \propto \exp\left\{-\frac{(x-\mu)^2}{2\sigma^2}\right\} I_{(x>a)}.$$

When $a < \mu$, we continuously generate i.i.d. samples from $N(\mu, \sigma^2)$ until a sample satisfying $X > a$ occurs. In the worst case, the efficiency of this method is 50%.

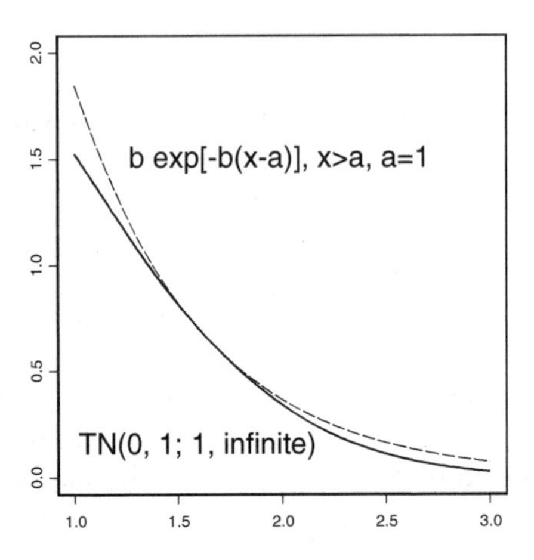

Figure 2.4 A truncated exponential envelope for the truncated normal distribution $TN(0, 1; 1, +\infty)$.

When $a > \mu$, especially when $a \gg \mu$, the above strategy is very inefficient. Without loss of generality, let $\mu = 0$ and $\sigma = 1$. We consider a truncated exponential envelope family with density $be^{-b(x-a)} I_{(x>a)}$ indexed by b (Robert, 1995). From (2.61), it is easy to obtain

$$c_b = \max_{x>a} \frac{f(x)}{be^{-b(x-a)}} = \begin{cases} (bc)^{-1} \exp(0.5b^2 - ba), & \text{if } b > a, \\ (bc)^{-1} \exp(-0.5a^2), & \text{if } b \le a, \end{cases}$$

where $c = \sqrt{2\pi}(1 - \Phi(a))$. The first bound is minimized at

$$b^* = (a + \sqrt{a^2 + 4})/2,$$

whereas $\hat{b} = a$ minimizes the second bound. The optimal choice of b is therefore b^*. ||

2.2.3 The sampling/importance resampling method

Finding a good or optimal envelope constant c is a vital step for the use of rejection methods. In general, this is not an easy task, especially, for high-dimensional cases. Another criticism on the rejection method is that it generates "useless" samples when rejecting. As a **noniterative** sampling procedure, the *sampling/importance resampling* (SIR) method proposed by Rubin (1987b, 1988) can bypass the two problems.

(a) The SIR without replacement

The SIR method generates an approximate i.i.d. sample of size m from the **target density** $f(x)$, $x \in \mathcal{S}_X \subseteq \mathbb{R}^d$. It consists of two steps: a sampling step and an importance resampling step. Specifically, it starts by simulating J i.i.d. samples $\{X^{(j)}\}_{j=1}^J$ from an **importance sampling density** or proposal density $g(x)$ with the same support $\mathcal{S}_X$ and constructing weights

$$\mathrm{w}(X^{(j)}) = \frac{f(X^{(j)})}{g(X^{(j)})} \tag{2.62}$$

and probabilities

$$\omega_j = \frac{\mathrm{w}(X^{(j)})}{\sum_{j'=1}^J \mathrm{w}(X^{(j')})}, \quad j = 1, \ldots, J. \tag{2.63}$$

Then, a second sample of size m ($m \le J$) is drawn from the discrete distribution on $\{X^{(j)}\}$ with probabilities $\{\omega_j\}$. Figure 2.5(a) depicts the relationship between f and g. We summarize it as follows.

THE SIR WITHOUT REPLACEMENT:

Step 1. Generate $X^{(1)}, \ldots, X^{(J)} \overset{\text{iid}}{\sim} g(\cdot)$;

Step 2. Select a subset $\{X^{(k_i)}\}_{i=1}^m$ from $\{X^{(j)}\}_{j=1}^J$ via resampling **without replacement** from the discrete distribution on $\{X^{(j)}\}$ with probabilities $\{\omega_j\}$.

As expected, the SIR algorithm is more effective if g is closer to f or if J/m is large. A good choice of J should depend on how close g is to f. If $g = f$, we can set $J = m$. The poorer is g as an approximation to f, the larger is J compared to m. Rubin (1988) showed that the SIR algorithm is exact when $J/m \to \infty$. In practice, Rubin (1987b) suggested $J/m = 20$ and Smith & Gelfand (1992) recommended $J/m \ge 10$ in their examples.

Example 2.16 (*Simulation from a density defined in the unit interval*). Let r be a known positive integer and $X \sim f(x)$, where

$$f(x) = \frac{\pi \sin^r(\pi x)}{B(\frac{1}{2}, \frac{r+1}{2})}, \quad 0 < x < 1. \tag{2.64}$$

For example, when $r = 6$, we consider a skew beta density, say $\mathrm{Beta}(x|2,4)$, as the importance sampling density $g(x)$, see Figure

2.5(a). Thus, the importance weight $\text{w}(x) = f(x)/\text{Beta}(x|2,4)$. We run the SIR algorithm by setting $J = 200{,}000$ and $m = 20{,}000$. Figure 2.5(b) shows that the histogram entirely recovers the target density function $f(x)$.

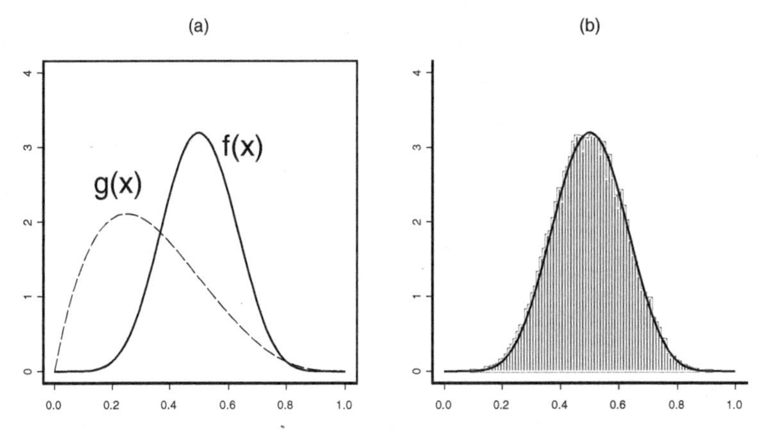

Figure 2.5 The SIR method. (a) The target density $f(x)$ is defined by (2.64) with $r = 6$ and the importance sampling density $g(x) = \text{Beta}(x|2,4)$; (b) The histogram of $f(x)$ is obtained by using the SIR method with $J = 200{,}000$ and $m = 20{,}000$. ||

An important feature of the SIR method is that it is noniterative (Rubin, 1988, p.396). Another advantage is its simplicity. In addition, the SIR method allows f to be known only up to a normalizing constant since the weights $\{\omega_j\}$ do not alter. The SIR method can be easily understood and used as a general tool for full Bayesian analysis (Albert, 1993). Besides Bayesian computation, the SIR method has been successfully applied to many statistical problems, including weighted likelihood bootstrap (Newton & Raftery, 1994), population dynamics model (Raftery *et al.*, 1995), stock assessment (McAllister *et al.*, 1994; McAllister & Ianelli, 1997). Givens & Raftery (1996) considered adaptive versions of the SIR. Skare *et al.* (2003) proposed an improved SIR algorithm.

(b) Theoretical justification

To verify that the SIR method generates samples having approximate density f, let X^* denote a draw from the discrete distribution over $\{X^{(j)}\}$ placing mass ω_j on $X^{(j)}$. The cdf of X^* is

$$\Pr(X^* \le x^*) = \sum_{j=1}^{J} \omega_j I_{(X^{(j)} \le x^*)} = \frac{\sum_{j=1}^{J} \text{w}(X^{(j)}) I_{(X^{(j)} \le x^*)}}{\sum_{j=1}^{J} \text{w}(X^{(j)})}.$$

When $J \to \infty$, a large quantity of $X^{(j)}$ are available with frequencies according to g and sums become integrals weighted by g, i.e.,

$$\Pr(X^* \leq x^*) \to \frac{\int \mathrm{w}(x) I_{(x \leq x^*)} g(x)\, dx}{\int \mathrm{w}(x) g(x)\, dx} = \int_{-\infty}^{x^*} f(x)\, dx,$$

which is the cdf associated with the density f.

(c) Determination of J and m for the SIR with replacement

If g is a poor approximation to f, resampling **with replacement** is preferable (Rubin, 1988). Li (2007) stated the SIR algorithm with replacement as follows.

THE SIR WITH REPLACEMENT:

Step 1. Generate $X^{(1)}, \ldots, X^{(J)} \stackrel{\text{iid}}{\sim} g(\cdot)$;

Step 2. Draw m values $\{Y^{(i)}\}_{i=1}^m$ from $\{X^{(j)}\}_{j=1}^J$ in such a way that $E(q_j | X^{(1)}, \ldots, X^{(J)}) = m\omega_j$, where q_j is the number of copies of $X^{(j)}$ in $\{Y^{(i)}\}_{i=1}^m$.

Li (2007) called $\{X^{(j)}\}_{j=1}^J$ a pool of inputs, $\{Y^{(i)}\}_{i=1}^m$ a resample, J the pool size, m the resample size, and $\mathrm{w}(X)$ defined in (2.62) the importance weight/ratio of X. Smith & Gelfand (1992) used simple weighted random sampling **with replacement** in Step 2 and called their method the **weighted bootstrap**.

A difficulty with the SIR is the determination of J. A theoretical determination of J requires a concrete objective function. Lee (1997) suggested using J to control the mean squared error of the probability estimate. McAllister & Ianelli (1997) required that the maximum $\mathrm{w}(X)$ be less than 0.04 of the total importance weight. As some inputs may be selected more than once in the unequal probability sampling step, we encounter a duplication problem. Many copies of a value in the output will lead to significant underestimation of standard error in the subsequent analysis when the outputs are used as if they are i.i.d.. For this reason, Li (2004) proposed using J to keep the maximum number of duplicates in the output at a tolerably low level. Li (2007) gave a general relation between J and m and showed that

- $J = O(m)$ iff the importance weight $\mathrm{w}(X)$ is bounded above.
- If the importance weight $\mathrm{w}(X)$ has a moment generating function, the suggested J is of order $O(m \log(m))$.

- J may need to be as large as $O(m^{r/(r-1)})$ if the importance weight $\mathrm{w}(X)$ has finite r-th moment for an $r > 1$.

2.2.4 The stochastic representation method

(a) The "$\stackrel{d}{=}$" operator

Let X and $\{Y_j\}_{j=1}^n$ be r.v.'s and g a function. If X and $g(Y_1, \ldots, Y_n)$ have the same distribution, denoted by

$$X \stackrel{d}{=} g(Y_1, \ldots, Y_n), \tag{2.65}$$

we say (2.65) is a one-to-many *stochastic representation* (SR) of X. The operator "$\stackrel{d}{=}$" has the following basic properties.

- If the cdf X is symmetric about the origin, i.e., $F(x) = 1 - F(-x)$ for every $x \in \mathcal{X}$, then $X \stackrel{d}{=} -X$.
- Let X and Y be two r.v.'s, then $X|Y \stackrel{d}{=} X$ iff X and Y are independent.
- The fact $X = Y$ implies $X \stackrel{d}{=} Y$, but the inverse is not true.

For instance, if $X \sim N(0, 1)$, then $X \stackrel{d}{=} -X$, but $X \neq -X$ in general. Another example is $U \stackrel{d}{=} 1 - U$, where $U \sim U[0, 1]$.

(b) Univariate SR: one-to-many

The **one-to-many** SR (2.65) implies that there is a simple approach to generate the r.v. X provided that the distributions of $\{Y_j\}_{j=1}^n$ are easy to generate. SR methods are sometimes called **transformation** methods. In fact, the inversion method in §2.2.1 can be viewed as a special case of the SR methods. For example, let $U \sim U(0, 1)$, then

$$X \stackrel{d}{=} -\log U/\beta \sim \text{Exponential}(\beta).$$

Another example is on gamma variate. Let $\{Y_j\} \stackrel{\text{iid}}{\sim} \text{Exponential}(\beta)$, then

$$X \stackrel{d}{=} Y_1 + \cdots + Y_n \sim \text{Gamma}(n, \beta).$$

Other examples include: beta distribution can be generated via independent gamma distributions; inverse gamma via gamma; chi-squared and log-normal via normal; Student's t- and F-distribution via normal and chi-squared (cf. Appendix A.2).

(c) Univariate SR: many-to-one

Let X have a difficult-sampling density $f_X(x)$, but Y have an easy-sampling density $f_Y(y)$, and they have the following relationship

$$G(X) \stackrel{d}{=} Y.$$

When G is a one-to-one map, X can then be generated via $X \stackrel{d}{=} G^{-1}(Y)$. However, there are important examples in which the map G is **many-to-one** so that the inverse is not uniquely defined. Without loss of generality, we assume that $G(X) = Y$ has two solutions $X_i = h_i(Y)$, $i = 1, 2$. Hence, $G(X)$ has density

$$f_Y(y) = \sum_{i=1}^{2} f_X(h_i(y))|\nabla h_i(y)|.$$

Michael *et al.* (1976) suggested the following algorithm: given an r.v. Y with density f_Y, we can obtain an r.v. X with density f_X by choosing $X = h_1(Y)$ with probability

$$\frac{f_X(h_1(Y))|\nabla h_1(Y)|}{f_Y(Y)} = \left\{1 + \frac{f_X(X_2)}{f_X(X_1)}\left|\frac{\nabla G(X_1)}{\nabla G(X_2)}\right|\right\}^{-1}$$

and choosing $X = h_2(Y)$ otherwise. This method can be summarized as follows.

MANY-TO-ONE TRANSFORMATION METHOD:

Step 1. Draw $U \sim U(0, 1)$ and independently draw $Y \sim f_Y(\cdot)$;

Step 2. Set $X_1 = h_1(Y)$ and $X_2 = h_2(Y)$;

Step 3. If $U \leq \left\{1+\frac{f_X(X_2)}{f_X(X_1)}\left|\frac{\nabla G(X_1)}{\nabla G(X_2)}\right|\right\}^{-1}$, return $X = X_1$, else return $X = X_2$.

Example 2.17 (*Generation of inverse Gaussian distribution*). Let $X \sim \text{IGaussian}(\mu, \lambda)$, see Appendix A.2.13, then (Shuster, 1968)

$$G(X) \hat{=} \frac{\lambda(X-\mu)^2}{\mu^2 X} \sim \chi^2(1).$$

Note that $G(X) = Y$ has two solutions

$$X_1 = \mu + \frac{\mu^2 Y}{2\lambda} - \frac{\mu}{2\lambda}\sqrt{4\mu\lambda Y + \mu^2 Y^2}, \quad X_2 = \frac{\mu^2}{X_1}.$$

One can verify that

$$\frac{f_X(X_2)}{f_X(X_1)} = \left(\frac{X_1}{\mu}\right)^3 \quad \text{and} \quad \frac{\nabla G(X_1)}{\nabla G(X_2)} = -\left(\frac{\mu}{X_1}\right)^2.$$

Thus, X_1 is chosen with probability $\mu/(\mu + X_1)$. The corresponding S-plus code for generating X is given in Appendix A.2.13. ||

(d) Multivariate SR

Suppose we want to simulate a random vector $X = (X_1, \dots, X_d)^\top$, but it meets complexity of the computation or difficulty of theoretic aspect. If we can find an SR of X as follows:

$$X_i \stackrel{d}{=} g_i(Y_1, \dots, Y_n), \quad i = 1, \dots, d,$$

where $\{Y_j\}_{j=1}^n$ are independent and are easily generated by a routine approach, then, this SR can be used to generate X. For example, Dirichlet distribution can be generated via independent gamma distributions; multinormal via uninormal, multivariate t-distribution via multinormal and chi-squared; Wishart via multinormal (cf. Appendix A.2).

Example 2.18 (*Uniform distribution in d-dimensional ball*). Let $X = (X_1, \dots, X_d)^\top \sim U(\mathbb{B}_d(r))$, where $\mathbb{B}_d(r)$ is the d-dimensional ball with radius r defined by

$$\mathbb{B}_d(r) = \{(x_1, \dots, x_d)^\top : x_1^2 + \cdots + x_d^2 \le r^2\}. \tag{2.66}$$

It can be verified that X has the following SR (see Problem 2.12)

$$\begin{aligned}
X_1 &\stackrel{d}{=} rY_1 \cos(\pi Y_2), \\
X_2 &\stackrel{d}{=} rY_1 \sin(\pi Y_2) \cos(\pi Y_3), \\
&\;\;\vdots \\
X_{d-2} &\stackrel{d}{=} rY_1 \sin(\pi Y_2) \cdots \sin(\pi Y_{d-2}) \cos(\pi Y_{d-1}), \\
X_{d-1} &\stackrel{d}{=} rY_1 \sin(\pi Y_2) \cdots \sin(\pi Y_{d-1}) \cos(2\pi Y_d), \\
X_d &\stackrel{d}{=} rY_1 \sin(\pi Y_2) \cdots \sin(\pi Y_{d-1}) \sin(2\pi Y_d),
\end{aligned}$$

where $Y_1, \dots, Y_d$ are mutually independent, and $Y_i \in (0, 1)$ has pdf

$$f_i(y) = \begin{cases} dy^{d-1}, & \text{when } i = 1, \\ \frac{\pi \sin^{d-i}(\pi y)}{B(\frac{1}{2}, \frac{d-i+1}{2})}, & \text{when } i = 2, \dots, d-1, \\ 1, & \text{when } i = d. \end{cases}$$

In Ex.2.16, we apply the SIR method to draw samples from $f_i(y)$. $\|$

(e) Mixture representation

Sometimes, it is quite difficult if we directly generate a random vector $X \sim f_X(x)$, but the augmented vector $(X, Z) \sim f_{(X,Z)}(x, z)$ is relatively easy to generate. In this situation, we may first generate the augmented vector and then pick up the desired components (Bulter, 1958). Statistically, we can represent f_X as the marginal distribution of $f_{(X,Z)}$ in the form

$$f_X(x) = \int_{\mathcal{Z}} f_{(X,Z)}(x, z)\, dz. \tag{2.67}$$

Alternatively, we can rewrite (2.67) in mixture form

$$f_X(x) = \int_{\mathcal{Z}} f_{(X|Z)}(x|z) f_Z(z) dz, \quad \text{or} \quad f_X(x) = \sum_{k \in \mathcal{Z}} p_k f_k(x),$$

depending on if Z is continuous or discrete (cf. Appendix A.3).

Example 2.19 (*Standard normal distribution*). Let $X \sim N(0, 1)$. Since the inverse of cdf for X does not have an explicit expression, the inversion method is not a good strategy to simulate X. A well-known approach for generating X is (Box & Muller, 1958):

$$\begin{aligned} X &\stackrel{d}{=} \sqrt{-2 \log U_1} \cos(2\pi U_2), \qquad (2.68) \\ Z &\stackrel{d}{=} \sqrt{-2 \log U_1} \sin(2\pi U_2), \end{aligned}$$

where $U_1, U_2 \stackrel{\text{iid}}{\sim} U(0, 1)$, and $X, Z \stackrel{\text{iid}}{\sim} N(0, 1)$. Essentially, this approach is first to augment X with an independent standard Gaussian r.v. Z, and then to generate the joint distribution $(X, Z) \sim N_2(\mathbf{0}, \mathbf{I}_2)$ via the SR (2.68). $\|$

Example 2.20 (*From mixture representation to SR*). Suppose that we want to generate a positive r.v. X with density given by

$$f_X(x) = \int_x^{\infty} z^{-1} f_Z(z)\, dz, \quad x > 0. \tag{2.69}$$

This mixture can be represented equivalently by

$$Z \sim f_Z(z), \ z > 0, \quad \text{and} \quad X|(Z = z) \sim U(0, z).$$

Hence, $\frac{X}{Z}|(Z = z) \sim U(0, 1)$, not depending on z, so that $\frac{X}{Z} \stackrel{d}{=} U \sim U(0, 1)$. Therefore,

$$X \stackrel{d}{=} UZ \tag{2.70}$$

and U and Z are mutually independent. In addition, if $\nabla f_X(\cdot)$ exists and $f_X(\infty) \to 0$, then

$$f_X(x) = -\int_x^{\infty} \nabla f_X(z)\, dz. \tag{2.71}$$

By comparing (2.69) with (2.71), we obtain

$$f_Z(z) = -z\nabla f_X(z). \tag{2.72}$$

This is the well-known Khintchine's (1938) theorem.

The SR (2.70) provides a very simple way to simulate X. For instance, if $Z \sim \text{Gamma}(a, 1)$, then X follows **gamma-integral** distribution (Devroye, 1986, p.191). If $X \sim \text{Exponential}(\beta)$, from (2.72), then Z must be $\text{Gamma}(2, \beta)$. ||

Example 2.21 (*Multivariate t-distribution*). If $Z \sim \text{Gamma}(\frac{\nu}{2}, \frac{\nu}{2})$ and $X|(Z = z) \sim N_d(\mu, z^{-1}\Sigma)$, then $X \sim t_d(\mu, \Sigma, \nu)$. Hence,

$$\sqrt{Z}(X - \mu)|(Z = z) \sim N_d(\mathbf{0}, \Sigma),$$

not depending on z, so that $\sqrt{Z}(X - \mu) \stackrel{d}{=} W \sim N_d(\mathbf{0}, \Sigma)$. Therefore, we have the following SR:

$$X \stackrel{d}{=} \mu + \frac{W}{\sqrt{Z}} \stackrel{d}{=} \mu + \frac{N_d(\mathbf{0}, \Sigma)}{\sqrt{\chi^2(\nu)/\nu}},$$

where W and Z are mutually independent. ||

2.2.5 The conditional sampling method

The **conditional sampling method** due to the prominent Rosenblatt transformation is particularly appealing when the joint distribution of a d-vector is very difficult to generate but one marginal distribution and $d - 1$ univariate conditional distributions are easy to simulate.

Let $X = (X_1, \ldots, X_d)^\top$ and its density $f(x)$ can be factorized as

$$f(x) = \left\{ \prod_{k=1}^{d-1} f_k(x_k | x_{k+1}, x_{k+2}, \ldots, x_d) \right\} \times f_d(x_d). \tag{2.73}$$

To generate X from $f(x)$, we only need to generate x_d from the marginal density $f_d(x_d)$, then to generate x_k sequentially from the conditional density $f_k(x_k|x_{k+1}, x_{k+2}, \ldots, x_d)$.

Rosenblatt (1952) further suggested that the above steps can be accomplished by using the inversion method. Let $F_d(x_d)$ be the cdf of X_d, and $F_k(x_k|x_{k+1}, \ldots, x_d)$ the conditional cdf of X_k given $X_{k+1} = x_{k+1}, \ldots, X_d = x_d$, we have

$$\begin{aligned} X_d &\stackrel{d}{=} F_d^{-1}(U_d), \\ (X_k|X_{k+1}, \ldots, X_d) &\stackrel{d}{=} F_k^{-1}(U_k|X_{k+1}, \ldots, X_d), \end{aligned} \tag{2.74}$$

for $k = d-1, \ldots, 1$, where $U_1, \ldots, U_d \stackrel{\text{iid}}{\sim} U(0,1)$. Note that the decomposition of (2.73) is not unique. In fact, there are $d!$ different representations. A better representation will result in a more efficient sampling scheme. As an illustration, consider the following example.

Example 2.22 (*Dirichlet distribution*). Let bivariate random vector $X = (X_1, X_2)^\top \sim \text{Dirichlet}(2, 1; 1)$, its pdf is

$$f(x_1, x_2) = \begin{cases} 6x_1, & \text{if } x_1, x_2 \geq 0,\ x_1 + x_2 \leq 1, \\ 0, & \text{otherwise.} \end{cases}$$

First, we factorize $f(x_1, x_2)$ into $f_2(x_2)f_1(x_1|x_2)$. It is easy to show that $X_2 \sim \text{Beta}(1, 3)$ and $\frac{X_1}{1-X_2}|X_2 \sim \text{Beta}(2, 1)$. Therefore the corresponding cdfs are given by

$$\begin{aligned} F_2(x_2) &= 1 - (1 - x_2)^3, \quad 0 \leq x_2 \leq 1, \\ F_1(x_1|x_2) &= (1 - x_2)^{-2}x_1^2, \quad 0 \leq x_1 \leq 1 - x_2. \end{aligned}$$

By (2.74), it follows that

$$X_2 \stackrel{d}{=} 1 - U_2^{1/3}, \quad X_1 \stackrel{d}{=} U_2^{1/3}U_1^{1/2}. \tag{2.75}$$

Second, we factorize $f(x_1, x_2)$ into $f_1(x_1)f_2(x_2|x_1)$. Similarly, $X_1 \sim \text{Beta}(2, 2)$ and $\frac{X_2}{1-X_1}|X_1 \sim \text{Beta}(1, 1)$. Their cdfs are given by

$$\begin{aligned} F_1(x_1) &= 3x_1^2 - 2x_1^3, \quad 0 \leq x_1 \leq 1, \\ F_2(x_2|x_1) &= (1 - x_1)^{-1}x_2, \quad 0 \leq x_2 \leq 1 - x_1, \end{aligned}$$

respectively. Hence

$$3X_1^2 - 2X_1^3 \stackrel{d}{=} U_1, \quad (1 - X_1)^{-1}X_2 \stackrel{d}{=} U_2. \tag{2.76}$$

Comparing (2.75) with (2.76), we know that (2.75) is more convenient than (2.76) for generating $X = (X_1, X_2)^\top$. ‖

Example 2.23 (*Truncated binormal distribution*). Let $(X, Y)^\top \sim TN_2(\mu, \Sigma; a, b)$, then the marginal density of X is given by (2.57) and the conditional distribution of $Y|(X = x)$ follows truncated uninormal distribution

$$TN(\mu_2 + \rho\sigma_2\sigma_1^{-1}(x - \mu_1),\ \sigma_2^2(1 - \rho^2);\ a_2, b_2).$$

Thus, we first use the grid method presented in Ex.2.13 to simulate X, and then use the rejection method described in Ex.2.15 to simulate Y for given $X = x$. ‖

2.2.6 The vertical density representation method

Troutt (1991, 1993) and Kotz & Troutt (1996) proposed a so-called *vertical density representation* (VDR) method to generate a univariate distribution. Kotz *et al.* (1997) studied systematically the multivariate VDR method.

Let X have a joint density $f(x)$ and $V = f(X)$ have a density $g(\cdot)$, then the conditional distribution of X given $V = v$ is the uniform distribution, $U(\mathbb{S}(v))$, over the set

$$\mathbb{S}(v) = \{x : x \in \mathbb{R}^d,\ f(x) \geq v\}. \tag{2.77}$$

Troutt (1991) showed that the density of V is given by

$$g(v) = -v\nabla A(v), \tag{2.78}$$

where $A(v)$ is the Lebesgue measure of the set $\mathbb{S}(v)$ and $\nabla A(v)$ denotes the derivative of $A(v)$ whose existence is postulated. To generate X, we only need to generate $V = v$ according to g and then to generate $X|(V = v)$ according to $U(\mathbb{S}(v))$. Therefore, essentially, the VDR method is a conditional sampling method, see Figure 2.6 for illustration. We summarize it as follows.

THE VDR METHOD:

Step 1. Generate $V \sim g(\cdot)$;

Step 2. Generate $X|(V = v) \sim U(\mathbb{S}(v))$.

Example 2.24 (*Spherical and multivariate t-distributions*). Fang *et al.* (1990, Ch.2) described several ways to define spherical distribution. Here we assume that X follows a spherical distribution with

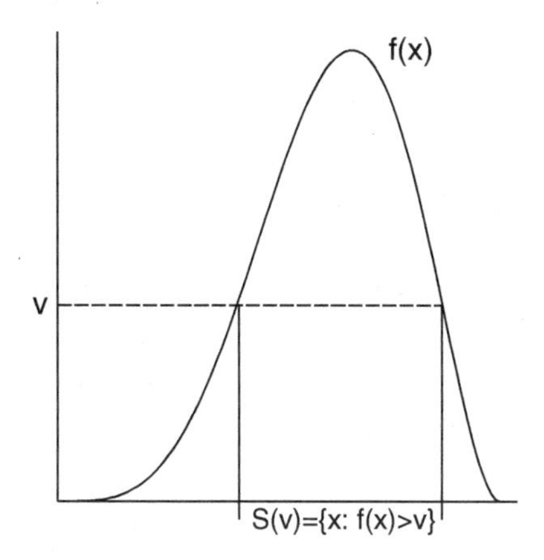

Figure 2.6 The VDR method.

density $f(x) = h(x^\top x)$, $x \in \mathbb{R}^d$, where h is strictly decreasing and differentiable. Let h^{-1} denote the inverse function of h, then from (2.77) we have

$$\mathbb{S}(v) = \{x : x \in \mathbb{R}^d, x^\top x \le h^{-1}(v)\}.$$

Note that the Lebesgue measure of $\mathbb{S}(v)$ is the volume of the d-dimensional ball with radius $\sqrt{h^{-1}(v)}$. From Problem 2.13, we have

$$A(v) = \frac{2\pi^{d/2}}{\Gamma(d/2)d}\Big(h^{-1}(v)\Big)^{d/2}.$$

By (2.78), the density of $V = f(X)$ is given by

$$g(v) = -\frac{v\pi^{d/2}}{\Gamma(d/2)}\Big(h^{-1}(v)\Big)^{d/2-1}\nabla h^{-1}(v).$$

Now, let $X \sim t_d(0, \mathbf{I}_d, m)$ (cf. Appendix A.3.6), the density of X is

$$f(x) = c\Big(1 + \frac{x^\top x}{m}\Big)^{-\frac{m+d}{2}}, \quad x \in \mathbb{R}^d,$$

where $c = \Gamma(\frac{m+d}{2})/\{(m\pi)^{d/2}\Gamma(\frac{m}{2})\}$. In this case, we have

$$h^{-1}(v) = m\Big(\Big(\frac{c}{v}\Big)^{\frac{2}{m+d}} - 1\Big), \tag{2.79}$$

$$g(v) = \frac{2(m\pi)^{d/2}}{(m+d)\Gamma(d/2)}\Big(\frac{c}{v}\Big)^{\frac{2}{m+d}}\Big(\Big(\frac{c}{v}\Big)^{\frac{2}{m+d}} - 1\Big)^{\frac{d}{2}-1}.$$

It is easy to verify the following SR,

$$V \stackrel{d}{=} cW^{\frac{m+d}{2}},$$

where $W \sim \text{Beta}(m/2, d/2)$. Therefore, we have an alternative algorithm for generating multivariate t-distribution as follows: (i) generate $W = w$ according to $\text{Beta}(m/2, d/2)$; (ii) calculate $V = v = cw^{\frac{m+d}{2}}$; (iii) generate X according to the uniform distribution in the d-dimensional ball with radius $\sqrt{h^{-1}(v)}$, where $h^{-1}(v)$ is given by (2.79), see Ex.2.18. ||

Example 2.25 (ℓ_1*-norm and Dirichlet distributions*). Assume that X has an ℓ_1-norm distribution with density $f(x) = h(\|x\|_1)$, where $x \in \mathbb{R}^d_+$, $\|x\|_1 = \sum_{i=1}^d x_i$, and $h(\cdot)$ is a strictly decreasing and differentiable function (Fang *et al.*, 1990, Ch.5). Let

$$\mathbb{S}(v) = \{x : x \in \mathbb{R}^d_+, \|x\|_1 \le h^{-1}(v)\}.$$

The Lebesgue measure of the $\mathbb{S}(v)$ equals its volume (see Problem 2.14), i.e., $A(v) = (h^{-1}(v))^d/d!$. Hence $V = f(X)$ has a density

$$g(v) = -\frac{v}{(d-1)!}\Big(h^{-1}(v)\Big)^{d-1} \nabla h^{-1}(v).$$

If $(X_1, \dots, X_d)^\top \sim \text{Dirichlet}(1, \dots, 1; a)$, $a > 0$, the joint pdf is

$$f(x_1, \dots, x_d) = c\left(1 - \sum_{i=1}^d x_i\right)^{a-1}, \quad c = \frac{\Gamma(d+a)}{\Gamma(a)}.$$

Obviously, it is an ℓ_1-norm distribution. Now we have

$$\begin{aligned} h^{-1}(v) &= 1 - \left(\frac{v}{c}\right)^{\frac{1}{a-1}}, &(2.80)\\ g(v) &= \frac{1}{(a-1)(d-1)!}\left(\frac{v}{c}\right)^{\frac{1}{a-1}}\left(1 - \left(\frac{v}{c}\right)^{\frac{1}{a-1}}\right)^{d-1}. \end{aligned}$$

Therefore, we obtain $V \stackrel{d}{=} cW^{a-1}$ and $W \sim \text{Beta}(a, d)$. The algorithm for generating $\text{Dirichlet}(1, \dots, 1; a)$ is as follows: (i) generate $W = w$ from $\text{Beta}(a, d)$; (ii) set $V = v = cw^{a-1}$; (iii) generate X from the uniform distribution in the d-dimensional simplex $\mathbb{S}(v)$ with $h^{-1}(v)$ given by (2.80). ||

2.3 Numerical Integration

In this section, we introduce four basic tools for evaluating integrals often encountered in Bayesian inferences. The Laplace approximation is an **analytic** approach to approximate integral based on the Taylor expansion around the mode of the log-integrand. Thus algorithms for finding the mode of a unimodal function presented in §2.1 will be helpful here. Riemannian simulation, importance sampling and entropy approximations are three **simulation-based** approaches to approximate integral based on i.i.d. samples from the target density or the proposal density. The previous section has illustrated a number of methods for the generation of r.v.'s with any given distribution and, hence, provides a basis for the three simulation-based approaches.

2.3.1 Laplace approximations

Suppose that we are interested in evaluating the integral

$$I(f) = \int_{\mathcal{X}} f(x)\, dx,$$

where the f is nonnegative and integrable (Robert & Casella, 1999). Let n be the sample size or a parameter which can go to infinity. We define $h(x) \hat{=} \frac{1}{n} \log f(x)$ that has a mode denoted by $\tilde{x}$. A third-order Taylor expansion of $h(x)$ around its mode $\tilde{x}$ gives

$$\begin{aligned} h(x) &= h(\tilde{x}) + (x-\tilde{x})\nabla h(\tilde{x}) + \frac{(x-\tilde{x})^2}{2!}\nabla^2 h(\tilde{x}) \\ &\quad + \frac{(x-\tilde{x})^3}{3!}\nabla^3 h(\tilde{x}) + R_n(x). \end{aligned}$$

Note that

$$\nabla h(\tilde{x}) = 0, \qquad \lim_{x \to \tilde{x}} R_n(x)/(x-\tilde{x})^3 = 0,$$

and $e^y = 1 + y + y^2/2! + R_n'$, we have

$$\begin{aligned} I(f) &\doteq e^{nh(\tilde{x})} \int_{\mathcal{X}} e^{0.5n(x-\tilde{x})^2 \nabla^2 h(\tilde{x})} e^{n\frac{(x-\tilde{x})^3}{3!}\nabla^3 h(\tilde{x})}\, dx \\ &= e^{nh(\tilde{x})} \int_{\mathcal{X}} e^{0.5n(x-\tilde{x})^2 \nabla^2 h(\tilde{x})} \left[1 + \frac{n(x-\tilde{x})^3}{6}\nabla^3 h(\tilde{x}) \right. \\ &\qquad \left. + \frac{n^2(x-\tilde{x})^6}{72}[\nabla^3 h(\tilde{x})]^2 + R_n'\right] dx. \end{aligned}$$

Therefore, the first- and second-order approximations to $I(f)$ are

$$\begin{aligned} I_1(f) &= e^{nh(\tilde{x})} \int_{\mathcal{X}} e^{0.5n(x-\tilde{x})^2 \nabla^2 h(\tilde{x})}\, dx, \quad \text{and} \\ I_2(f) &= e^{nh(\tilde{x})} \int_{\mathcal{X}} e^{0.5n(x-\tilde{x})^2 \nabla^2 h(\tilde{x})} \left[1 + \frac{n(x-\tilde{x})^3}{6} \nabla^3 h(\tilde{x}) \right] dx, \end{aligned}$$

respectively. Tierney & Kadane (1986) further considered the extension to the case of vector.

We note that the integrand in the first-order approximation is the kernel of a normal density with mean $\tilde{x}$ and variance $\sigma^2 = -1/n\nabla^2 h(\tilde{x})$. Let $\mathcal{X} = [a, b]$, then

$$\int_a^b f(x)\, dx \doteq f(\tilde{x})\sqrt{2\pi}\sigma \left\{ \Phi\Big(\frac{b-\tilde{x}}{\sigma}\Big) - \Phi\Big(\frac{a-\tilde{x}}{\sigma}\Big) \right\}. \tag{2.81}$$

Example 2.26 (*The first-order Laplace approximation to incomplete beta integral*). To illustrate the Laplace approximation, we consider evaluating the following incomplete beta integral

$$\int_a^b \frac{x^{\alpha-1}(1-x)^{\beta-1}}{B(\alpha, \beta)}\, dx.$$

The mode of $f(x) = \text{Beta}(x|\alpha, \beta)$ is given by $\tilde{x} = \frac{\alpha-1}{\alpha+\beta-2}$ and

$$\sigma = 1 \Big/ \sqrt{\frac{\alpha-1}{\tilde{x}^2} + \frac{\beta-1}{(1-\tilde{x})^2}}.$$

Table 2.6 *The first-order Laplace approximation to incomplete beta integral for* $\alpha = \beta = 3$

Interval $[a, b]$	Exact	Approximation
$[0.50, 0.55]$	0.09312	0.09313
$[0.45, 0.65]$	0.35795	0.35837
$[0.30, 0.70]$	0.67384	0.67712
$[0.20, 0.80]$	0.88416	0.90457
$[0.10, 0.90]$	0.98288	1.04621

For $\alpha = \beta = 3$, we obtain $\tilde{x} = 0.5$ and $\sigma = 0.25$. In Table 2.6, we see that the first-order Laplace approximation (2.81) works better in the central interval of the density, but the accuracy is not very high when the interval is enlarged. ||

2.3.2 Riemannian simulation

The Laplace method has at least two limitations. First, the integrand f must be unimodal or nearly so. Second, although the second- or third-order approximation provides better accuracy than the first-order approximation, numerical computation of the associated Hessian matrices will be prohibitively difficult anyway, especially, for x of moderate- to high-dimension (e.g., greater than 10). For these reasons, practitioners often turn to Monte Carlo methods.

(a) Classical Monte Carlo integration

Suppose we are interested in evaluating

$$\mu = E_f\{h(X)\} = \int_{\mathcal{X}} h(x)f(x)\,dx, \tag{2.82}$$

where the support of the random vector X is denoted by $\mathcal{X}$ and $h(x) \geq 0$. If we can draw i.i.d. random samples $X^{(1)}, \ldots, X^{(m)}$ from the density f, an approximation to μ can be obtained as the empirical average

$$\bar{\mu}_m = \frac{1}{m}\sum_{i=1}^{m} h(X^{(i)}). \tag{2.83}$$

This estimator is often referred to as the Monte Carlo integration,[1] following Metropolis & Ulam (1949). The **strong law of large numbers** states that $\bar{\mu}_m$ converges **almost surely** (a.s.) to μ. Its convergence rate can be assessed by the **Central Limit Theorem**:

$$\frac{\bar{\mu}_m - \mu}{\sigma/\sqrt{m}} \to N(0,1) \text{ in distribution,}$$

or equivalently,

$$\Pr\{|\bar{\mu}_m - \mu| \leq 1.96\sigma m^{-1/2}\} = 0.95,$$

where

$$\begin{aligned} \sigma^2 &= \text{Var}_f\{h(X)\} \\ &= \int_{\mathcal{X}} (h(x) - \mu)^2 f(x)\,dx. \end{aligned}$$

[1] Sometimes, this Monte Carlo integration is also called **classical**, **crude**, **standard**, **native**, **regular**, or **naïve** Monte Carlo integration in order to distinguish it from Monte Carlo integrations via **importance sampling** presented in §2.3.3.

Hence, the **theoretical rate of convergence**[2] is $O(m^{-1/2})$, regardless of the dimensionality of x. Note that the variance of $\bar{\mu}_m$ can be estimated by

$$\widehat{\text{Var}}(\bar{\mu}_m) = \frac{\hat{\sigma}^2}{m} = \frac{1}{m^2}\sum_{i=1}^{m}[h(X^{(i)}) - \bar{\mu}_m]^2,$$

we say the **speed of convergence** of $\bar{\mu}_m$ is of order $O(m^{-1})$.

(b) Motivation for Riemannian simulation

Although (2.83) is rather attractive for practical users because of its simplicity, the speed of convergence is very low. The approach of **Riemannian simulation** or **simulation by Riemann sums** (Yakowitz *et al.*, 1978; Philippe, 1997a, 1997b) shares the same simplicity as the classical Monte Carlo integration, while speeding up the convergence from $O(m^{-1})$ to $O(m^{-2})$ for the one-dimensional setting. To motivate the approach, we first consider the one-dimensional case of (2.82). Let $\mathcal{X} = [a, b]$ and $a = a_1 < \cdots < a_{m+1} = b$, then when $m \to \infty$, the Riemann sum

$$\sum_{i=1}^{m} h(a_i)f(a_i)[a_{i+1} - a_i] \to \int_a^b h(x)f(x)\,dx.$$

By replacing the deterministic points $\{a_i\}_{i=1}^{m+1}$ by stochastic points $\{X_{(i)}\}_{i=1}^{m+1}$, the ordered statistics of i.i.d. samples $X^{(1)}, \ldots, X^{(m+1)}$ from $f(x)$, the approach of Riemannian simulation approximates the integral (2.82) by

$$\hat{\mu}^R = \sum_{i=1}^{m} h(X_{(i)})f(X_{(i)})[X_{(i+1)} - X_{(i)}]. \tag{2.84}$$

We call $\hat{\mu}^R$ the **Riemannian sum estimator** of μ. When f is known only up to a normalizing constant, that is, $f(x) = c^{-1}f^*(x)$

[2]The theoretical rate of convergence of the Monte Carlo integration is $O(m^{-1/2})$ in the sense of **probability** and not the usual sense of **absolute error**. The law of the iterated logarithm shows that with probability one,

$$\lim_{m\to\infty} \sup \sqrt{\frac{m}{2\log(\log m)}}|\bar{\mu}_m - \mu| = \sigma^2.$$

Therefore, the theoretical rate of convergence of the Monte Carlo integration is in no case worse than $O(\sqrt{\log(\log m)/m})$.

with c being unknown, (2.84) can be replaced by

$$\frac{\sum_{i=1}^{m} h(X_{(i)}) f^*(X_{(i)})[X_{(i+1)} - X_{(i)}]}{\sum_{i=1}^{m} f^*(X_{(i)})[X_{(i+1)} - X_{(i)}]}.$$

(c) Variance of the Riemannian sum estimator

Let F denote the cdf of r.v. $X \sim f(x)$ and F^{-1} the inverse function of F. The integral (2.82) can be rewritten as

$$\mu = \int h(x) dF(x) = \int_0^1 H(u)\, du,$$

where $H(u) = h(F^{-1}(u))$. Further, let $U_{(1)}, \ldots, U_{(m+1)}$ be an ordered sample from $U[0,1]$, then we have

$$\begin{aligned} X_{(i+1)} - X_{(i)} &= F^{-1}(U_{(i+1)}) - F^{-1}(U_{(i)}) \\ &= (U_{(i+1)} - U_{(i)}) \nabla F^{-1}(U_{(i)}) + \text{Remainder}. \end{aligned}$$

As the remainder is negligible and $\nabla F^{-1}(x) = 1/f(F^{-1}(x))$, from (2.84), we obtain

$$\begin{aligned} \hat{\mu}^R &= \sum_{i=1}^{m} h(F^{-1}(U_{(i)})) f(F^{-1}(U_{(i)}))[X_{(i+1)} - X_{(i)}] \\ &\doteq \sum_{i=1}^{m} H(U_{(i)})[U_{(i+1)} - U_{(i)}] \\ &= \delta(U) - H(0)U_{(1)} - H(U_{(m+1)})[1 - U_{(m+1)}], \end{aligned}$$

where $\delta(U)$ is defined by (2.97). Problem 2.15 shows that

$$\text{Var}\{\delta(U)\} = O(m^{-2}).$$

Similarly, we can verify that (See Philippe, 1987a, 1987b for more details)

$$\begin{aligned} \text{Var}\{H(0)U_{(1)}\} &= O(m^{-2}) \quad \text{and} \\ \text{Var}\{H(U_{(m+1)})[1 - U_{(m+1)}]\} &= O(m^{-2}) \end{aligned}$$

so that $\text{Var}\{\hat{\mu}^R\} = O(m^{-2})$.

When compared with the classical Monte Carlo estimator $\bar{\mu}_m$, the Riemannian sum estimator $\hat{\mu}^R$ improves the approximation by reducing the variance from $O(m^{-1})$ to $O(m^{-2})$. Unfortunately, this improvement fails to extend to the case of multidimensional integrals due to the "curse of dimensionality."

Example 2.27 (*Comparison of empirical average with Riemannian sum estimator*). Let $X \sim \text{Beta}(a, b)$ with $a = 3$, $b = 7$ and

$$h(x) = x^2 + \log(x + 1)$$

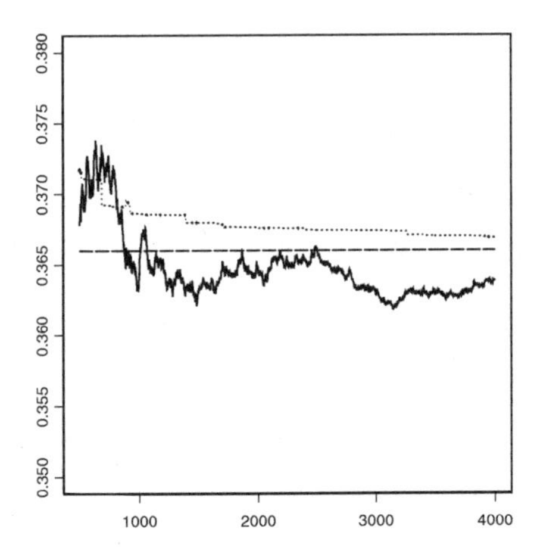

Figure 2.7 Comparison between the convergence of the empirical average $\bar{\mu}_m$ (solid line) and the Riemannian sum estimator $\hat{\mu}^R$ (dotted line) for $a = 3$ and $b = 7$. The final values are 0.363785 and 0.366862, respectively, for a true value of 0.366 (dashed line).

be the function of interest. We generate $m = 4{,}000$ i.i.d. samples $X^{(1)}, \ldots, X^{(m)}$ from $\text{Beta}(a, b)$ and compare the empirical average $\bar{\mu}_m$ defined by (2.83) with the Riemannian sum estimator given by

$$\hat{\mu}^R = \sum_{i=1}^{m-1} h(X_{(i)}) \frac{X_{(i)}^2 (1 - X_{(i)})^6}{B(3, 7)} [X_{(i+1)} - X_{(i)}].$$

Figure 2.7 illustrates that $\hat{\mu}^R$ has much greater stability and faster speed of convergence than $\bar{\mu}_m$. ∥

2.3.3 The importance sampling method

The main reason for low efficiency associated with the **classical Monte Carlo integration** is that it wastes a lot of effort in evaluating random samples located in regions where the function values are almost zero. The **importance sampling** idea (Marshall, 1956) suggests that one should focus on the regions of "importance" so as to save computational resources. The importance sampling method has a close relationship with the SIR method in §2.2.3.

(a) The formulation of the importance sampling method

Suppose that we want to evaluate the integral (2.82), the procedure can be summarized as follows.

THE IMPORTANCE SAMPLING METHOD:

Step 1. Generate i.i.d. samples $\{X^{(i)}\}_{i=1}^m$ from a proposal density[3] $g(\cdot)$ with the same support of $f(\cdot)$;

Step 2. Construct importance weights

$$\mathrm{w}(X^{(i)}) = f(X^{(i)})/g(X^{(i)})$$

for $i = 1, \dots, m$ and approximate μ by

$$\tilde{\mu}_m = \frac{1}{m} \sum_{i=1}^{m} \mathrm{w}(X^{(i)}) h(X^{(i)}). \tag{2.85}$$

We call (2.85) the **importance sampling estimator**. It enjoys good frequentist properties such as (Gamerman, 1997):

- It is an unbiased estimator, i.e., $E_g(\tilde{\mu}_m) = \mu$;
- $\mathrm{Var}(\tilde{\mu}_m) = \sigma^2/m$ with $\sigma^2 = \mathrm{Var}_g\{\mathrm{w}(X)h(X)\}$;
- The strong law of large numbers states $\tilde{\mu}_m \to \mu$ a.s.;
- The central limit theorem states $\sqrt{m}(\tilde{\mu}_m - \mu)/\sigma \to N(0,1)$ in distribution.

By properly choosing g, one can reduce the variance of the estimator $\tilde{\mu}_m$ substantially. A good candidate for g is the one that is close to the shape of $h(x)f(x)$.

Example 2.28 (*Comparison of classical Monte Carlo integration with importance sampling estimator*). Consider to evaluate the integral $\mu = \int_{\mathcal{X}} f(x)\, dx$, where $x = (x_1, x_2)^\top$, $\mathcal{X} = [-1, 1]^2$ and

$$f(x) = e^{-90(x_1-0.5)^2 - 10(x_2+0.1)^4}.$$

[3]The proposal density $g(\cdot)$ has various names such as **importance (sampling) density**, **trial density**, **instrumental density**, **generating density**, etc.

We first generate $m = 6{,}000$ i.i.d. random samples $\{X^{(i)}\}_{i=1}^m$ from uniform distribution $U(\mathcal{X})$ and estimate μ by the empirical mean

$$\bar{\mu}_m = \frac{4}{m}\sum_{i=1}^{m} f(X^{(i)}).$$

Then, we choose $g(x)$ proportional to

$$e^{-90(x_1-0.5)^2-10(x_2+0.1)^2} I_{(x\in\mathcal{X})}$$

as a proposal density. In fact, $g(x)$ is a product of two independent truncated normal distributions (cf. Problem 1.1):

$$g(x) = TN\left(x_1 \middle| 0.5, \frac{1}{180}; -1, 1\right) \cdot TN\left(x_2 \middle| -0.1, \frac{1}{20}; -1, 1\right).$$

We also generate $m = 6{,}000$ i.i.d. random samples $\{X^{(i)}\}_{i=1}^m$ from $g(x)$ and estimate μ by importance sampling estimator

$$\tilde{\mu}_m = \frac{1}{m}\sum_{i=1}^{m} \frac{f(X^{(i)})}{g(X^{(i)})}.$$

Figure 2.8 illustrates that $\tilde{\mu}_m$ has much greater stability and faster speed of convergence than $\bar{\mu}_m$.

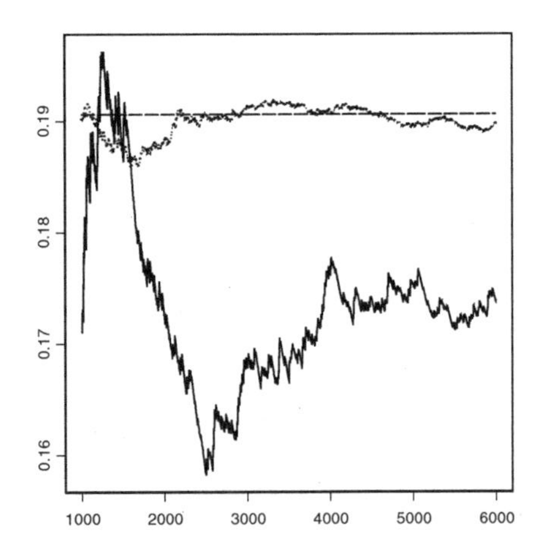

Figure 2.8 Comparison between the convergence of the empirical mean $\bar{\mu}_m$ (solid line) and the importance sampling estimator $\tilde{\mu}_m$ (dotted line). The final values are 0.1739 and 0.1898, respectively, for a true value of 0.1906 (dashed line). ||

(b) The weighted estimator

A practical alternative to the importance sampling estimator $\tilde{\mu}_m$ is to use the **weighted estimator**

$$\hat{\mu}_m = \sum_{i=1}^{m} \omega_i h(X^{(i)}), \tag{2.86}$$

where

$$\omega_i = \frac{\mathrm{w}(X^{(i)})}{\sum_{j=1}^m \mathrm{w}(X^{(j)})} = \frac{f(X^{(i)})/g(X^{(i)})}{\sum_{j=1}^m f(X^{(j)})/g(X^{(j)})}.$$

A major advantage of using $\hat{\mu}_m$ instead of the unbiased estimator $\tilde{\mu}_m$ is that we need only to know the **weight function** $\mathrm{w}(x) = f(x)/g(x)$, i.e., both f and g could be known up to constants. The weighted estimator $\hat{\mu}_m$ is only **asymptotically unbiased** (cf. Eq. (2.87)) but it often has a smaller *mean squared error* (MSE) than the unbiased estimator $\tilde{\mu}_m$ (Casella & Robert, 1998).

To verify the above facts, let $Y = \mathrm{w}(X)h(X)$ and $W = \mathrm{w}(X)$, and let $\bar{Y}$ and $\bar{W}$ be the corresponding sample means. We rewrite $\hat{\mu}_m$ as

$$\hat{\mu}_m = \frac{\tilde{\mu}_m}{\bar{W}} = \tilde{\mu}_m[1 - (\bar{W} - 1) + (\bar{W} - 1)^2 - \cdots].$$

Hence, we obtain (Liu, 2001, p.35–36)

$$\begin{aligned} E_g(\hat{\mu}_m) &\doteq \mu - \frac{\mathrm{Cov}_g(W,Y)}{m} + \frac{\mu \mathrm{Var}_g(W)}{m}, \\ \mathrm{Var}_g(\hat{\mu}_m) &\doteq \frac{1}{m}\Big[\mu^2 \mathrm{Var}_g(W) - 2\mu \mathrm{Cov}_g(W,Y) + \mathrm{Var}_g(Y)\Big]. \end{aligned} \tag{2.87}$$

Note that the MSE of $\tilde{\mu}_m$ is

$$\mathrm{MSE}(\tilde{\mu}_m) = E_g(\tilde{\mu}_m - \mu)^2 = \mathrm{Var}_g(Y)/m,$$

so that we have

$$\begin{aligned} \mathrm{MSE}(\hat{\mu}_m) &= \mathrm{Var}_g(\hat{\mu}_m) + [E_g(\hat{\mu}_m) - \mu]^2 \\ &= \mathrm{MSE}(\tilde{\mu}_m) + \frac{1}{m}\Big[\mu^2 \mathrm{Var}_g(W) - 2\mu \mathrm{Cov}_g(W,Y)\Big] \\ &\quad + O(m^{-2}). \end{aligned}$$

Without loss of generality, we assume that $\mu > 0$, then $\mathrm{MSE}(\hat{\mu}_m) < \mathrm{MSE}(\tilde{\mu}_m)$ when $\mu < 2\mathrm{Cov}_g(W,Y)/\mathrm{Var}_g(W)$.

2.3.4 The cross-entropy method

A major drawback for the **importance sampling method** is that the optimal **proposal density** (or the optimal **reference parameter** in the family of proposal densities) is usually very difficult to obtain. Deriving the name from **cross-entropy** distance (or Kullback–Leibler divergence), the CE method is a valuable tool for Monte Carlo integration. The method was motivated by an adaptive algorithm for estimating probabilities of **rare event** in complex stochastic networks (Rubinstein, 1997), which involves variance minimization. The advantage of the CE method is that it provides a simple and fast adaptive procedure for estimating the optimal reference parameters. Moreover, under mild regularity conditions, the CE method terminates with probability 1 in a finite number of iterations and delivers a consistent and asymptotically normal estimator for the optimal reference parameters.

(a) Efficiency of classical Monte Carlo estimator

Consider estimation of the tail probability

$$p = \Pr(X > \gamma) = \int I_{(x>\gamma)} f(x)\, dx$$

for a large number γ, where the random variable X has pdf $f(x)$. If p is very small, we call $\{X > \gamma\}$ the **rare event**, and p the **rare-event probability**. Let $X^{(1)}, \ldots, X^{(m)}$ be a random sample from the pdf of X, then the classical Monte Carlo estimator of p is given by

$$\hat{p} = \frac{1}{m} \sum_{i=1}^{m} I_{(X^{(i)}>\gamma)}.$$

If we define a new r.v. $Y = I_{(X>\gamma)}$, then $E(Y) = E(Y^2) = p$ and $\text{Var}(Y) = p(1 - p)$. Obviously, $E(\hat{p}) = p$ and $\text{Var}(\hat{p}) = p(1-p)/m$. The *coefficient of variation* (CV) of $\hat{p}$ defined by

$$\text{CV}(\hat{p}) = \frac{\sqrt{\text{Var}(\hat{p})}}{E(\hat{p})} = \sqrt{\frac{1-p}{mp}}$$

is often used in the simulation literature as an accuracy measure for the estimator $\hat{p}$ (Rubinstein & Kroese, 2004, p.9). When p is very small, we have $\text{CV}(\hat{p}) \doteq 1/\sqrt{mp}$. As an illustration, suppose $p = 10^{-6}$ and $\text{CV}(\hat{p}) = 0.01$, then the sample size $N \doteq 10^{10}$, implying that estimating small probabilities via classical Monte Carlo simulation is computationally prohibitive.

(b) Basic idea of the CE algorithm for rare-event simulation

Let X be a d-dimensional random vector taking values in some space $\mathcal{X}$ and $f(x;\theta_0)$ be the pdf of X, where $\theta_0 \in \Theta$ is a **given** parameter vector. Let $T(\cdot)$ be some real function on $\mathcal{X}$ and we are interested in the calculation of

$$q = \Pr_{\theta_0}\{T(X) > \gamma\} = E_{\theta_0}[I_{\{T(X)>\gamma\}}] = \int I_{\{T(x)>\gamma\}} f(x;\theta_0)\,dx.$$

Since the classical Monte Carlo method is not applicable for rare-event simulations, we consider importance sampling method presented in §2.3.3. We first generate i.i.d. samples $\{X_g^{(i)}\}_{i=1}^m$ from a proposal density $g(\cdot)$ and then estimate q using the importance sampling estimator

$$\hat{q} = \frac{1}{m}\sum_{i=1}^m I_{\{T(X_g^{(i)})>\gamma\}} \frac{f(X_g^{(i)};\theta_0)}{g(X_g^{(i)})}.$$

The best choice of g that minimizes the variance of the estimator $\hat{q}$ is (Geweke, 1989; Robert & Casella, 1999, p.84)

$$g^*(x) = \frac{I_{\{T(x)>\gamma\}} f(x;\theta_0)}{q}. \tag{2.88}$$

Note that g^* depends on the unknown quantity q. Moreover, it is often convenient to select a g in the family of pdfs $\{f(x;\theta) : \theta \in \Theta\}$. The idea now is to choose an **optimal reference parameter** θ^{opt} such that the "distance" between the g^* and $f(x;\theta^{\text{opt}})$ is minimal. Considering the Kullback–Leibler divergence as the measure of the "distance" (cf. §1.6.2), we obtain

$$\begin{aligned}
\theta^{\text{opt}} &= \arg\min_{\theta\in\Theta} \text{KL}(g^*, f(x;\theta)) \\
&= \arg\max_{\theta\in\Theta} \int g^*(x) \log f(x;\theta)\,dx \\
&\overset{(2.88)}{=} \arg\max_{\theta\in\Theta} E_{\theta_0}[I_{\{T(X)>\gamma\}} \log f(X;\theta)] \\
&= \arg\max_{\theta\in\Theta} E_{\theta'}[I_{\{T(X)>\gamma\}} R(X;\theta_0,\theta') \log f(X;\theta)], \quad (2.89)
\end{aligned}$$

for **any** reference parameter θ', where $R(x;\theta_0,\theta') = f(x;\theta_0)/f(x;\theta')$ is the likelihood ratio at x between $f(\cdot;\theta_0)$ and $f(\cdot;\theta')$. Note that θ_0 is a known constant, we define two new functions

$$\begin{aligned}
Q_{\gamma,x}(\theta|\theta') &= I_{\{T(x)>\gamma\}} R(x;\theta_0,\theta') \log f(x;\theta), \\
Q_\gamma(\theta|\theta') &= E_{\theta'}[Q_{\gamma,X}(\theta|\theta')].
\end{aligned}$$

Therefore, (2.89) can be rewritten as

$$\begin{aligned} \theta^{\text{opt}} &= \arg\max_{\theta\in\Theta} Q_\gamma(\theta|\theta'), \\ &\doteq \arg\max_{\theta\in\Theta} \frac{1}{m}\sum_{i=1}^{m} Q_{\gamma,X^{(i)}}(\theta|\theta'), \end{aligned} \tag{2.90}$$

where $\{X^{(i)}\}_{i=1}^m \stackrel{\text{iid}}{\sim} f(x;\theta')$. In other words, θ^{opt} can be obtained by solving (with respect to θ) the following system of equations

$$\sum_{i=1}^{m} \nabla^{10} Q_{\gamma,X^{(i)}}(\theta|\theta') = 0. \tag{2.91}$$

The advantage of this approach is that the solution to (2.91) can often be calculated analytically, at least for the case that f belongs to the exponential family.

(c) The CE algorithm

The idea of the CE algorithm is to construct a sequence of levels $\{\gamma^{(t)}, t \ge 1\}$ and a sequence of reference parameters $\{\theta^{(t)}, t \ge 0\}$ and iterate in both $\gamma^{(t)}$ and $\theta^{(t)}$. Specifically, by selecting a not very small δ (say $\delta = 0.01$) and by setting $\theta^{(0)} = \theta_0$, we let $\gamma^{(1)}$ ($< \gamma$) be the level such that the probability

$$q^{(1)} = E_{\theta^{(0)}}\left[I_{\{T(X)>\gamma^{(1)}\}}\right] = \int I_{\{T(x)>\gamma^{(1)}\}} f(x;\theta^{(0)})\, dx$$

is at least δ. Then we let $\theta^{(1)}$ be the optimal CE reference parameter for estimating $q^{(1)}$, and repeat the two steps iteratively with the goal of estimating the pair (q, θ^{opt}). Each iteration of the CE algorithm consists of a **quantile step** (or Q-step) and a **maximization step** (or M-step).[4]

- *Q-step: estimate the quantile $\gamma^{(t)}$ by (2.92).* Given $\theta^{(t-1)}$, let $\gamma^{(t)}$ be a $(1-\delta)$-quantile of $T(X)$ in the sense that

$$\Pr_{\theta^{(t-1)}}\{T(X) > \gamma^{(t)}\} \ge \delta,\ \Pr_{\theta^{(t-1)}}\{T(X) \le \gamma^{(t)}\} \ge 1-\delta,$$

where $X \sim f(\cdot;\theta^{(t-1)})$. An estimator $\hat{\gamma}^{(t)}$ of $\gamma^{(t)}$ can be obtained as

$$\hat{\gamma}^{(t)} = T_{(\lceil(1-\delta)m\rceil)}, \tag{2.92}$$

[4]One alternative name to the CE algorithm is maybe the QM algorithm, mimicking the acronym of the EM/MM algorithm.

where $\lceil x \rceil$ denotes the smallest integer larger than x, $T_{(1)} \le \cdots \le T_{(m)}$ represent the order statistics of $\{T(X^{(i)})\}_{i=1}^{m}$, and

$$X^{(1)}, \ldots, X^{(m)} \overset{\text{iid}}{\sim} f(\cdot; \theta^{(t-1)}). \tag{2.93}$$

- *M-step: update* $\theta^{(t)}$. Given $\gamma^{(t)}$ and $\theta^{(t-1)}$, using (2.90), we find

$$\theta^{(t)} = \arg\max_{\theta \in \Theta} Q_{\gamma^{(t)}}(\theta | \theta^{(t-1)}).$$

  Based on $\hat{\gamma}^{(t)}$ and $\hat{\theta}^{(t-1)}$, using the same samples specified by (2.93), we estimate $\theta^{(t)}$ with $\hat{\theta}^{(t)}$, which can be obtained by solving (with respect to θ) the following system of equations:

$$\sum_{i=1}^{m} \nabla^{10} Q_{\hat{\gamma}^{(t)}, X^{(i)}}(\theta | \hat{\theta}^{(t-1)}) = 0. \tag{2.94}$$

The two-step process is repeated until $\hat{\gamma}^{(t)} = \gamma$. The corresponding $\hat{\theta}^{(t)} = \theta^{\text{opt}}$. Finally, let $\{X^{(i)}\}_{i=1}^{M} \overset{\text{iid}}{\sim} f(x; \theta^{\text{opt}})$, we estimate the rare-event probability q by

$$\hat{q} = \frac{1}{M} \sum_{i=1}^{M} I_{\{T(X^{(i)}) > \gamma\}} R(X^{(i)}; \theta_0, \theta^{\text{opt}}). \tag{2.95}$$

Example 2.29 (*A rare-event simulation associated with exponential distributions*). Consider the weighted graph of Figure 2.9 with random weights $X_1, \ldots, X_5$. Let $\{X_j\}_{j=1}^{5}$ be independent and exponentially distributed with means $\theta_{10}, \ldots, \theta_{50}$, respectively. Let

$$\theta_0 = (\theta_{10}, \ldots, \theta_{50})^\top = (0.25, 0.4, 0.1, 0.3, 0.2)^\top,$$

the joint pdf of $X = (X_1, \ldots, X_5)^\top$ is

$$f(x; \theta_0) = \left(\prod_{j=1}^{5} \theta_{j0}^{-1} \right) \exp\left(- \sum_{j=1}^{5} \frac{x_j}{\theta_{j0}} \right).$$

Let

$$T(X) = \min\{X_1 + X_4, X_2 + X_5, X_1 + X_3 + X_5, X_2 + X_3 + X_4\}$$

denote the length of the shortest path from node A to node B. We wish to estimate $q = \Pr_{\theta_0}\{T(X) > \gamma\}$ with $\gamma = 2$. Note that the likelihood ratio is given by

$$\begin{aligned} R(x;\theta_0,\theta') &= \frac{f(x;\theta_0)}{f(x;\theta')} \\ &= \left(\prod_{j=1}^{5}\frac{\theta'_j}{\theta_{j0}}\right)\exp\left(-\sum_{j=1}^{5}x_j\left(\frac{1}{\theta_{j0}}-\frac{1}{\theta'_j}\right)\right). \end{aligned}$$

It is easy to obtain

$$\frac{\partial \log f(x;\theta)}{\partial \theta_j} = x_j\theta_j^{-2} - \theta_j^{-1}$$

so that the j-th equation of (2.91) becomes

$$\sum_{i=1}^{m} I_{\{T(X^{(i)})>\gamma\}}R(X^{(i)};\theta_0,\theta')(X_j^{(i)}\theta_j^{-2}-\theta_j^{-1}) = 0, \quad 1 \le j \le 5.$$

Therefore, the j-th component of θ^{opt} is

$$\theta_j = \frac{\sum_{i=1}^{m} I_{\{T(X^{(i)})>\gamma\}}R(X^{(i)};\theta_0,\theta')X_j^{(i)}}{\sum_{i=1}^{m} I_{\{T(X^{(i)})>\gamma\}}R(X^{(i)};\theta_0,\theta')}.$$

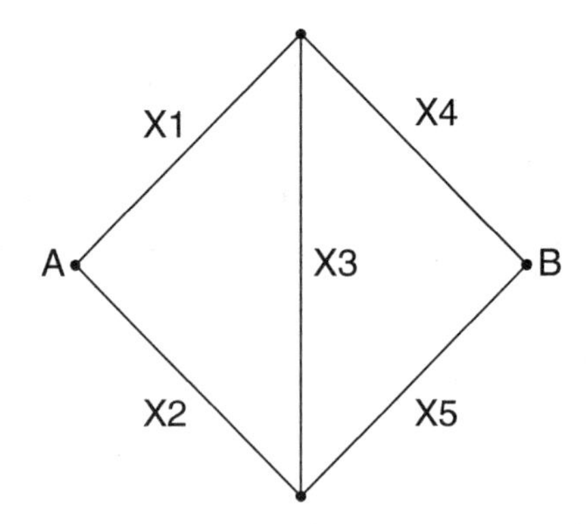

Figure 2.9 Shortest path from node A to node B (Source: Rubinstein & Kroese, 2004, p.31).

Rubinstein & Kroese (2004, p.33) reported the following results. The classical Monte Carlo with 10^7 samples gave an estimate 1.65×10^{-5} with an estimated *coefficient of variation* (CV) of 0.165 and the *central processing unit* (CPU) time is 630 seconds.[5] With 10^8 samples they got the estimate 1.30×10^{-5} with CV 0.03 and the CPU time is 6350 seconds. Table 2.7 displays the results of the CE algorithm, using $m = 1000$ and $\delta = 0.1$. This table was computed in less than half a second.

Table 2.7 *Evolution of the sequence* $\{(\hat{\gamma}^{(t)}, \hat{\theta}^{(t)})\}$

t	$\hat{\gamma}^{(t)}$	$\hat{\theta}^{(t)}$				
0		0.250	0.400	0.100	0.300	0.200
1	0.575	0.513	0.718	0.122	0.474	0.335
2	1.032	0.873	1.057	0.120	0.550	0.436
3	1.502	1.221	1.419	0.121	0.707	0.533
4	1.917	1.681	1.803	0.132	0.638	0.523
5	2.000	1.692	1.901	0.129	0.712	0.564

Source: Rubinstein & Kroese (2004, p.33).

Using the estimated optimal reference parameter vector $\theta^{\text{opt}} = \hat{\theta}^{(5)} = (1.692, 1.901, 0.129, 0.712, 0.564)^\top$, the final step of (2.95) with $M = 10^5$ gave an estimate of 1.34×10^{-5} with an estimated CV of 0.03 and the CPU time was only 3 seconds. ||

Problems

2.1 Derivative of a vector. Let x and a be two $n \times 1$ vectors, b an $m \times 1$ vector, A an $m \times n$ matrix and B an $n \times n$ matrix. Define

$$\frac{\partial b^\top}{\partial x} = \left(\frac{\partial b_1}{\partial x}, \ldots, \frac{\partial b_m}{\partial x}\right).$$

Show that

$$\begin{aligned}
\frac{\partial (a^\top x)}{\partial x} &= \frac{\partial (x^\top a)}{\partial x} = a, \\
\frac{\partial (Ax)}{\partial x^\top} &= A, \qquad \frac{\partial (Ax)^\top}{\partial x} = A^\top, \\
\frac{\partial (x^\top Bx)}{\partial x} &= (B + B^\top)x, \qquad \frac{\partial^2 (x^\top Bx)}{\partial x \partial x^\top} = B + B^\top.
\end{aligned}$$

[5]Rubinstein & Kroese implemented the calculation by using a MATLAB on a Pentium III 500 MHz processor.

2.2 The delta method. Let $\hat{\theta} - \theta \dot{\sim} N_d(\mathbf{0}, C)$ and $h(\cdot)$ be a differentiable function. Prove that

$$h(\hat{\theta}) - h(\theta) \dot{\sim} N(0, (\nabla h(\hat{\theta}))^{\top} C \nabla h(\hat{\theta})).$$

2.3 Truncated normal distribution (Johnson & Kotz, 1970). Let $X \sim TN(\mu, \sigma^2; a, b)$ (cf. Problem 1.1), show that

$$\begin{aligned} E(X) &= \mu + \sigma \frac{\phi(\frac{a-\mu}{\sigma}) - \phi(\frac{b-\mu}{\sigma})}{\Phi(\frac{b-\mu}{\sigma}) - \Phi(\frac{a-\mu}{\sigma})}, \\ \mathrm{Var}(X) &= \sigma^2 \left[1 + \frac{\frac{a-\mu}{\sigma}\phi(\frac{a-\mu}{\sigma}) - \frac{b-\mu}{\sigma}\phi(\frac{b-\mu}{\sigma})}{\Phi(\frac{b-\mu}{\sigma}) - \Phi(\frac{a-\mu}{\sigma})} \right] - [EX - \mu]^2. \end{aligned}$$

2.4 Prove that the function $Q(\theta|\theta^{(t)})$ defined in (2.39) minorizes $\ell(\theta|Y_{\text{obs}})$ at $\theta^{(t)}$.

2.5 (Böhning & Lindsay, 1988). Let $p = (p_1, \dots, p_n)^{\top} \in \{p : p_j \geq 0, \sum_{j=1}^{n} p_j = 1\}$, then

$$\mathrm{diag}(p) - pp^{\top} \leq \frac{1}{2}\left(\mathbf{I}_n - \frac{1}{n}\mathbf{1}_n\mathbf{1}_n^{\top}\right).$$

2.6 Multinomial logistic regression (Böhning, 1992). Consider baseline-category logit model for nominal responses. Let Y be a categorical response with K categories and $p_k(x) = \Pr\{Y = k|x\}$ the response probability at a fixed vector $x_{n\times 1}$ of covariates so that $\sum_{k=1}^{K} p_k(x) = 1$. A baseline-category logit model often assumes $\log[p_k(x)/p_K(x)] = x^{\top}\theta_k$ for $k = 1, \dots, K-1$, or equivalently,

$$p_k(x) = \frac{\exp(x^{\top}\theta_k)}{1 + \sum_{h=1}^{K-1} \exp(x^{\top}\theta_h)}, \qquad k = 1, \dots, K$$

where $\theta_K = \mathbf{0}$ and $\theta_k = (\theta_{k1}, \dots, \theta_{kn})^{\top}$ denote parameters for the k-th category. Consider m independent observations and let $y_i = (y_{i1}, \dots, y_{iK})^{\top}$ denote the observation for subject i ($i = 1, \dots, m$), where $y_{ik} = 1$ when the response is in category k and $y_{ik} = 0$ otherwise while $\sum_{k=1}^{K} y_{ik} = 1$. Let $x_i = (x_{i1}, \dots, x_{in})^{\top}$ denote covariates for subject i and $\theta = (\theta_1^{\top}, \dots, \theta_{K-1}^{\top})^{\top}$ the $n(K-1)$-vector of parameters, then the log-likelihood is

$$\ell(\theta|Y_{\text{obs}}) = \sum_{i=1}^{m} \left\{ \sum_{k=1}^{K-1} y_{ik}(x_i^{\top}\theta_k)) - \log\left[1 + \sum_{k=1}^{K-1} e^{x_i^{\top}\theta_k}\right] \right\}.$$

Prove that

(a) The score vector is

$$\nabla \ell(\theta|Y_{\rm obs}) = \sum_{i=1}^{m} \left\{ \left[y_i^{(-K)} - p^{(-K)}(x_i) \right] \otimes x_i \right\},$$

and the observed information $-\nabla^2 \ell(\theta|Y_{\rm obs})$ is given by

$$\sum_{i=1}^{m} \left\{ \left[\text{diag}\left(p^{(-K)}(x_i)\right) - \left(p^{(-K)}(x_i)\right)^{\otimes 2} \right] \otimes x_i x_i^{\top} \right\},$$

where $y_i^{(-K)} = (y_{i1}, \ldots, y_{i,K-1})^{\top}$ and

$$p^{(-K)}(x_i) = (p_1(x_i), \ldots, p_{K-1}(x_i))^{\top}.$$

(b) $-\nabla^2 \ell(\theta|Y_{\rm obs}) \le \frac{1}{2}(\mathbf{I}_{K-1} - \frac{1}{K}\mathbf{1}\mathbf{1}^{\top}) \otimes \sum_{i=1}^{m} x_i x_i^{\top} \hat{=} B$ and $B^{-1} = 2(\mathbf{I}_{K-1} + \mathbf{1}\mathbf{1}^{\top}) \otimes (\sum_{i=1}^{m} x_i x_i^{\top})^{-1}$.

(c) Devise a QLB algorithm to find the MLEs of θ.

2.7 Prove that the function $Q(\theta|\theta^{(t)})$ defined in (2.49) minorizes $\ell(\theta|Y_{\rm obs})$ at $\theta^{(t)}$.
(*Hint*: Note that

$$x_{(i)}^{\top}\theta = \sum_{j \in \mathbb{J}_i} \lambda_{ij} [\lambda_{ij}^{-1} x_{ij} (\theta_j - \theta_j^{(t)}) + x_{(i)}^{\top} \theta^{(t)}]$$

and using the concavity inequality, i.e., the reverse of inequality (e) in Problem 1.10.)

2.8 Let $r = 1$, show that (2.56) can be rewritten in matrix form as

$$\theta^{(t+1)} = \theta^{(t)} + X^{\top}(y - e^{X\theta^{(t)}})/Z^{\top} e^{X\theta^{(t)}},$$

where $X = (x_{ij}) = (x_{(1)}, \ldots, x_{(m)})^{\top}$, $Y = (|x_{ij}|) = \text{abs}(X)$ and $Z = \text{diag}(Y\mathbf{1}_q)Y$.

2.9 Let r.v. X have the following pdf

$$f(x) = \frac{a}{2\sinh(a)} \sin(x) \exp\{a\cos(x)\},$$

where $0 < x < \pi$, $a > 0$, $\sinh(a) = (e^a - e^{-a})/2$. Prove that

$$X \stackrel{d}{=} \arccos\left\{ a^{-1} \log\left[(1-U)e^a + Ue^{-a} \right] \right\}, \quad U \sim U(0,1).$$

2.10 Generation of truncated distribution. Let $X \sim F(\cdot)$ and $Y \sim G(\cdot)$, where

$$G(y) = 0I_{(y<a)} + \frac{F(y) - F(a)}{F(b) - F(a)} I_{(a \le y \le b)} + 1I_{(y>b)},$$

$-\infty \le a < b \le +\infty$. Show that

$$Y \stackrel{d}{=} F^{-1}(F(a) + U[F(b) - F(a)]), \quad U \sim U(0, 1).$$

2.11 Positively correlated bivariate beta distribution (Albert & Gupta, 1983, 1985). A two-dimensional random vector $(X_1, X_2)^\top$ is said to have a **positively correlated bivariate beta distribution**, if the joint density is

$$\int_0^1 \frac{z^{a-1}(1-z)^{b-1}}{B(a,b)} \prod_{i=1}^{2} \frac{x_i^{\gamma_i z - 1}(1 - x_i)^{\gamma_i(1-z)-1}}{B(\gamma_i z, \gamma_i(1-z))} \, dz.$$

Show how to use the mixture method to simulate $(X_1, X_2)^\top$. (*Hint*: Consider the augmented vector $(X_1, X_2, Z)^\top$ with $Z \sim \text{Beta}(a, b)$ and $X_i|(Z = z) \sim \text{Beta}(\gamma_i z, \gamma_i(1-z))$ for $i = 1, 2$.)

2.12 Verify the fact on the SR of X stated in Ex.2.18.

2.13 Let $\mathbb{B}_d(r)$ denote the d-dimensional ball with radius r, see (2.66). Verify that the volume of $\mathbb{B}_d(r)$ is $2\pi^{d/2} r^d / [\Gamma(d/2)d]$.

2.14 Let $\mathbb{V}_d(r)$ denote the d-dimensional ℓ_1-ball,

$$\mathbb{V}_d(r) = \{(x_1, \dots, x_d)^\top : x_i \ge 0, \; x_1 + \cdots + x_d \le r\}. \tag{2.96}$$

Verify that the volume of $\mathbb{V}_d(r)$ is $r^d/d!$.

2.15 (Yakowitz *et al.*, 1978). Let $U = (U_{(1)}, \dots, U_{(m+1)})$ be an ordered sample from $U[0, 1]$. If the derivative $\nabla H(x)$ is bounded on $[0, 1]$, the estimator

$$\delta(U) = \sum_{i=0}^{m+1} H(U_{(i)})(U_{(i+1)} - U_{(i)}) \tag{2.97}$$

has a variance of order $O(m^{-2})$, where $U_{(0)} \hat{=} 0$ and $U_{(m+2)} \hat{=} 1$.

CHAPTER 3

Exact Solutions

Exact or closed-form solutions, if available, to statistical problems are favored in statistical theory and practice for obvious reasons. For example, its simplicity facilitates the communication of statistical analysis to a wider audience and thus make the contribution of statistics visible. Unfortunately, it may not be possible to obtain exact solutions in many practical statistical models. However, surprisingly the IBF approach allows such solutions in a variety of nontrivial statistical problems (Ng, 1997a; Tian, 2000; Tian & Tan, 2003). In this chapter, we first demonstrate that the IBF can be used to derive closed-form solutions to various Bayesian missing data problems including sample surveys with nonresponse, misclassified multinomial model, genetic linkage model, Weibull process with missing data, prediction problem, bivariate normal model, the 2×2 crossover trial with missing data and hierarchical models. We will show how to derive the explicit posterior density of the parameter of interest given the observed data. With this, subsequent statistical inference is straightforward. Then we extend the IBF in *product measurable space* (PMS) to *nonproduct measurable space* (NPMS) and focus on their applications in obtaining exact solutions in multivariate distributions.

3.1 Sample Surveys with Nonresponse

Suppose that a mail survey is conducted to determine the attitudes of individuals in a certain population towards a particular proposal (Tian *et al.*, 2003). Let n denote the sample size of the questionnaire. Assume that n_1 individuals respond but $n_2 = n - n_1$ do not. Of these n_1 respondents, there are y_i individuals whose answers are classified into category A_i, $i = 1, \dots, k$. Denote the respondents and nonrespondents by R and NR, respectively. The observed counts and the cell probabilities are summarized in Table 3.1 with $\{\theta_{i\cdot}\}_{i=1}^k$ being the parameters of interest.

The observed data are $Y_{\text{obs}} = \{y_1, \dots, y_k, n_2\}$ with $n_2 = n - \sum_{i=1}^k y_i$ and the parameter vector is $\theta = (\theta_{11}, \dots, \theta_{k1}, \theta_{12}, \dots, \theta_{k2})^\top$, while $Z = (Z_1, \ldots, Z_k)^\top$ denote the missing data with $n_2 = \sum_{i=1}^k Z_i$.

Table 3.1 *$k \times 2$ observed frequencies and cell probabilities*

Categories	R	NR	Total	Categories	R	NR	Total
A_1	y_1	Z_1		A_1	θ_{11}	θ_{12}	$\theta_{1\cdot}$
$\vdots$	$\vdots$	$\vdots$		$\vdots$	$\vdots$	$\vdots$	$\vdots$
A_k	y_k	Z_k		A_k	θ_{k1}	θ_{k2}	$\theta_{k\cdot}$
Total	n_1	n_2	n	Total	$\theta_{\cdot 1}$	$\theta_{\cdot 2}$	1

Source: Tian *et al.* (2003).

Then, we have

$$Z|(Y_{\text{obs}}, \theta) \sim \text{Multinomial}\left(n_2; \frac{\theta_{12}}{\theta_{\cdot 2}}, \ldots, \frac{\theta_{k2}}{\theta_{\cdot 2}}\right)$$

and

$$\mathcal{S}_{(Z|Y_{\text{obs}})} = \left\{(z_1, \ldots, z_k)^\top \colon \sum_{i=1}^k z_i = n_2,\ 0 \le z_i \le n_2,\ 1 \le i \le k\right\}.$$

The likelihood for the complete-data $\{Y_{\text{obs}}, Z\}$ is proportional to

$$\prod_{i=1}^k \theta_{i1}^{y_i} \theta_{i2}^{z_i}.$$

Using Dirichlet(α_1, α_2) as the prior distribution of θ, where $\alpha_1 = (\alpha_{11}, \ldots, \alpha_{k1})^\top$ and $\alpha_2 = (\alpha_{12}, \ldots, \alpha_{k2})^\top$, we have

$$\theta|(Y_{\text{obs}}, Z = z) \sim \text{Dirichlet}(y + \alpha_1,\ z + \alpha_2),$$

where $y = (y_1, \ldots, y_k)^\top$ and $z = (z_1, \ldots, z_k)^\top$. From (1.36), we obtain

$$f(\theta|Y_{\text{obs}}) = c^{-1}(\alpha_1, \alpha_2) \times \left\{\prod_{i=1}^k \theta_{i1}^{y_i + \alpha_{i1} - 1} \theta_{i2}^{\alpha_{i2} - 1}\right\} \times \theta_{\cdot 2}^{n_2},$$

where

$$c(\alpha_1, \alpha_2) = \sum_{z \in \mathcal{S}_{(Z|Y_{\text{obs}})}} \binom{n_2}{z_1, \ldots, z_k} B(y + \alpha_1,\ z + \alpha_2).$$

From the property of beta function and Dirichlet-multinomial density, we have

$$B(y+\alpha_1,\ z+\alpha_2) = B(y+\alpha_1)B(z+\alpha_2)B\Big(\mathbf{1}_k^\top(y+\alpha_1),\ \mathbf{1}_k^\top(z+\alpha_2)\Big)$$

and (cf. Problem 3.1)

$$\sum_{z\in\mathcal{S}_{(Z|Y_{\rm obs})}} \binom{n_2}{z_1,\dots,z_k} B(z+\alpha_2) = B(\alpha_2). \tag{3.1}$$

Hence,

$$c(\alpha_1,\alpha_2) = B(y+\alpha_1)\times B(n_1+\alpha_{\cdot 1},\ n_2+\alpha_{\cdot 2})\times B(\alpha_2),$$

where $\alpha_{\cdot 1} = \sum_{i=1}^k \alpha_{i1}$ and $\alpha_{\cdot 2} = \sum_{i=1}^k \alpha_{i2}$. The posterior mean of θ_{11} is equal to the ratio of $c(\alpha_1+(1,0,\dots,0)^\top,\alpha_2)$ to $c(\alpha_1,\alpha_2)$, i.e.,

$$E(\theta_{11}|Y_{\rm obs}) = \frac{y_1+\alpha_{11}}{n+\alpha_{\cdot\cdot}},$$

where $\alpha_{\cdot\cdot} = \alpha_{\cdot 1}+\alpha_{\cdot 2}$. Similarly,

$$E(\theta_{12}|Y_{\rm obs}) = \frac{(n_2+\alpha_{\cdot 2})\alpha_{12}}{(n+\alpha_{\cdot\cdot})\alpha_{\cdot 2}}.$$

Thus, the Bayes estimator of $\theta_{1\cdot} = \theta_{11}+\theta_{12}$ is given by

$$E(\theta_{1\cdot}|Y_{\rm obs}) = \frac{y_1+\alpha_{11}+\alpha_{12}+n_2\alpha_{12}/\alpha_{\cdot 2}}{n+\alpha_{\cdot\cdot}}.$$

Therefore, the IBF provides a simple and exact solution for such a rather complicated missing data problem.

3.2 Misclassified Multinomial Model

Geng & Asano (1989) and Tian *et al.* (2003) considered a contingency table with dichotomous error-free variables A and B, and the corresponding error-prone variables a and b. Limited by cost, the complete 2^4 table is available for a sub-sample only, as shown in Table 3.2 with corresponding cell probabilities. The objective is to find posterior means of cell probabilities of error-free variables, i.e.,

$$\begin{aligned}
\Pr(A=1,B=1) &= \theta_1+\theta_5+\theta_9+\theta_{13},\\
\Pr(A=2,B=1) &= \theta_2+\theta_6+\theta_{10}+\theta_{14},\\
\Pr(A=1,B=2) &= \theta_3+\theta_7+\theta_{11}+\theta_{15}, \quad \text{and}\\
\Pr(A=2,B=2) &= \theta_4+\theta_8+\theta_{12}+\theta_{16}.
\end{aligned}$$

Table 3.2 *Counts and probabilities for main- and sub-sample*

Main-sample						Sub-sample					
		$a=1$		$a=2$				$a=1$		$a=2$	
b	B	A=1	A=2	A=1	A=2	b	B	$A=1$	$A=2$	$A=1$	$A=2$
1	1	m_1		m_2		1	1	$y_1\ (\theta_1)$	$y_2\ (\theta_2)$	$y_5\ (\theta_5)$	$y_6\ (\theta_6)$
	2						2	$y_3\ (\theta_3)$	$y_4\ (\theta_4)$	$y_7\ (\theta_7)$	$y_8\ (\theta_8)$
2	1	m_3		m_4		2	1	$y_9\ (\theta_9)$	$y_{10}(\theta_{10})$	$y_{13}(\theta_{13})$	$y_{14}(\theta_{14})$
	2						2	$y_{11}(\theta_{11})$	$y_{12}(\theta_{12})$	$y_{15}(\theta_{15})$	$y_{16}(\theta_{16})$

Source: Tian *et al.* (2003).

Let $\theta = (\theta_1, \dots, \theta_{16})^\top$ and $Y_{\text{obs}} = \{m_1, m_2, m_3, m_4; y\}$, where $y = (y_1, \dots, y_{16})^\top$. In the main sample, we introduce a latent vector $Z = (Z_1, \dots, Z_{16})^\top$ such that

$$\textstyle\sum_{k=1}^4 Z_{4(j-1)+k} = m_j, \quad j = 1, \dots, 4.$$

Partition Z into $(Z_{(1)}^\top, Z_{(2)}^\top, Z_{(3)}^\top, Z_{(4)}^\top)^\top$, where $Z_{(j)} = (Z_{4(j-1)+1}, \dots, Z_{4(j-1)+4})^\top$. Let θ, y, z and α have the same partition as Z. The conditional predictive density is

$$f_{(Z|Y_{\text{obs}},\theta)}(z|Y_{\text{obs}}, \theta) = \prod_{j=1}^4 \text{Multinomial}\left(z_{(j)} \,\middle|\, m_j;\ \frac{\theta_{(j)}}{\mathbf{1}_4^\top \theta_{(j)}}\right),$$

and

$$\mathcal{S}_{(Z_{(j)}|Y_{\text{obs}})} = \left\{z_{(j)}\colon\ \mathbf{1}_4^\top z_{(j)} = m_j,\ 0 \le z_{4(j-1)+k} \le m_j,\ 1 \le k \le 4\right\}.$$

The likelihood function for the complete-data is proportional to

$$\prod_{i=1}^{16} \theta_i^{y_i + z_i}.$$

Using Dirichlet(α) with $\alpha = (\alpha_1, \dots, \alpha_{16})^\top$ as the prior distribution of θ, we have

$$f_{(\theta|Y_{\text{obs}},Z)}(\theta|Y_{\text{obs}}, z) = \text{Dirichlet}(\theta|y + z + \alpha).$$

From (1.36), the observed posterior is

$$f(\theta|Y_{\text{obs}}) = c^{-1}(\alpha) \times \prod_{i=1}^{16} \theta_i^{y_i+\alpha_i-1} \times \prod_{j=1}^4 (\mathbf{1}_4^\top \theta_{(j)})^{m_j},$$

where

$$c(\alpha) = \sum_{\{z_{(j)} \in \mathcal{S}(Z_{(j)}|Y_{\text{obs}}), 1 \le j \le 4\}} \binom{m_1}{z_{(1)}} \binom{m_2}{z_{(2)}} \binom{m_3}{z_{(3)}} \binom{m_4}{z_{(4)}} B(y + z + \alpha).$$

By identity (3.1), we obtain

$$\begin{aligned} c(\alpha) &= B\Big(m_1 + \mathbf{1}_4^\top \alpha_{(1)}, m_2 + \mathbf{1}_4^\top \alpha_{(2)}, m_3 + \mathbf{1}_4^\top \alpha_{(3)}, m_4 + \mathbf{1}_4^\top \alpha_{(4)}\Big) \\ &\quad \times \prod_{j=1}^{4} B(y_{(j)} + \alpha_{(j)}). \end{aligned}$$

Let $a_i = y_i + \alpha_i$, $a. = \sum_{i=1}^{16}(y_i + \alpha_i)$ and $m. = \sum_{j=1}^{4} m_j$, then the posterior means of $\{\theta_i\}$ are given by

$$\begin{aligned} E(\theta_i|Y_{\text{obs}}) &= \frac{a_i}{a. + m.}\left(1 + \frac{m_1}{\sum_{j=1}^{4} a_j}\right), \quad i = 1, \cdots, 4, \\ E(\theta_i|Y_{\text{obs}}) &= \frac{a_i}{a. + m.}\left(1 + \frac{m_2}{\sum_{j=5}^{8} a_j}\right), \quad i = 5, \cdots, 8, \\ E(\theta_i|Y_{\text{obs}}) &= \frac{a_i}{a. + m.}\left(1 + \frac{m_3}{\sum_{j=9}^{12} a_j}\right), \quad i = 9, \cdots, 12, \\ E(\theta_i|Y_{\text{obs}}) &= \frac{a_i}{a. + m.}\left(1 + \frac{m_4}{\sum_{j=13}^{16} a_j}\right), \quad i = 13, \cdots, 16. \end{aligned}$$

3.3 Genetic Linkage Model

In this study (Rao, 1973; Tanner, 1996, p.66 & p.113; Lange, 2002), AB/ab animals are crossed to measure the recombination fraction (r) between loci with alleles A and a at the first locus and alleles B and b at the second locus. Then the offspring of an $AB/ab \times AB/ab$ mating falls into the four categories AB, Ab, aB and ab with cell probabilities

$$\frac{\theta+2}{4}, \ \frac{1-\theta}{4}, \ \frac{1-\theta}{4}, \ \frac{\theta}{4}, \quad 0 \le \theta \le 1,$$

where $\theta = (1-r)^2$. Observed frequencies $Y_{\text{obs}} = (y_1, y_2, y_3, y_4)^\top$ then follow a multinomial distribution with above cell probabilities. This data set has become a classic proof-of-principle example for several computation methods and algorithms. Augmenting the observed data Y_{obs} with a latent variable Z by splitting $y_1 = Z + (y_1 - Z)$, we have

$$Z|(Y_{\text{obs}}, \theta) \sim \text{Binomial}(y_1, \theta/(\theta+2)). \tag{3.2}$$

Using the usual Beta(a, b) as the prior distribution of θ, we have

$$\theta|(Y_{\text{obs}}, Z = z) \sim \text{Beta}(a + y_4 + z, b + y_2 + y_3). \tag{3.3}$$

Obviously, $\mathcal{S}_{(\theta,Z|Y_{\text{obs}})} = \mathcal{S}_{(\theta|Y_{\text{obs}})} \times \mathcal{S}_{(Z|Y_{\text{obs}})}$. Therefore, with the discrete version of the IBF (1.36), the observed posterior density of θ is given exactly by

$$f(\theta|Y_{\text{obs}}) = \frac{(\theta+2)^{y_1}\theta^{a+y_4-1}(1-\theta)^{b+y_2+y_3-1}}{\sum_{z=0}^{y_1}\binom{y_1}{z}B(a+y_4+z, b+y_2+y_3)2^{y_1-z}}. \tag{3.4}$$

Example 3.1 (*Genetic linkage data*). To obtain i.i.d. posterior samples from (3.4), we adopt the rejection method (cf. §2.2.2). With the observed frequencies $(y_1, y_2, y_3, y_4) = (125, 18, 20, 34)$ and the uniform prior (i.e., $a = b = 1$), (3.4) becomes

$$f(\theta|Y_{\text{obs}}) = c_{\text{G}}^{-1}(\theta+2)^{125}\theta^{34}(1-\theta)^{38}$$

where $c_{\text{G}} \approx 2.3577 \times 10^{28}$ is the normalizing constant. The mode of $f(\theta|Y_{\text{obs}})$ is $\tilde{\theta} \approx 0.62682$. Naturally we wish to select a member from Beta(α, β) as an envelope distribution for the rejection method. The Beta$(\theta|\alpha, \beta)$ that matches the mode of $f(\theta|Y_{\text{obs}})$ should satisfy $(\alpha-1)/(\alpha+\beta-2) = 0.62682$. This provides a clue for finding α and β. According to (2.61), let

$$c_{\alpha,\beta} = \max_{\theta\in[0,1]} f(\theta|Y_{\text{obs}})/\text{Beta}(\theta|\alpha, \beta),$$

then, the optimal α and β are such that $c_{\alpha,\beta}$ is minimized. The following are choices for α and β:

α	35	35	35	35	34	33	30	20	10
β	19	20	21	23	20.6	20	18.3	12.3	6.36
$c_{\alpha,\beta}$	1.55	1.35	1.27	1.43	1.29	1.30	1.37	1.68	2.38

So Beta$(\theta|35, 21)$ is the most efficient envelope density. With this envelope density, the rejection method can be implemented readily. The corresponding acceptance probability is $1/c_{\alpha,\beta} = 0.7830$. ‖

3.4 Weibull Process with Missing Data

A model widely used in industrial testing is the Weibull process, i.e., a nonhomogeneous Poisson process with mean function

$$m(t) = (t/\alpha)^{\beta}, \quad \alpha > 0,\ \beta > 0.$$

Suppose that the reliability growth testing for a repairable system is performed during time interval $(0,\ t]$, then, the number of failures in $(0,\ t]$, denoted by $N(t)$, is a Poisson random variable with

$$\Pr\{N(t) = n\} = \frac{\{m(t)\}^n}{n!} e^{-m(t)}.$$

The testing is called a **failure-truncated testing** if it is observed until the first n (n is pre-determined) failure times, $0 < x_1 < x_2 < \cdots < x_n$, have occurred. A **time-truncated testing** refers to the situation where observations are truncated after a pre-fixed time t, and the corresponding failure times are $0 < x_1 < x_2 < \cdots < x_n < t$. The likelihood function for both cases can be written as (Crowder *et al.*, 1991)

$$L(\alpha, \beta|\text{data}) = \beta^n \alpha^{-n\beta} \prod_{i=1}^{n} x_i^{\beta-1} \cdot e^{-(T/\alpha)^{\beta}}, \quad \alpha > 0,\ \beta > 0, \tag{3.5}$$

where $T = x_n$ if the testing is failure-truncated, and $T = t$ if it is time-truncated. Bayesian inference on α and β has been studied by Kuo & Yang (1996).

This section concerns the model where missing data may occur. Suppose the first $r-1$ failures $Z = \{x_1, \ldots, x_{r-1}\}$ are missing, and we only observed $Y_{\text{obs}} = \{x_r, \ldots, x_n\}$ for the failure-truncated testing or $Y_{\text{obs}} = \{x_r, \ldots, x_n, t\}$ for the time-truncated testing, where $1 < r < n$. The purpose is to obtain the observed posterior $f(\alpha, \beta|Y_{\text{obs}})$. The complete-data likelihood $L(\alpha, \beta|Y_{\text{obs}}, Z)$ is given by (3.5). Based on arguments in Box & Tiao (1973), Guida *et al.* (1989) suggested

$$f(\alpha, \beta) \propto (\alpha\beta)^{-1}, \quad \alpha > 0,\ \beta > 0,$$

as the noninformative prior for (α, β). The joint posterior for the complete-data is then given by

$$f(\alpha, \beta|Y_{\text{obs}}, Z) \propto \beta^{n-1} \alpha^{-n\beta-1} \prod_{i=1}^{n} x_i^{\beta-1} \cdot e^{-(T/\alpha)^{\beta}}.$$

It is well known that given $N(t) = r$, the first r failure times $x_1, \ldots, x_r$ have the same distribution as the order statistics corresponding to r independent r.v.'s with pdf $\beta x^{\beta-1}/t^\beta$, $0 \le x \le t$. That is,

$$f(x_1, \ldots, x_r | N(t) = r) = r! \beta^r \prod_{i=1}^{r} (x_i^{\beta-1}/t^\beta).$$

Consequently, the conditional predictive density is

$$\begin{aligned} f(Z|Y_{\text{obs}}, \alpha, \beta) &= f(x_1, \ldots, x_{r-1}|x_r, \alpha, \beta) \\ &= (r-1)! \beta^{r-1} \prod_{i=1}^{r-1} (x_i^{\beta-1}/x_r^\beta). \end{aligned}$$

From (1.38), we have the following exact expression

$$f(\alpha, \beta|Y_{\text{obs}}) = \frac{(w_0\beta)^{n-r}\alpha^{-n\beta-1}}{\Gamma(n)\Gamma(n-r)} \left(x_r^{r-1} \prod_{i=r}^{n} x_i \right)^{\beta} \cdot e^{-(T/\alpha)^\beta},$$

where $w_0 \hat{=} \sum_{i=r+1}^{n} \ln(T/x_i) + r\ln(T/x_r)$. For purpose of sampling, we note that the conditional pdf is

$$f(\alpha|Y_{\text{obs}}, \beta) \propto f(\alpha, \beta|Y_{\text{obs}}) \propto \alpha^{-n\beta-1} e^{-(T/\alpha)^\beta}$$

and $f(\beta|Y_{\text{obs}}) = f(\alpha, \beta|Y_{\text{obs}})/f(\alpha|Y_{\text{obs}}, \beta)$, and hence we obtain

$$\alpha^\beta|(Y_{\text{obs}}, \beta) \sim \text{IGamma}(n, T^\beta), \quad \text{and} \tag{3.6}$$

$$\beta|Y_{\text{obs}} \sim \text{Gamma}(n-r, w_0). \tag{3.7}$$

This provides a conditional sampling method (cf. §2.2.5) to obtain i.i.d. posterior samples of α and β.

Example 3.2 (*Engine failure data*). A total of 40 failure times (in (0, 8063]) for some engine undergoing development testing was reported (Zhou & Weng, 1992, p.51–52) as follows: $*$, $*$, $*$, 171, 234, 274, 377, 530, 533, 941, 1074, 1188, 1248, 2298, 2347, 2347, 2381, 2456, 2456, 2500, 2913, 3022, 3038, 3728, 3873, 4724, 5147, 5179, 5587, 5626, 6824, 6983, 7106, 7106, 7568, 7568, 7593, 7642, 7928, 8063 hours. Here, the exact failure times for the first three failures are unknown and are denoted by $*$. Because these data are failure-truncated, we have $n = 40$, $T = x_{40} = 8063$ and $r = 4$. Yu *et al.* (2008a) showed that the data are coming from a Weibull process with 95% confidence level. They further obtained the MLEs $\hat{\alpha} = 0.0914$, $\hat{\beta} = 0.6761$, and a 95% CI of β given by $[0.4607, 0.8894]$.

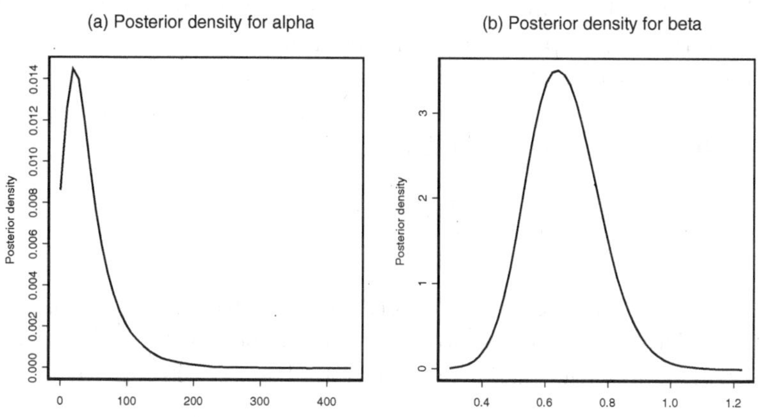

Figure 3.1 The posterior densities of α and β generated by the conditional sampling method with sample size 20,000 based on (3.6) and (3.7) for the engine failure data.

It is easy to obtain $w_0 = 54.73$. We generate 20,000 i.i.d. samples $\{\beta_j\}$ of β from (3.7), and the Bayes estimate of β is 0.6585. The 95% Bayes CI of β is then $[0.4609, 0.8922]$. Figure 3.1(b) shows that the posterior distribution of β is quite symmetric and can be approximated by a normal distribution. For a given β_j, we first generate

$$\gamma_j \sim \text{Gamma}(n, T^{\beta_j}),$$

then

$$\gamma_j^{-1} \sim \text{IGamma}(n, T^{\beta_j}).$$

By (3.6), we have

$$\alpha_j = (\gamma_j^{-1})^{1/\beta_j}.$$

Hence, $\{\alpha_j\}$ are i.i.d. posterior samples of α. Figure 3.1(a) shows that the posterior density of α is very skew. ‖

3.5 Prediction Problem with Missing Data

Prediction is the earliest form of statistical inference (e.g., Aitchison & Dunsmore, 1975; Geisser, 1993; West & Harrison, 1989). In this section, let $0 < x_{(1)} < \cdots < x_{(n)}$ denote the order statistics of nonnegative random variables from n i.i.d. samples from pdf $f(\cdot; \lambda)$ and continuous cdf $F(\cdot; \lambda)$, where λ is the parameter vector. Furthermore, we assume that only part of the data

$$0 < x_{(n_1)} < \cdots < x_{(n_k)}, \quad 1 \le n_1 < \cdots < n_k \le n, \quad 1 \le k \le n$$

are observed. The goal is to construct a prediction interval for the mean of a future sample, which is independent of the first sample and has the same pdf f. We denote this mean by $\bar{Y} = (1/m)\sum_{\ell=1}^{m} Y_\ell$. From a Bayesian point of view, the prediction interval of $\bar{Y}$ can be constructed via its prediction density:

$$f(\bar{Y}|\text{data}) = \int f(\bar{Y}|\lambda) \times f(\lambda|\text{data})\, d\lambda.$$

Since $f(\bar{Y}|\lambda)$ is relatively easy to get, it suffices to derive the posterior density $f(\lambda|\text{data})$, which is proportional to the product of the prior density $\pi(\lambda)$ and the likelihood function (David, 1981, p.10)

$$n! \prod_{j=1}^{k} f(x_{(n_j)}; \lambda) \times \prod_{j=0}^{k} \frac{\{F(x_{(n_{j+1})}; \lambda) - F(x_{(n_j)}; \lambda)\}^{n_{j+1}-n_j-1}}{(n_{j+1} - n_j - 1)!},$$

where $x_{(n_0)} = -\infty$, $x_{(n_{k+1})} = +\infty$, $n_0 = 0$, $n_{k+1} = n + 1$.

We can also derive $f(\lambda|\text{data})$ by the IBF. Without loss of generality, suppose $Y_{\text{obs}} = (x_{(1)}, \dots, x_{(r)}, x_{(s+1)}, \dots, x_{(n)})^\top$ denote the observed data and $Z = (x_{(r+1)}, \dots, x_{(s)})^\top$ consists of missing data, where $x_{(1)} < \cdots < x_{(r)} < x_{(r+1)} < \cdots < x_{(s)} < x_{(s+1)} < \cdots < x_{(n)}$. Further, if let

$$f(x; \lambda) = \text{Exponential}(x|\lambda) \quad \text{and} \quad \pi(\lambda) = \text{Gamma}(\lambda|\alpha_0, \beta_0),$$

then the likelihood is

$$n!\lambda^n \exp\left\{-\lambda \sum_{i=1}^{n} x_{(i)}\right\}$$

and

$$f(\lambda|Y_{\text{obs}}, Z) = \text{Gamma}\left(\lambda \,\middle|\, n + \alpha_0,\ \sum_{i=1}^{n} x_{(i)} + \beta_0\right).$$

On the other hand, given Y_{obs}, Z has the same distribution as the order statistics corresponding to $s - r$ independent random variables with pdf $f(\cdot; \lambda)/\{F(x_{(s+1)}; \lambda) - F(x_{(r)}; \lambda)\}$ (Lehmann, 1983, p.65), namely,

$$\begin{aligned} f(Z|Y_{\text{obs}}, \lambda) &= f(x_{(r+1)}, \dots, x_{(s)}|x_{(r)}, x_{(s+1)}, \lambda) \\ &= \frac{(s-r)!\lambda^{s-r} \exp\{-\lambda \sum_{i=r+1}^{s} x_{(i)}\}}{[\exp(-\lambda x_{(r)}) - \exp(-\lambda x_{(s+1)})]^{s-r}}. \end{aligned}$$

By the IBF (1.36), we obtain

$$f(\lambda|Y_{\text{obs}}) = c_{\text{P}}^{-1} \times \lambda^{N-1} e^{-\lambda X_+} \times \{e^{-\lambda x_{(r)}} - e^{-\lambda x_{(s+1)}}\}^{s-r},$$

where $N \hat{=} n + \alpha_0 + r - s$, $X_+ \hat{=} \sum_{i=1}^{r} x_{(i)} + \sum_{i=s+1}^{n} x_{(i)} + \beta_0$ and

$$c_{\text{P}} = \sum_{j=0}^{s-r} \binom{s-r}{j} (-1)^j \frac{\Gamma(N)}{\{X_+ + (s-r)x_{(r)} + j(x_{(s+1)} - x_{(r)})\}^N}.$$

Finally, it is easy to show that $\bar{Y}|\lambda \sim \text{Gamma}(m,\ m\lambda)$.

3.6 Binormal Model with Missing Data

A bivariate normal sample with missing values on both variables is a classical missing data problem (Wilks, 1932). However, a closed-form solution cannot be obtained by either the EM (Dempster *et al.*, 1977; McLachlan & Krishnan, 1997, p.45–49 & p.91–94), the DA (Tanner & Wong, 1987), or the Gibbs sampling (Gelfand & Smith, 1990, p.404–405). In this section, we obtain a closed-form solution to this problem by means of the IBF.

Table 3.3 *Data from a bivariate normal distribution*

Variate 1:	1	1	–1	–1	2	2	–2	–2	*	*	*	*
Variate 2:	1	–1	1	–1	*	*	*	*	2	2	–2	–2

Source: Murray (1977). The * denotes a missing value.

Motivated by the 12 observations in Table 3.3 (Murray, 1977), let $x_i = (x_{1i}, x_{2i})^\top$, $i = 1, \ldots, n$, be a random sample of size n from $N_2(\mu_0, \Sigma)$ with known mean μ_0 and unknown covariance matrix

$$\Sigma = \begin{pmatrix} \sigma_1^2 & \rho\sigma_1\sigma_2 \\ \rho\sigma_1\sigma_2 & \sigma_2^2 \end{pmatrix}.$$

Without loss of generality, let $\mu_0 = \mathbf{0}_2$. Denote the observed data and the missing data by

$$\begin{aligned} Y_{\text{obs}} &= \{x_i\}_{i=1}^{n_1} \cup \{x_{1i}\}_{i=n_1+1}^{n_1+n_2} \cup \{x_{2i}\}_{i=n_1+n_2+1}^{n} \quad \text{and} \\ Z &= \{x_{2i}\}_{i=n_1+1}^{n_1+n_2} \cup \{x_{1i}\}_{i=n_1+n_2+1}^{n}, \end{aligned}$$

respectively. A standard prior of Σ originated in Box & Tiao (1973, p.426) is given by

$$\pi(\Sigma) \propto |\Sigma|^{-(p+1)/2} = (\sigma_1\sigma_2\sqrt{1-\rho^2})^{-(p+1)} \tag{3.8}$$

where p denotes the dimension of the multivariate normal distribution (for the current case, $p = 2$). Hence, the complete-data posterior $f(\Sigma|Y_{\text{obs}}, Z)$ is proportional to

$$\frac{1}{(\sigma_1\sigma_2\sqrt{1-\rho^2})^{n+p+1}} \exp\left\{-\frac{\sigma_2^2 s_1^2(n) - 2\rho\sigma_1\sigma_2 s_{12}(n) + \sigma_1^2 s_2^2(n)}{2\sigma_1^2\sigma_2^2(1-\rho^2)}\right\},$$

where $s_k^2(n) \hat{=} \sum_{i=1}^n x_{ki}^2$, $k = 1, 2$, and $s_{12}(n) = \sum_{i=1}^n x_{1i}x_{2i}$. On the other hand, the conditional prediction distribution is

$$f(Z|Y_{\text{obs}}, \Sigma) = \prod_{i=n_1+1}^{n_1+n_2} \frac{1}{\sqrt{2\pi}\sigma_2\sqrt{1-\rho^2}} \exp\left\{-\frac{(x_{2i} - \rho\sigma_2 x_{1i}/\sigma_1)^2}{2\sigma_2^2(1-\rho^2)}\right\}$$

$$\times \prod_{i=n_1+n_2+1}^{n} \frac{1}{\sqrt{2\pi}\sigma_1\sqrt{1-\rho^2}} \exp\left\{-\frac{(x_{1i} - \rho\sigma_1 x_{2i}/\sigma_2)^2}{2\sigma_1^2(1-\rho^2)}\right\}.$$

By the point-wise IBF (1.36), we obtain

$$\begin{aligned} f(\Sigma|Y_{\text{obs}}) \quad \propto \quad & \frac{1}{\sigma_1^{n-n_3+1+p}\sigma_2^{n-n_2+1+p}(1-\rho^2)^{(n_1+1+p)/2}} \\ & \times \exp\left\{-\frac{\sigma_2^2 s_1^2(n_1) - 2\rho\sigma_1\sigma_2 s_{12}(n_1) + \sigma_1^2 s_2^2(n_1)}{2\sigma_1^2\sigma_2^2(1-\rho^2)}\right\} \\ & \times \exp\left\{-\frac{\sum_{i=n_1+1}^{n_1+n_2} x_{1i}^2}{2\sigma_1^2} - \frac{\sum_{i=n_1+n_2+1}^{n} x_{2i}^2}{2\sigma_2^2}\right\}. \end{aligned} \tag{3.9}$$

Substituting the data in Table 3.3 into (3.9), we obtain

$$\begin{aligned} f(\sigma_1^2, \sigma_2^2, \rho|Y_{\text{obs}}) \quad \propto \quad & (\sigma_1\sigma_2)^{-(9+p)}(1-\rho^2)^{-(5+p)/2} \\ & \times \exp\left\{-\frac{2\sigma_1^2 + 2\sigma_2^2}{\sigma_1^2\sigma_2^2(1-\rho^2)} - \frac{8}{\sigma_1^2} - \frac{8}{\sigma_2^2}\right\}. \end{aligned} \tag{3.10}$$

Integrating (3.10) with respect to σ_1^2 and σ_2^2, we obtain

$$f(\rho|Y_{\text{obs}}) \propto \frac{(1-\rho^2)^{4.5+0.5p}}{(1.25-\rho^2)^{7+p}}.$$

Let $p = 2$, we have

$$f(\rho|Y_{\text{obs}}) \propto \frac{(1-\rho^2)^{5.5}}{(1.25-\rho^2)^{9}},$$

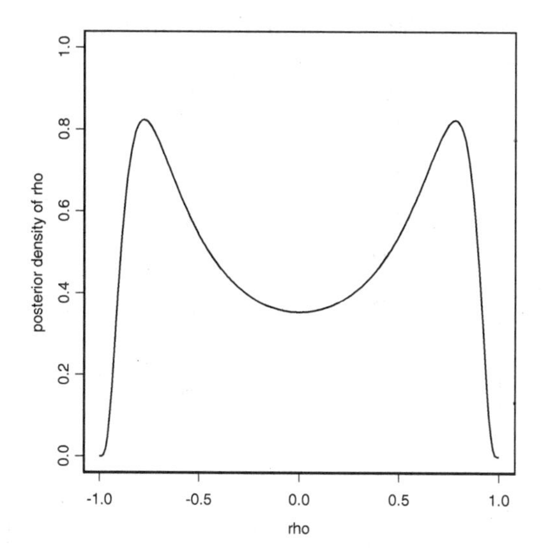

Figure 3.2 Posterior distribution of ρ defined in (3.11).

which is slightly different from the result in Tanner (1996, p.96). By numerical integration, the normalizing constant is

$$\int_{-1}^{1} \frac{(1-\rho^2)^{5.5}}{(1.25-\rho^2)^9}\, d\rho = 0.3798.$$

Thus, the posterior distribution of ρ is (see Figure 3.2)

$$f(\rho|Y_{\rm obs}) = \frac{(1-\rho^2)^{5.5}}{0.3798(1.25-\rho^2)^9}. \tag{3.11}$$

3.7 The 2 × 2 Crossover Trial with Missing Data

In a typical 2×2 crossover trial each subject receives two different treatments (e.g., a new drug A and a standard drug B). Half of the subjects receive A first and then, after a suitably chosen period of time,[1] receive (cross over to) B. The remaining subjects receive B first and then cross over to A. An example of such a trial is given by Maas *et al.* (1987). The data structure is listed in Table 3.4.

The standard random effects model for the 2×2 crossover trial is

$$y_{ijk} = \mu + (-1)^{j-1}\frac{\phi}{2} + (-1)^{k-1}\frac{\theta}{2} + \delta_i + \varepsilon_{ijk}, \tag{3.12}$$

[1]It means a wash-out period.

Table 3.4 *Data from a* 2×2 *crossover trial*

Subject	Sequence	Period 1	Period 2
1	AB	$*$	y_{112}
2	AB	y_{211}	y_{212}
3	AB	y_{311}	$*$
4	AB	y_{411}	y_{412}
5	AB	y_{511}	y_{512}
6	BA	y_{621}	$*$
7	BA	y_{721}	y_{722}
8	BA	y_{821}	y_{822}
9	BA	y_{921}	y_{922}
10	BA	$y_{10,21}$	$y_{10,22}$

NOTE: A and B are new and standard tablet formulations of Carbamazepine. The observations are logs of the maxima of concentration-time curves. The $*$ denotes a missing value.

where y_{ijk} is the response to the i-th subject ($i = 1, \dots, n$) receiving the j-th treatment ($j = 1, 2$, corresponding treatments A and B) in period k ($k = 1, 2$); μ is the grand mean; ϕ is the treatment effect; θ is the period effect; δ_i is the random effect of the i-th subject; ε_{ijk} is the random error. The δ_i and ε_{ijk} are assumed to be independent for all i, j, k with $\delta_i \sim N(0, \sigma_2^2)$ and $\varepsilon_{ijk} \sim N(0, \sigma_1^2)$.

The interest is to estimate all parameters. Using the Gibbs sampler, Gelfand *et al.* (1990) implemented a full Bayesian analysis of the data. Here we derive a closed-form solution using the IBF. Suppose that the first m subjects have observations missing at random from one of the two periods, and that the subjects $i = m+1, \dots, n$ have complete observations. Define

$$\mathbf{y}_i = \begin{pmatrix} z_i \\ v_i \end{pmatrix}, \quad X_i = \begin{pmatrix} x_{iu} \\ x_{iv} \end{pmatrix}, \quad i = 1, \dots, m,$$

where z_i is missing, v_i is the observed data, and X_i denotes the corresponding 2×3 design matrix. For subjects $i = m+1, \dots, n$, $\mathbf{y}_i$ denotes all the observed data. Hence, $Z = (z_1, \dots, z_m)^\top$ is missing and $Y_{\text{obs}} = (v_1, \dots, v_m, \mathbf{y}_{m+1}^\top, \dots, \mathbf{y}_n^\top)^\top$ is the observed data. The complete-data likelihood function is given by

$$L(\psi, \sigma_1^2, \sigma_3^2 | \mathbf{y}) = N_{2n}(\mathbf{y} | X\psi, S), \tag{3.13}$$

where

$$\begin{aligned}
\mathbf{y}_{2n\times 1} &= (\mathbf{y}_1^\top, \dots, \mathbf{y}_n^\top)^\top, \\
\psi &= (\mu, \phi, \theta)^\top, \\
\sigma_3^2 &= \sigma_1^2 + 2\sigma_2^2, \\
X_{2n\times 3} &= (X_1^\top, \dots, X_n^\top)^\top, \\
S_{2n\times 2n} &= \text{diag}(\Sigma, \Sigma, \dots, \Sigma), \\
\Sigma &= \begin{pmatrix} \sigma_1^2 + \sigma_2^2 & \sigma_2^2 \\ \sigma_2^2 & \sigma_1^2 + \sigma_2^2 \end{pmatrix},
\end{aligned}$$

and $|\Sigma| = \sigma_1^2 \times \sigma_3^2$.

When both σ_1^2 and σ_2^2 are known, the likelihood function $L(\psi|\mathbf{y})$ is given by (3.13). If the prior of ψ is $N_3(\eta_0, C_0)$, then the complete-data posterior is

$$f(\psi|Y_{\text{obs}}, Z) = N_3(\psi|D(X^\top S^{-1}\mathbf{y} + C_0^{-1}\eta_0),\ D), \tag{3.14}$$

where

$$\begin{aligned}
D &= (X^\top S^{-1} X + C_0^{-1})^{-1}, \\
X^\top S^{-1} X &= \sum_{i=1}^n X_i^\top \Sigma^{-1} X_i, \quad \text{and} \\
X^\top S^{-1} \mathbf{y} &= \sum_{i=1}^n X_i^\top \Sigma^{-1} \mathbf{y}_i.
\end{aligned}$$

Define

$$X_z = \begin{pmatrix} x_{1z} \\ \vdots \\ x_{mz} \end{pmatrix}, \quad X_v = \begin{pmatrix} x_{1v} \\ \vdots \\ x_{mv} \end{pmatrix}, \quad \text{and} \quad \mathbf{v} = \begin{pmatrix} v_1 \\ \vdots \\ v_m \end{pmatrix}.$$

Since $(z_i, v_i)^\top$ is distributed as bivariate normal with mean $X_i\psi$ and variance Σ for $i = 1, \dots, m$, we obtain

$$\begin{aligned}
f(Z|Y_{\text{obs}}, \psi) &= f(Z|\mathbf{v}, \psi) = \prod_{i=1}^m f(z_i|v_i, \psi) \qquad (3.15) \\
&= N_m\left(Z \middle| X_z\psi + \frac{\sigma_2^2}{\sigma_{12}^2}(\mathbf{v} - X_v\psi), \left(\sigma_{12}^2 - \frac{\sigma_2^4}{\sigma_{12}^2}\right) \mathbf{I}_m \right),
\end{aligned}$$

where $\sigma_{12}^2 = \sigma_1^2 + \sigma_2^2$. By the function-wise IBF (1.37), the posterior density of the parameter vector $\psi = (\mu, \phi, \theta)^\top$ is exactly given by

$$f(\psi|Y_{\text{obs}}) = N_3(\psi|\tau, P), \tag{3.16}$$

where

$$\begin{aligned}
\tau &= P(C_0^{-1}\eta_0 + \textstyle\sum_{i=m+1}^n X_i^\top \Sigma^{-1}\mathbf{y}_i + \sigma_{12}^{-2} X_v^\top \mathbf{v}), \quad \text{and} \\
P &= \left(D^{-1} - \frac{\sigma_{12}^2}{\sigma_{12}^4 - \sigma_2^4}\left(X_z - \frac{\sigma_2^2}{\sigma_{12}^2}X_v\right)^\top \left(X_z - \frac{\sigma_2^2}{\sigma_{12}^2}X_v\right)\right)^{-1}.
\end{aligned}$$

3.8 Hierarchical Models

Hierarchical models are widely used in practice for data analysis. In this section, for simplicity, we analyze a simple hierarchical model (Ex.3.3) by the IBF. Another example is presented in Problem 3.6. More complicated generalized linear mixed effects model can be implemented by the IBF sampling (see Chapter 5 or Tan, Tian & Ng, 2003, 2006; Tan, Tian & Fang, 2007). Consider a Bayesian hierarchical model with three stages: $f(Y_{\text{obs}}|\theta)$, $f(\theta|\alpha)$ and $f(\alpha)$, where Y_{obs} denotes the observed data, θ unknown parameter vector and α unknown hyperparameter. The joint density is

$$f(Y_{\text{obs}}, \theta, \alpha) = f(Y_{\text{obs}}|\theta) \times f(\theta|\alpha) \times f(\alpha).$$

The primary interest here is on the observed posterior $f(\theta|Y_{\text{obs}})$. Treating α as the missing data, the explicit expressions can be obtained by the IBF via the following two conditional distributions:

$$f(\alpha|Y_{\text{obs}}, \theta) \propto f(\theta|\alpha) \times f(\alpha), \tag{3.17}$$

$$f(\theta|Y_{\text{obs}}, \alpha) \propto f(Y_{\text{obs}}|\theta) \times f(\theta|\alpha). \tag{3.18}$$

Example 3.3 (*Normal means model*). Let $Y_{\text{obs}} = (y_1, \ldots, y_n)^\top$ and $\theta = (\theta_1, \ldots, \theta_n)^\top$. Suppose that

$$y_i|\theta_i \sim N(\theta_i, \sigma_{i0}^2)$$

with known variances σ_{i0}^2, $i = 1, \ldots, n$. The conjugate prior of $\theta_i|\alpha$ for $i = 1, \ldots, n$ are assumed to be i.i.d. $N(0, \alpha)$. Furthermore, we assume that α has a conjugate inverse gamma prior IGamma$(\frac{q_0}{2}, \frac{\lambda_0}{2})$ with known $q_0 > 0$ and $\lambda_0 \geq 0$. Now, we obtain

$$\begin{aligned}
f(Y_{\text{obs}}|\theta) &= \prod_{i=1}^n N(y_i|\theta_i, \sigma_{i0}^2), \\
f(\theta|\alpha) &= \prod_{i=1}^n N(\theta_i|0, \alpha), \\
f(\alpha) &= \text{IGamma}(\alpha|q_0/2, \lambda_0/2).
\end{aligned}$$

Formulae (3.17) and (3.18) yield

$$
\begin{aligned}
f(\alpha|Y_{\text{obs}}, \theta) &= \text{IGamma}\left(\alpha \left| \frac{n+q_0}{2}, \frac{\theta^\top\theta + \lambda_0}{2}\right.\right), \\
f(\theta|Y_{\text{obs}}, \alpha) &= \prod_{i=1}^{n} N\left(\theta_i \left| \frac{\alpha y_i}{\alpha + \sigma_{i0}^2}, \frac{\alpha\sigma_{i0}^2}{\alpha + \sigma_{i0}^2}\right.\right).
\end{aligned}
$$

Using (1.36), we obtain

$$
f(\theta|Y_{\text{obs}}) = c_{\text{N}}^{-1} \times \left(\frac{\theta^\top\theta + \lambda_0}{2}\right)^{-\frac{n+q_0}{2}} \exp\left\{-\sum_{i=1}^{n} \frac{(\theta_i - y_i)^2}{2\sigma_{i0}^2}\right\}, \quad (3.19)
$$

where the normalizing constant c_{N} only involves a one-dimensional integral, i.e.,

$$
c_{\text{N}} = \frac{(2\pi)^{\frac{n}{2}} \prod_{i=1}^{n} \sigma_{i0}}{\Gamma(\frac{n+q_0}{2})} \int_0^\infty \alpha^{-1-\frac{q_0}{2}} \frac{\exp\{-\frac{\lambda_0}{2\alpha} - \frac{1}{2}\sum_{i=1}^{n} \frac{y_i^2}{\alpha+\sigma_{i0}^2}\}}{\prod_{i=1}^{n}(\alpha + \sigma_{i0}^2)^{1/2}} \, d\alpha.
$$

Had (1.38) been used, we would have to encounter an n-fold integral. This shows the advantage of the point-wise IBF (1.36) where the conditional densities are used to reduce the dimensionality of the involved integral (cf. Ex.1.3). To generate i.i.d. samples from (3.19) is then relatively easy and is left to Problem 3.5. ||

3.9 Nonproduct Measurable Space (NPMS)

So far we have only dealt with PMS and have shown many statistical models involve only PMS. In §1.3.1, we especially distinguished the PMS from NPMS which is a difficult issue. We will present some theoretically interesting results in this section. This will also raise awareness of the problem of NPMS in practice.

In the case of PMS, we derived three IBF (1.3), (1.4) and (1.5). Following the identity (1.1), we now consider the case of NPMS, i.e., $\mathcal{S}_Y \neq \mathcal{S}_{(Y|X)}(x)$. For any given $x \in \mathcal{S}_X$, we have $y \in \mathcal{S}_{(Y|X)}(x)$ and

$$
\int_{\mathcal{S}_{(Y|X)}(x)} f_Y(y)dy \neq 1.
$$

Therefore, a counterpart of the point-wise IBF cannot be achieved. However, we can obtain a similar function-wise IBF and a similar sampling IBF. For an arbitrary $y_0 \in \mathcal{S}_Y$ and all $x \in \mathcal{S}_{(X|Y)}(y_0)$, we have

$$f_X^{y_0}(x) \propto \frac{f_{(X|Y)}(x|y_0)}{f_{(Y|X)}(y_0|x)}, \tag{3.20}$$

$$f_X^{y_0}(x) = \left\{ \int_{\mathcal{S}_{(X|Y)}(y_0)} \frac{f_{(X|Y)}(x|y_0)}{f_{(Y|X)}(y_0|x)} \, dx \right\}^{-1} \frac{f_{(X|Y)}(x|y_0)}{f_{(Y|X)}(y_0|x)}. \tag{3.21}$$

We call $f_X^{y_0}(x)$ specified by (3.20) or (3.21) a **transition marginal density** of X with transition point $y_0 \in \mathcal{S}_Y$. Note the arbitrariness of the transition point y_0, we may find a point, y^*, which may not belong to $\mathcal{S}_Y$, such that

$$\mathcal{S}_{(X|Y)}(y_0) = \mathcal{S}_{(X|Y)}(y^*) = \mathcal{S}_X \tag{3.22}$$

when $y_0 = y^*$ or $y_0 \to y^*$. Hence the marginal density $f_X(x) = f_X^{y^*}(x)$, $x \in \mathcal{S}_X$.

In multivariate distribution theory, we usually know the joint pdf and want to find the marginals and conditionals. It is quite easy to obtain the conditionals since the conditional pdf is proportional to the joint pdf, however, one must face an integration in order to obtain the marginals. The following Ex.3.4 shows that such integration can be avoided by using the IBF. Different from Ex.3.4, both Ex.3.5 and Problem 3.8 show that the joint pdf can be derived by IBF from two known conditionals.

Example 3.4 (*Uniform distribution on an ordered domain*). Let (X, Y) be uniformly distributed on

$$\mathcal{S}_{(X,Y)} = \{(x, y) \colon 0 < x < y < 1\},$$

as shown in Figure 3.3. Noting that $\mathcal{S}_{(X,Y)} \neq \mathcal{S}_X \times \mathcal{S}_Y = (0,1)^2$, $\mathcal{S}_{(Y|X)}(x) = (x, 1) \subset \mathcal{S}_Y$ and $\mathcal{S}_{(X|Y)}(y) = (0, y) \subset \mathcal{S}_X$, we have

$$\begin{aligned} X|(Y = y) &\sim U(0, y), \quad \text{and} \\ Y|(X = x) &\sim U(x, 1), \end{aligned}$$

where $U(a, b)$ denotes the uniform distribution on interval (a, b). It is easy to verify that

$$\begin{aligned} f_X(x) &= 2(1 - x), \quad 0 < x < 1, \quad \text{and} \\ f_Y(y) &= 2y, \qquad\quad\; 0 < y < 1. \end{aligned}$$

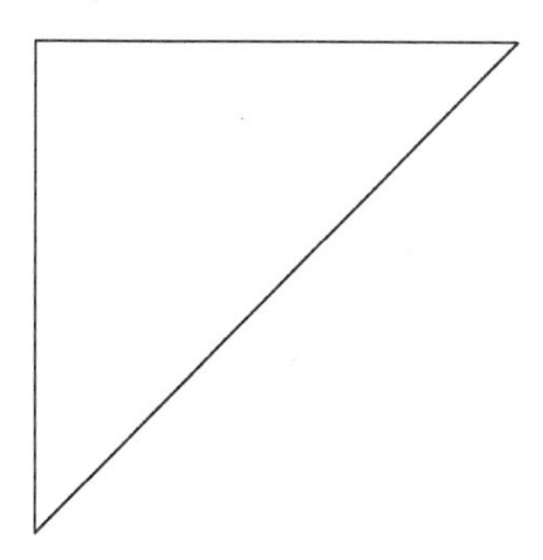

Figure 3.3 The joint support $\mathcal{S}_{(X,Y)} = \{(x, y)\colon\ 0 < x < y < 1\}$.

For some transition point $y_0 \in (0,1) = \mathcal{S}_Y$, from (3.21) we have

$$\frac{f_{(X|Y)}(x|y_0)}{f_{(Y|X)}(y_0|x)} = \frac{1-x}{y_0}, \quad 0 < x < y_0$$

and

$$\left\{\int_0^{y_0} \frac{f_{(X|Y)}(x|y_0)}{f_{(Y|X)}(y_0|x)}\,dx\right\}^{-1} = \frac{2}{2-y_0}.$$

Therefore, the transition marginal density of X with transition point $y_0 \in (0,1)$ is

$$f_X^{y_0}(x) = \frac{2(1-x)}{y_0(2-y_0)}, \quad 0 < x < y_0.$$

Set $y^* = 1$ ($y^* \notin \mathcal{S}_Y$). When $y_0 \to y^* = 1$, we have $f_X(x) = f_X^1(x) = 2(1-x)$, $x \in (0,1) = \mathcal{S}_X$. ‖

Example 3.5 (*Distribution in the unit ball*). Let $(X_1, \ldots, X_d)^\top$ be a random vector with support $\mathcal{S}_{(X_1,\ldots,X_d)} = \mathbb{B}_d$, where $\mathbb{B}_d \hat{=} \mathbb{B}_d(1)$ and $\mathbb{B}_d(r)$ denotes the d-dimensional ball with radius r defined in (2.66). Partition $(X_1, \ldots, X_d)^\top$ into two parts: $X = (X_1, \ldots, X_k)^\top$ and $Y = (X_{k+1}, \ldots, X_d)^\top$, $1 \le k < d$. The supports of X and Y are $\mathcal{S}_X = \mathbb{B}_k$ and $\mathcal{S}_Y = \mathbb{B}_{d-k}$, respectively. Let

$$\begin{aligned} X|(Y=y) &\sim U\Big(\mathbb{B}_k(\sqrt{1-y^\top y}\,)\Big), \\ Y|(X=x) &\sim U\Big(\mathbb{B}_{d-k}(\sqrt{1-x^\top x}\,)\Big). \end{aligned}$$

Our objective is to find the joint distribution of (X, Y). Note that $\mathcal{S}_{(X|Y)}(y) = \mathbb{B}_k(\sqrt{1-y^\top y})$ and $\mathcal{S}_{(Y|X)}(x) = \mathbb{B}_{d-k}(\sqrt{1-x^\top x})$, thus

$\mathcal{S}_{(X,Y)} \neq \mathcal{S}_X \times \mathcal{S}_Y$. For some arbitrary transition point $y_0 \in \mathbb{B}_{d-k} = \mathcal{S}_Y$, from (3.20), the transition marginal density of X is

$$f_X^{y_0}(x) \propto \frac{(1 - x^\top x)^{(d-k)/2}}{(1 - y_0^\top y_0)^{k/2}}, \quad x \in \mathcal{S}_{(X|Y)}(y_0).$$

Set $y^* = (0, \dots, 0)^\top$ ($y^* \in \mathcal{S}_Y$). When taking $y_0 = y^*$, the marginal pdf of X is

$$f_X(x) = f_X^{y^*}(x) \propto (1 - x^\top x)^{(d-k)/2}, \quad x \in \mathbb{B}_k = \mathcal{S}_X.$$

Therefore the joint distribution of (X, Y) is equal to

$$f_X(x) \cdot f_{(Y|X)}(y|x) \propto 1,$$

i.e., (X, Y) is uniformly distributed in the unit ball $\mathbb{B}_d$. ‖

Problems

3.1 Prove the identity (3.1) by using the property of Dirichlet multinomial distribution (cf. Appendix A.3.4).

3.2 Compare the true curve $f(\theta|Y_{\text{obs}})$ exactly given by (3.4) with the estimated curve by a kernel density smoother based on i.i.d. samples generated via the rejection method (cf. Ex.3.1).

3.3 Consider a more general missing pattern for the Weibull process presented in §3.4. Suppose that we only observed $Y_{\text{obs}} = \{x_{i_1}, \dots, x_{i_s}, t\}$ for the failure-truncated testing and the other failure times are missing.

(a) Derive the observed posterior $f(\alpha, \beta|Y_{\text{obs}})$ by using the IBF.

(b) Try to give a conditional sampling method similar to (3.6) and (3.7).

3.4 **Bivariate normal model with known covariance matrix** (Tian, 2000). Let $(u_{1i}, u_{2i})^\top$, $i = 1, \dots, n_1$, $(v_{1j}, v_{2j})^\top$, $j = 1, \dots, n_2$, and $(w_{1k}, w_{2k})^\top$, $k = 1, \dots, n_3$ be i.i.d. from a common bivariate normal $N_2(\theta, \Delta)$ with $\theta = (\theta_1, \theta_2)^\top \sim N_2(\mu, \Sigma)$, where θ is not observable but Δ, $\mu = (\mu_1, \mu_2)^\top$, and Σ are assumed to be known. Define

$$\begin{aligned} u &= \begin{pmatrix} u_1 \\ u_2 \end{pmatrix} = \begin{pmatrix} u_{11}, \ldots, u_{1n_1} \\ u_{21}, \ldots, u_{2n_1} \end{pmatrix}, \\ \bar{u} &= \begin{pmatrix} \bar{u}_1 \\ \bar{u}_2 \end{pmatrix} = \frac{1}{n_1} u \mathbf{1}_{n_1} = \begin{pmatrix} u_1 \mathbf{1}_{n_1}/n_1 \\ u_2 \mathbf{1}_{n_1}/n_1 \end{pmatrix}, \end{aligned}$$

with similar notations for v and w. Let $y = (w_2, u_1, u_2, v_1)^\top$ be the known data and $z = (v_2, w_1)^\top$ be unobserved so that $x_{2\times n} = (u, v, w) = \{y, z\}$, where $n = \sum_{\ell=1}^{3} n_\ell$. Prove that

(a) $f(\theta|\bar{y}, \bar{z}) = N_2(\theta|\eta, \Omega)$, where $\bar{y} = (\bar{w}_2, \bar{u}_1, \bar{u}_2, \bar{v}_1)^\top$, $\bar{z} = (\bar{v}_2, \bar{w}_1)^\top$, $\bar{x} = x\mathbf{1}_n/n$, $\Omega = (n\Delta^{-1} + \Sigma^{-1})^{-1}$, and $\eta = \Omega(n\Delta^{-1}\bar{x} + \Sigma^{-1}\mu)$.

(b) The conditional pdf of $\bar{z}|(\bar{y}, \theta)$ is

$$N_2\left(\begin{pmatrix} \theta_2 + \Delta_{21}\Delta_{11}^{-1}(\bar{v}_1 - \theta_1) \\ \theta_1 + \Delta_{12}\Delta_{22}^{-1}(\bar{w}_2 - \theta_2) \end{pmatrix}, \begin{pmatrix} \frac{\Delta_{22\cdot 1}}{n_2} & 0 \\ 0 & \frac{\Delta_{11\cdot 2}}{n_3} \end{pmatrix} \right),$$

where $\Delta_{11\cdot 2} = \Delta_{11} - \Delta_{12}\Delta_{22}^{-1}\Delta_{21}$,

$$\Delta_{22\cdot 1} = \Delta_{22} - \Delta_{21}\Delta_{11}^{-1}\Delta_{12}, \quad \Delta = \begin{pmatrix} \Delta_{11} & \Delta_{12} \\ \Delta_{21} & \Delta_{22} \end{pmatrix}.$$

(c) $f(\theta|y) = N_2(\theta|\delta, Q)$, where

$$Q = \left(\Omega^{-1} - (n_2 + n_3)\Delta^{-1} + \begin{pmatrix} n_2\Delta_{11}^{-1} & 0 \\ 0 & n_3\Delta_{22}^{-1} \end{pmatrix} \right)^{-1},$$

$$\delta = Q\left\{ \Delta^{-1} \begin{pmatrix} n_1\bar{u}_1 + n_2\bar{v}_1 + \Delta_{12}\Delta_{22}^{-1} \cdot n_3\bar{w}_2 \\ n_1\bar{u}_2 + \Delta_{21}\Delta_{11}^{-1} \cdot n_2\bar{v}_1 + n_3\bar{w}_2 \end{pmatrix} + \Sigma^{-1}\mu \right\}.$$

3.5 Generate i.i.d. samples from (3.19) by the rejection method with (a) the multivariate normal distribution with mean vector $(y_1, \ldots, y_n)^\top$ and covariance matrix $\text{diag}(\sigma_{10}^2, \ldots, \sigma_{n0}^2)$, and (b) the multivariate t-distribution $t_n(0, \lambda_0\mathbf{I}_n, q_0)$ as the envelope function.

3.6 **Hierarchical Poisson model.** Let $y_i|\theta_i \overset{\text{ind}}{\sim} \text{Poisson}(\theta_i t_i)$, where $\{t_i\}$ are known constants, $i = 1, \ldots, n$. Let $\theta_i|\alpha \overset{\text{iid}}{\sim}$

Gamma(β_0, α^{-1}) with known β_0, and $\alpha \sim$ IGamma(q_0, λ_0) with known $q_0 > 0$ and $\lambda_0 \geq 0$. Prove that

$$\begin{aligned} f(\alpha|Y_{\rm obs}, \theta) &= \text{IGamma}(\alpha|n\beta_0 + q_0, \textstyle\sum_{i=1}^n \theta_i + \lambda_0), \\ f(\theta|Y_{\rm obs}, \alpha) &= \textstyle\prod_{i=1}^n \text{Gamma}(\theta_i|y_i + \beta_0, t_i + \alpha^{-1}), \\ f(\theta|Y_{\rm obs}) &= \frac{1}{c_{\rm P}(\sum_{i=1}^n \theta_i + \lambda_0)^{n\beta_0+q_0}} \prod_{i=1}^n \frac{\theta_i^{y_i+\beta_0-1} e^{-\theta_i t_i}}{\Gamma(y_i + \beta_0)}, \end{aligned}$$

where

$$c_{\rm P} = \frac{1}{\Gamma(n\beta_0 + q_0)} \int_0^\infty \frac{e^{-\lambda_0/\alpha}}{\alpha^{1+n\beta_0+q_0}} \prod_{i=1}^n (t_i + 1/\alpha)^{-y_i-\beta_0} \, d\alpha.$$

3.7 Finite-mixture models. Using the EM algorithm, McLachlan & Krishnan (1997) discussed the estimation of the proportions and parameters in finite-mixture models. By using the Gibbs sampler, Gelman & King (1990), Smith & Roberts (1993), Diebolt & Robert (1994), Chib (1995), Escobar & West (1995) and Robert (1996) considered the same problem. Suppose the underlying population consists of d distinct subpopulations with unknown proportions $\theta_1, \ldots, \theta_d$ such that $0 \leq \theta_i \leq 1$, $\sum_{i=1}^d \theta_i = 1$, and its pdf is $f(x;\theta) = \sum_{i=1}^d \theta_i f_i(x)$, x: $m \times 1$, where $\theta = (\theta_1, \ldots, \theta_{d-1})^\top$. Let $\{y_j\}_{j=1}^n \stackrel{\rm iid}{\sim} f(x;\theta)$ and $y = (y_1^\top, \ldots, y_n^\top)^\top$ denote the observed data. In Table 3.5, we introduce an nd-dimensional latent vector $z = (z_1^\top, \ldots, z_n^\top)^\top$ with $z_j = (z_{1j}, \ldots, z_{dj})^\top$ and for $1 \leq i \leq d$, $1 \leq j \leq n$, $z_{ij} = 1$ if y_j draws from the i-th component and $= 0$ otherwise. If the prior $f(\theta) =$ Dirichlet$(\theta|\alpha_1, \ldots, \alpha_d)$, verify the following facts:

(a) The complete-data posterior is $f(\theta|y, z) =$ Dirichlet$(\theta|\alpha_1 + n_1, \ldots, \alpha_d + n_d)$, where $n_i = \sum_{j=1}^n z_{ij}$ represents the number of $\{y_j\}_{j=1}^n$ drawing from the i-th component. (*Hint*: $z_{ij} \sim$ Binomial$(1, \theta_i f_i(y_j))$, and the complete-data likelihood is $n!\Pi_{i=1}^d \Pi_{j=1}^n (\theta_i f_i(y_j))^{z_{ij}}/z_{ij}!$.)

(b) The conditional prediction distribution is

$$f(z|y, \theta) = \left\{ \prod_{j=1}^n f^{-1}(y_j; \theta) \right\} \cdot \prod_{i=1}^d \left\{ \theta_i^{n_i} \prod_{j=1}^n \frac{(f_i(y_j))^{z_{ij}}}{z_{ij}!} \right\}.$$

(*Hint*: $z_{ij}|(y_j, \theta) \sim$ Binomial$(1, \frac{\theta_i f_i(y_j)}{f(y_j;\theta)})$ and $\sum_{i=1}^d z_{ij} = 1$.)

(c) The observed posterior is

$$f(\theta|y) = c_{\mathrm{F}}^{-1} \cdot \Gamma(\alpha_+ + n)\theta_1^{\alpha_1 - 1} \cdots \theta_d^{\alpha_d - 1} \prod_{j=1}^{n} f(y_j; \theta),$$

where $\alpha_+ \hat{=} \sum_{i=1}^d \alpha_i$,

$$c_{\mathrm{F}} = \sum_{z_1} \cdots \sum_{z_n} \left\{ \prod_{i=1}^{d} \Gamma(\alpha_i + n_i) \right\} \prod_{i=1}^{d} \prod_{j=1}^{n} \frac{(f_i(y_j))^{z_{ij}}}{z_{ij}!},$$

and $\sum_{z_1}$ denotes the summation over all values of $z_{11}, \ldots, z_{d1}$ such that $z_{11} + \cdots + z_{d1} = 1$.

Table 3.5 *Latent variables array*

	1	$\cdots$	n	Freq.	MP	CD
1	z_{11}	$\cdots$	z_{1n}	$\Sigma_j z_{1j} = n_1$	θ_1	f_1
$\vdots$	$\vdots$	$\vdots$	$\vdots$	$\vdots$	$\vdots$	$\vdots$
i	z_{i1}	$\cdots$	z_{in}	$\Sigma_j z_{ij} = n_i$	θ_i	f_i
$\vdots$	$\vdots$	$\vdots$	$\vdots$	$\vdots$	$\vdots$	$\vdots$
d	z_{d1}	$\cdots$	z_{dn}	$\Sigma_j z_{dj} = n_d$	θ_d	f_d
Freq.	$\Sigma_i z_{i1} = 1$	$\cdots$	$\Sigma_i z_{in} = 1$	$\Sigma_i n_i = n$		
Marg. Prob.	$f(y_1;\theta)$	$\cdots$	$f(y_n;\theta)$		1	
Obs. Data	y_1	$\cdots$	y_n			
Mis. Data	z_1	$\cdots$	z_n			

MP: marginal probability. CD: component density.

3.8 Distribution in the unit ℓ_1-ball (Tian & Tan, 2003). Let $(X_1, \ldots, X_d)^\top$ be a random vector with support $\mathcal{S}_{(X_1,\ldots,X_d)} = \mathbb{V}_d$, where $\mathbb{V}_d \hat{=} \mathbb{V}_d(1)$ and $\mathbb{V}_d(r)$ denotes the d-dimensional ℓ_1-ball defined in (2.96). Partition it into two parts: $X = (X_1, \ldots, X_k)^\top$ and $Y = (X_{k+1}, \ldots, X_d)^\top$, $1 \le k < d$. The supports of X and Y are $\mathcal{S}_X = \mathbb{V}_k$ and $\mathcal{S}_Y = \mathbb{V}_{d-k}$. Let

$$X|(Y = y) \sim U\Big(\mathbb{V}_k(\sqrt{1 - \mathbf{1}_{n-k}^\top y}\,)\Big),$$
$$Y|(X = x) \sim U\Big(\mathbb{V}_{d-k}(\sqrt{1 - \mathbf{1}_k^\top x}\,)\Big).$$

Prove that

(a) For some arbitrary transition point $y_0 \in \mathbb{V}_{d-k}$, the transition marginal density of X is

$$f_X^{y_0}(x) \propto \frac{(1 - \mathbf{1}_k^\top x)^{(d-k)/2}}{(1 - \mathbf{1}_{d-k}^\top y_0)^{k/2}}, \quad x \in \mathcal{S}_{(X|Y)}(y_0).$$

(b) The marginal pdf of X is proportional to $(1 - \mathbf{1}_k^\top x)^{(d-k)/2}$.

(c) $(X, Y)^\top \sim U(\mathbb{V}_d)$.

CHAPTER 4

Discrete Missing Data Problems

Many statistical problems can be formulated as discrete *missing data problems* (MDPs), e.g., Dawid & Skene (1979) may be the first to apply the EM algorithm to find MLEs of observed error rates in the absence of a golden/well-accepted standard by treating the disease status as the missing data. Other examples include change-point problems (Carlin *et al.*, 1992; Pievatolo & Rotondi, 2000), capture and recapture models (George & Robert, 1992; Robert & Casella, 1999, p.307), finite mixture models (McLachlan, 1997), normal mixture model with left censoring (Lyles *et al.*, 2001), sample survey with nonresponse (Albert & Gupta, 1985; Chiu & Sedransk, 1986), crime survey (Kadane, 1985), misclassified multinomial models (Tian *et al.*, 2003), inference from nonrandomly missing categorical data (Nordheim, 1984), zero-inflated Poisson models (Lambert, 1992; Rodrigues, 2003), medical screening/diagnostic tests (Johnson & Gastwirth, 1991; Joseph *et al.*, 1995; Zhou *et al.*, 2002) and bioassay (Qu *et al.*, 1996).

In this chapter, we focus on discrete MDPs where the latent variable (or missing data) is a discrete random variable/vector. In §4.1, we introduce a noniterative sampling procedure, called exact IBF sampling, to obtain i.i.d. samples exactly from the observed posterior distribution for discrete MDPs (Tian, Tan & Ng, 2007). The exact IBF sampling is essentially a conditional sampling, thus completely avoiding convergence and slow convergence problems in iterative algorithms such as MCMC. Different from the general IBF sampler of Tan, Tian & Ng (2003), the implementation of this algorithm does not involve the EM nor the SIR methods. The key idea is to first utilize the sampling IBF to derive the conditional distribution of the missing data given the observed data, and then to draw i.i.d. samples from the complete-data posterior distribution. In §4.2–§4.8, we illustrate the noniterative algorithm with the genetic linkage model, contingency tables with one/two supplemental margin(s), the hidden sensitivity model for surveys with two sensitive questions, a zero-inflated Poisson model, changepoint problems, a capture-recapture model and several related real datasets.

4.1 The Exact IBF Sampling

Let $Y_{\rm obs}$ denote the observed data, Z the missing or latent data and θ the parameter vector of interest. Consider a DA structure with complete-data posterior distribution $f(\theta|Y_{\rm obs}, Z)$ and conditional predictive distribution $f(Z|Y_{\rm obs}, \theta)$. The goal is to obtain i.i.d. samples from the observed posterior distribution $f(\theta|Y_{\rm obs})$.

The conditional sampling method (cf. §2.2.5) states that: If we could obtain independent samples $\{Z^{(\ell)}\}_{\ell=1}^L$ from $f(Z|Y_{\rm obs})$ and generate $\theta^{(\ell)} \sim f(\theta|Y_{\rm obs}, Z^{(\ell)})$ for $\ell = 1, \dots, L$, then $\{\theta^{(\ell)}\}_1^L$ are i.i.d. samples from $f(\theta|Y_{\rm obs})$. Therefore, the key is to be able to generate independent samples from $f(Z|Y_{\rm obs})$.

Let $\mathcal{S}_{(\theta|Y_{\rm obs})}$ and $\mathcal{S}_{(Z|Y_{\rm obs})}$ denote conditional supports of $\theta|Y_{\rm obs}$ and $Z|Y_{\rm obs}$, respectively. By exchanging the role of θ and Z, the sampling IBF (1.37) becomes

$$f(Z|Y_{\rm obs}) \propto \frac{f(Z|Y_{\rm obs}, \theta_0)}{f(\theta_0|Y_{\rm obs}, Z)}, \tag{4.1}$$

for an arbitrary $\theta_0 \in \mathcal{S}_{(\theta|Y_{\rm obs})}$ and all $Z \in \mathcal{S}_{(Z|Y_{\rm obs})}$. When Z is a discrete r.v. or random vector taking finite values on the domain, without loss of generality, we denote the conditional support of $Z|(Y_{\rm obs}, \theta)$ by

$$\mathcal{S}_{(Z|Y_{\rm obs}, \theta)} = \{z_1, \dots, z_K\}.^{1}$$

Since the $f(Z|Y_{\rm obs}, \theta)$ is available, first, we can directly identify $\{z_k\}_1^K$ from the model specification and thus all $\{z_k\}_1^K$ are known. Second, we assume that $\{z_k\}_1^K$ does not depend on the value of θ, therefore we have

$$\mathcal{S}_{(Z|Y_{\rm obs})} = \mathcal{S}_{(Z|Y_{\rm obs}, \theta)} = \{z_1, \dots, z_K\}.$$

Because of the discreteness of Z, the notation $f(z_k|Y_{\rm obs})$ will be used to denote the pmf, i.e., $f(z_k|Y_{\rm obs}) = \Pr\{Z = z_k|Y_{\rm obs}\}$. Therefore, the key is to find $p_k = f(z_k|Y_{\rm obs})$ for $k = 1, \dots, K$. For some $\theta_0 \in \mathcal{S}_{(\theta|Y_{\rm obs})}$, let

$$q_k = q_k(\theta_0) = \frac{\Pr\{Z = z_k|Y_{\rm obs}, \theta_0\}}{f(\theta_0|Y_{\rm obs}, z_k)}, \quad k = 1, \dots, K. \tag{4.2}$$

As both $f(Z|Y_{\rm obs}, \theta)$ and $f(\theta|Y_{\rm obs}, Z)$ are available, the computation of (4.2) is straightforward. Observing that all $\{q_k\}_{k=1}^K$ depend on

[1]In §4.8, we will discuss the case that Z is a discrete, but not finite (e.g., a Poisson or negative binomial) random variable.

θ_0, we then denote q_k by $q_k(\theta_0)$ to emphasize its dependency on θ_0. From the sampling IBF (4.1), we immediately obtain

$$p_k = \frac{q_k(\theta_0)}{\sum_{k'=1}^K q_{k'}(\theta_0)}, \quad k = 1, \dots, K, \tag{4.3}$$

where $\{p_k\}_1^K$ do not depend on θ_0. Thus, it is easy to draw from $f(Z|Y_{\text{obs}})$ since it is a discrete distribution with probability p_k on z_k for $k = 1, \dots, K$ (cf. Appendix A.1.1). The sampling procedure is summarized as follows.

THE EXACT IBF SAMPLING:

Given both the complete-data posterior distribution $f(\theta|Y_{\text{obs}}, Z)$ and the conditional predictive distribution $f(Z|Y_{\text{obs}}, \theta)$,

Step 1. Identify $\mathcal{S}_{(Z|Y_{\text{obs}})} = \{z_1, \dots, z_K\}$ from $f(Z|Y_{\text{obs}}, \theta)$ and calculate $\{p_k\}_1^K$ according to (4.3) and (4.2);

Step 2. Generate i.i.d. samples $\{Z^{(\ell)}\}_{\ell=1}^L$ of Z from the probability mass fuunction $f(Z|Y_{\text{obs}})$ with probabilities $\{p_k\}_1^K$ on $\{z_k\}_1^K$;

Step 3. Generate $\theta^{(\ell)} \sim f(\theta|Y_{\text{obs}}, Z^{(\ell)})$ for $\ell = 1, \dots, L$, then $\{\theta^{(\ell)}\}_1^L$ are i.i.d. samples from the observed posterior distribution $f(\theta|Y_{\text{obs}})$.

4.2 Genetic Linkage Model

To illustrate the exact IBF sampler, we consider the following small sample data set for the genetic linkage model (see §3.3): $Y_{\text{obs}} = (y_1, y_2, y_3, y_4)^\top = (14, 0, 1, 5)^\top$. From (3.2), obviously Z is discrete and takes values on

$$\mathcal{S}_{(Z|Y_{\text{obs}}, \theta)} = \mathcal{S}_{(Z|Y_{\text{obs}})} = \{0, 1, \dots, y_1\}.$$

Let $a = b = 1$ (i.e., the uniform prior) and $\theta_0 = 0.5$, then $q_k(\theta_0)$ and p_k can be calculated according to (4.2) and (4.3). These results are listed in Table 4.1.

If we choose $\theta_0 = 0.8$, then $\{q_k(\theta_0)\}_{k=1}^K$ will vary but $\{p_k\}_{k=1}^K$ remains the same. Hence, the exact IBF sampling is as follows: (i) Draw $L = 30{,}000$ independent samples $\{Z^{(\ell)}\}_1^L$ of Z from the discrete distribution $f(Z|Y_{\text{obs}})$ with $p_k = \Pr\{Z = z_k|Y_{\text{obs}}\}$ given in Table 4.1; (ii) Generate $\theta^{(\ell)} \sim f(\theta|Y_{\text{obs}}, Z^{(\ell)})$ defined in (3.3) for $\ell = 1, \dots, L$,

Table 4.1 *The values of* $\{q_k(\theta_0)\}$ *with* $\theta_0 = 0.5$ *and* $\{p_k\}$

k	z_k	$q_k(\theta_0)$	p_k	k	z_k	q_k	p_k
1	0	0.0670	0.0094	9	8	1.572×10^{-1}	2.200×10^{-2}
2	1	0.3518	0.0493	10	9	4.580×10^{-2}	6.400×10^{-3}
3	2	0.8894	0.1245	11	10	1.012×10^{-2}	1.416×10^{-3}
4	3	1.4230	0.1992	12	11	1.635×10^{-3}	2.289×10^{-4}
5	4	1.6010	0.2241	13	12	1.829×10^{-4}	2.560×10^{-5}
6	5	1.3340	0.1868	14	13	1.266×10^{-5}	1.772×10^{-6}
7	6	0.8466	0.1185	15	14	4.090×10^{-7}	5.727×10^{-8}
8	7	0.4147	0.0581				

Source: Tian, Tan & Ng (2007).

then $\{\theta^{(\ell)}\}_1^L$ are i.i.d. samples from the observed posterior distribution $f(\theta|Y_{\text{obs}})$.

The accuracy of the exact IBF sampling is shown in Figure 4.1(a), where the hardly visible dotted curve is estimated by a kernel density smoother based on the i.i.d. IBF samples and the solid line is exactly given by (3.4). In addition, the histogram based on these samples is plotted in Figure 4.1(b), which shows that the exact IBF sampling has recovered the density completely as expected.

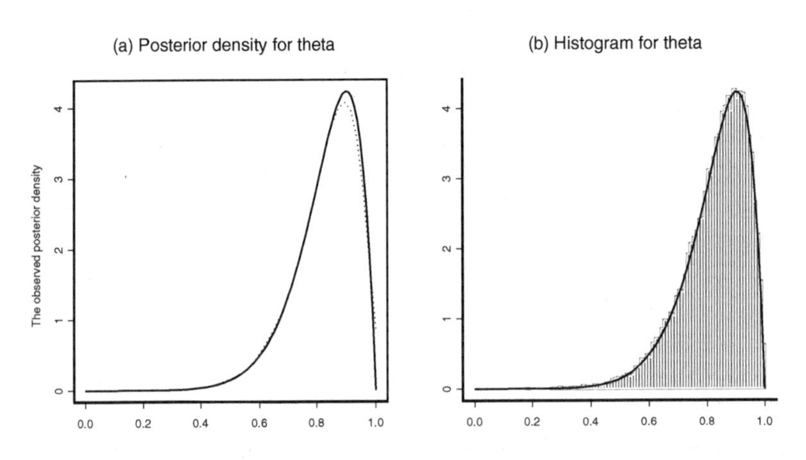

Figure 4.1 (a) The comparison between the observed posterior density of θ (solid curve) exactly given by (3.4) with the dotted curve estimated by a kernel density smoother based on $L = 30{,}000$ i.i.d. samples generated via the exact IBF sampling. (b) The histogram of θ based on $L = 30{,}000$ i.i.d. samples generated via the exact IBF sampling.

4.3 Contingency Tables with One Supplemental Margin

Strauss *et al.* (2001) reported an HIV study which examines the relationship between self-reported HIV status and history of exchanging sex for drugs and money. All participants were drug-dependent women offenders mandated to treatment through the criminal justice system of New York City. The data were collected as part of an evaluation study of prison-based, jailed-based, community-based residential and community-based outpatient drug treatment programs. The data reflect baseline responses from 325 clients interviewed at the four treatment programs from May, 1995 to December, 1996. Table 4.2 gives the cross-classification of history of sex exchange (no or yes, denoted by $X = 0$ or $X = 1$) and HIV status (negative or positive, denoted by $Y = 0$ or $Y = 1$) as reported by the women. Generally, a sizable proportion of the data would be missing (i.e., a quarter in this example) in AIDS studies that measure HIV status from self-report or biological data. For this example, it is assumed to be MAR, which allows missingness in HIV status to depend on the observed sex exchange history (Rubin, 1976; Little & Rubin, 2002, p.12). The objective was to examine if HIV status is associated with exchanging sex for drugs and money.

Let $Y_{\text{obs}} = \{(n_1, \dots, n_4); (n_{12}, n_{34})\}$ denote the observed frequencies, $\theta = (\theta_1, \dots, \theta_4)^\top \in \mathbb{T}_4$ the cell probability vector and $\psi = \theta_1\theta_4/(\theta_2\theta_3)$ the odds ratio. Under the assumption of MAR, the observed-data likelihood function of θ is given by[2]

$$L(\theta|Y_{\text{obs}}) \propto \left(\prod_{i=1}^{4} \theta_i^{n_i}\right) \times (\theta_1 + \theta_2)^{n_{12}} (\theta_3 + \theta_4)^{n_{34}}. \tag{4.4}$$

By writing $n_{12} = Z_1 + Z_2$ with $Z_2 \hat{=} n_{12} - Z_1$ and $n_{34} = Z_3 + Z_4$ with $Z_4 \hat{=} n_{34} - Z_3$, a natural latent vector $Z = (Z_1, Z_3)^\top$ can be introduced so that the likelihood function for the complete-data $\{Y_{\text{obs}}, Z\}$ is proportional to

$$\prod_{i=1}^{4} \theta_i^{n_i + Z_i}.$$

[2]Note that (4.4) has the same functional form as a GDD (cf. Problem 4.1). If the conjugate prior (4.11) is chosen, then the posterior of θ is a GDD. The SR (4.43) provides a straightforward procedure for generating i.i.d. samples from a GDD. Therefore, the data augmentation for this example is not necessary (see Problem 4.2).

Table 4.2 *Human immunodeficiency virus (HIV) data*

Sex exchange	$Y=0$ (HIV$-$)	$Y=1$ (HIV$+$)	Supplement on X
$X=0$ (no)	$108\,(n_1,\ \theta_1)$	$18\ (n_2,\ \theta_2)$	$44\ (n_{12},\ \theta_1+\theta_2)$
$X=1$ (yes)	$93\ (n_3,\ \theta_3)$	$23\ (n_4,\ \theta_4)$	$39\ (n_{34},\ \theta_3+\theta_4)$

NOTE: X denotes women's history of sex exchange and Y denotes woman's HIV status, "supplement on X" means that women only reported their history of sex exchange but didn't report their HIV status. The observed frequencies and the corresponding probabilities are in parentheses.

The prior for θ is assumed to be of the Dirichlet$(\alpha_1, \dots, \alpha_4)$, a conjugate prior for θ. Thus, the complete-data posterior is

$$\theta|(Y_{\text{obs}}, Z) \sim \text{Dirichlet}(n_1 + Z_1 + \alpha_1, \dots, n_4 + Z_4 + \alpha_4). \qquad (4.5)$$

Note that given Y_{obs} and θ, Z_1 and Z_3 are independent binomially distributed. Thus, the conditional predictive distribution is

$$\begin{aligned} f(Z|Y_{\text{obs}}, \theta) &= \text{Binomial}(Z_1|n_{12},\ \theta_1/(\theta_1+\theta_2)) \\ &\quad \times \text{Binomial}(Z_3|n_{34},\ \theta_3/(\theta_3+\theta_4)). \end{aligned} \qquad (4.6)$$

To apply the exact IBF sampling, we first need to identify the conditional support of $Z|(Y_{\text{obs}}, \theta)$. From (4.6), we have

$$\begin{aligned} \mathcal{S}_{(Z|Y_{\text{obs}})} &= \mathcal{S}_{(Z|Y_{\text{obs}},\theta)} = \{z_1, \dots, z_K\} \\ &= \left\{ \begin{array}{cccc} (0,0) & (0,1) & \cdots & (0, n_{34}) \\ (1,0) & (1,1) & \cdots & (1, n_{34}) \\ \vdots & \vdots & \ddots & \vdots \\ (n_{12},0) & (n_{12},1) & \cdots & (n_{12}, n_{34}) \end{array} \right\}, \end{aligned}$$

where $K = (n_{12}+1)(n_{34}+1)$. We then calculate $\{p_k\}_{k=1}^K$ according to (4.3) and (4.2) with $\theta_0 = (0.25, \dots, 0.25)^\top$. Third, we draw $L =$ 100,000 i.i.d. samples $\{Z^{(\ell)}\}_{\ell=1}^L$ of Z from the pmf $f(Z|Y_{\text{obs}})$ with probabilities $\{p_k\}_1^K$ on $\{z_k\}_1^K$. Finally, we draw $\theta^{(\ell)} \sim f(\theta|Y_{\text{obs}}, Z^{(\ell)})$ via (4.5) for $\ell = 1, \dots, L$, then $\{\theta^{(\ell)}\}_1^L$ are i.i.d. samples from the observed posterior distribution $f(\theta|Y_{\text{obs}})$.

For the HIV data, we adopt the uniform prior, i.e., $\alpha_1 = \cdots = \alpha_4 = 1$. The Bayes estimates of θ and the odds ratio ψ are given in Table 4.3. Since the Bayes CIs include the value of 1, there is no association between sex exchange and HIV status.

Table 4.3 *Bayesian estimates of parameters for the HIV data*

Parameters	Bayesian mean	Bayesian std	95% Bayesian CI
θ_1	0.4453	0.0286	[0.3893, 0.5012]
θ_2	0.0776	0.0168	[0.0478, 0.1136]
θ_3	0.3800	0.0281	[0.3253, 0.4360]
θ_4	0.0969	0.0185	[0.0636, 0.1361]
$\psi = \frac{\theta_1\theta_2}{\theta_3\theta_4}$	1.5610	0.5549	[0.7593, 2.8959]

Source: Tian, Tan & Ng (2007).

4.4 Contingency Tables with Two Supplemental Margins

4.4.1 Neurological complication data

Choi & Stablein (1982) reported a neurological study in which 33 young meningitis patients at the St. Louis Children's Hospital were given neurological tests at the beginning and the end of a standard treatment on neurological complication. The response to each test is the absence (denoted by 0) or the presence (denoted by 1) of any neurological complications. The data are reported in Table 4.4. The primary objective of this study is to assess if the proportion of patients having neurological complications would be different before and after the treatment.

Table 4.4 *Neurological complication data*

	$Y = 0$	$Y = 1$	Supplement on X
$X = 0$	6 (n_1, θ_1)	3 (n_2, θ_2)	2 $(n_{12}, \theta_1 + \theta_2)$
$X = 1$	8 (n_3, θ_3)	8 (n_4, θ_4)	4 $(n_{34}, \theta_3 + \theta_4)$
Supplement on Y	2 $(n_{13}, \theta_1+\theta_3)$	0 $(n_{24}, \theta_2+\theta_4)$	

NOTE: "$X = 1(0)$" means that a patient does (not) have any complications at the beginning of the treatment, "$Y = 1(0)$" means that a patient does (not) have any complications at the end of the treatment. The observed frequencies and probabilities are in parentheses.

4.4.2 MLEs via the EM algorithm

Let $Y_{\rm obs} = \{(n_1, \ldots, n_4); (n_{12}, n_{34}); (n_{13}, n_{24})\}$ denote the observed frequencies and $\theta = (\theta_1, \ldots, \theta_4)^{\top} \in \mathbb{T}_4$ the cell probability vector.

The parameter of interest is

$$\theta_{23} = \Pr(Y=1) - \Pr(X=1) = \theta_2 - \theta_3,$$

the difference between the proportions of patients with neurological complications before and after the treatment. Under the assumption of MAR, the observed-data likelihood function is

$$\begin{aligned} L(\theta|Y_{\rm obs}) &\propto \left\{\prod_{i=1}^4 \theta_i^{n_i} \times (\theta_1+\theta_2)^{n_{12}}(\theta_3+\theta_4)^{n_{34}}\right\} \\ &\quad \times (\theta_1+\theta_3)^{n_{13}}(\theta_2+\theta_4)^{n_{24}}, \quad \theta \in \mathbb{T}_4. \end{aligned}$$

Writing $n_{13} = Z_1+(n_{13}-Z_1)$ and $n_{24} = Z_2+(n_{24}-Z_2)$, we introduce a latent vector $Z = (Z_1, Z_2)^{\top}$, and obtain the following augmented-likelihood function

$$L(\theta|Y_{\rm obs}, Z) \propto \left(\prod_{i=1}^4 \theta_i^{n_i+Z_i}\right) \times (\theta_1+\theta_2)^{n_{12}}(\theta_3+\theta_4)^{n_{34}}, \tag{4.7}$$

where $Z_3 \hat{=} n_{13} - Z_1$ and $Z_4 \hat{=} n_{24} - Z_2$. Note that this augmented-likelihood has the same functional form of (4.42) and thus from Problem 4.1(b), we obtain the following MLEs of θ:

$$\begin{cases} \theta_i = \dfrac{n_i+Z_i}{N}\left(1+\dfrac{n_{12}}{n_1+Z_1+n_2+Z_2}\right), & i=1,\ 2, \\[2ex] \theta_i = \dfrac{n_i+Z_i}{N}\left(1+\dfrac{n_{34}}{n_3+Z_3+n_4+Z_4}\right), & i=3,\ 4, \end{cases} \tag{4.8}$$

where $N \hat{=} \Sigma_{i=1}^4 n_i + n_{12} + n_{34} + n_{13} + n_{24}$. Similar to (4.6), the conditional predictive distribution is

$$\begin{aligned} f(Z|Y_{\rm obs}, \theta) &= \text{Binomial}(Z_1|n_{13},\ \theta_1/(\theta_1+\theta_3)), \\ &\quad \times \text{Binomial}(Z_2|n_{24},\ \theta_2/(\theta_2+\theta_4)). \end{aligned} \tag{4.9}$$

Hence, the E-step of the EM is to compute

$$E(Z_1|Y_{\rm obs}, \theta) = \frac{n_{13}\theta_1}{\theta_1+\theta_3}, \quad \text{and} \quad E(Z_2|Y_{\rm obs}, \theta) = \frac{n_{24}\theta_2}{\theta_2+\theta_4}. \tag{4.10}$$

The M-step updates (4.8) by replacing $\{Z_\ell\}_{\ell=1}^2$ with their conditional expectations. The MLE of θ_{23} is then given by $\hat{\theta}_{23} = \hat{\theta}_2 - \hat{\theta}_3$. The 95% asymptotic CI for θ_{23} is given by

$$[\hat{\theta}_{23} - 1.96 \times \text{Se}(\hat{\theta}_{23}),\ \hat{\theta}_{23} + 1.96 \times \text{Se}(\hat{\theta}_{23})],$$

where

$$\text{Se}(\hat{\theta}_{23}) = \{\text{Var}(\hat{\theta}_2) + \text{Var}(\hat{\theta}_3) - 2\text{Cov}(\hat{\theta}_2, \hat{\theta}_3)\}^{1/2}.$$

For the data in Table 4.4, using $\theta^{(0)} = \mathbf{1}_4/4$ as initial values, the EM algorithm based on (4.8) and (4.10) converged at the 6-th iteration. The resultant MLEs are

$$(\hat{\theta}_1, \hat{\theta}_2, \hat{\theta}_3, \hat{\theta}_4)^\top = (0.2495,\ 0.1094,\ 0.3422,\ 0.2989)^\top,$$

and $\hat{\theta}_{23} = -0.2328$. The corresponding standard errors are given by (0.0819, 0.0585, 0.0925, 0.0865) and 0.1191. Therefore, the 95% asymptotic CI of θ_{23} is $[-0.4663, 0.0007]$. Since the asymptotic CI includes the value of 0, we conclude that the incidence rates of neurological complication before and after the standard treatment are essentially the same. However, such a CI depends on the large-sample theory and the sample size in this case is not that large.

4.4.3 Generation of i.i.d. posterior samples

For Bayesian analysis, the *grouped Dirichlet distribution* (GDD)

$$\theta \sim \text{GD}_{4,2,2}\Big((n_1^*, \ldots, n_4^*)^\top,\ (n_{12}^*, n_{34}^*)^\top\Big) \tag{4.11}$$

is a natural conjugate prior distribution of θ. Hence, the complete-data posterior of θ is still a GDD:

$$\begin{aligned} \theta|(Y_{\text{obs}}, Z) \ \sim\ & \text{GD}_{4,2,2}\Big((n_1 + n_1^* + Z_1, \ldots, n_4 + n_4^* + Z_4)^\top, \\ & (n_{12} + n_{12}^*, n_{34} + n_{34}^*)^\top\Big). \end{aligned} \tag{4.12}$$

The SR (4.43) provides a straightforward procedure for generating i.i.d. samples from a GDD. To apply the exact IBF sampling, we first need to identify the support of $Z|Y_{\text{obs}}$. From (4.9), we have $\mathcal{S}_{(Z|Y_{\text{obs}})} = \{z_1, \ldots, z_K\}$ with $K = (n_{13}+1)(n_{24}+1)$. For the purpose of illustration, in Table 4.4, let $n_{24} = 3$ instead. Thus, the corresponding $\{z_k\}_{k=1}^K$ are listed in the second column of Table 4.5. The last column of Table 4.5 displays $\{p_k\}_{k=1}^K$ based on (4.3) and (4.2). Next, we draw $L = 10{,}000$ i.i.d. samples $\{Z^{(\ell)}\}_{\ell=1}^L$ of Z from the pmf $f(Z|Y_{\text{obs}})$ with probabilities $\{p_k\}_1^K$ on $\{z_k\}_1^K$. Finally, we draw $\theta^{(\ell)} \sim f(\theta|Y_{\text{obs}}, Z^{(\ell)})$ via (4.12) for $\ell = 1, \ldots, L$, then $\{\theta^{(\ell)}\}_1^L$ are i.i.d. samples from $f(\theta|Y_{\text{obs}})$.

Table 4.5 *The values of $\{q_k(\theta_0)\}$ with various θ_0 and $\{p_k\}$*

k	z_k	$q_k(\theta_0)$	$q_k(\theta_0')$	p_k
1	(0,0)	0.003350222	0.2648067	0.12314502
2	(1,0)	0.004690310	0.3707294	0.17240303
3	(2,0)	0.002042891	0.1614732	0.07509110
4	(0,1)	0.003654787	0.2888800	0.13434002
5	(1,1)	0.005014368	0.3963434	0.18431451
6	(2,1)	0.002142892	0.1693775	0.07876689
7	(0,2)	0.001790846	0.1415512	0.06582661
8	(1,2)	0.002410754	0.1905497	0.08861275
9	(2,2)	0.001011552	0.0799546	0.03718188
10	(0,3)	0.000382659	0.0302460	0.01406552
11	(1,3)	0.000505776	0.0399773	0.01859094
12	(2,3)	0.000208441	0.0164755	0.00766172

Note: $\theta_0 = (0.25, 0.25, 0.25, 0.25)^{\top}$ and $\theta_0' = (0.2, 0.2, 0.5, 0.1)^{\top}$.

Again, we assume no prior information and adopt the uniform prior, i.e., $n_1^* = \cdots = n_4^* = 1$ and $n_{12}^* = n_{34}^* = 0$. The Bayes estimates of θ and θ_{23} are given by (0.2280, 0.1411, 0.3007, 0.3302) and -0.1594. Their corresponding standard deviations are (0.0691, 0.0614, 0.0783, 0.0804) and 0.1087. The 95% Bayes CI of θ_{23} is $[-0.3664, 0.0538]$, which includes the value of 0. This lends support to the belief that neurological complication rates are essentially the same before and after the standard treatment.

4.5 The Hidden Sensitivity (HS) Model for Surveys with Two Sensitive Questions

4.5.1 Randomized response models

In questionnaires for political and sociological surveys, respondents sometimes encounter sensitive questions about, e.g., their normative charges to a certain service and their involvement in potentially embarrassing behaviors such as visiting pornographic web sites, or illegal activities such as tax evasion (Elffers *et al.*, 1992). Similarly, individuals may be asked if they have had abortion experience, drug abuse history, homosexual activities and AIDS in some medical and epidemiological questionnaires. The individuals may choose not to answer or may intentionally provide wrong answers, according to whether the choice is to their advantage. Many techniques have been proposed to encourage greater cooperation from the respondents and *randomized response* (RR) sampling is amongst the most popular method to overcome such a nonresponse issue (Fox & Tracy, 1986; Chaudhuri & Mukerjee, 1988; Lee, 1993).

Warner (1965) introduced the RR model as a survey methodology for sensitive questions to reduce response error, protect the privacy of respondents and increase response rates. Under Warner's model, respondents are drawn using simple random sampling with replacement from the population. It requires the respondent to give a "Yes" or "No" reply either to the sensitive question or to the complement of the question depending on the outcome of a *randomizing device* (RD) not reported to the interviewer. Horvitz *et al.* (1967) and Greenberg *et al.* (1969) developed an unrelated question RR model by introducing a nonsensitive and unrelated question. Since then, other investigators proposed various alternatives to the RR strategy.

Fox & Tracy (1984) considered the estimation of correlation between two sensitive questions. Lakshmi & Raghavarao (1992) also discussed a 2×2 contingency table based on binary randomized responses. Christofides (2005) presented an RR technique for two sensitive characteristics at the same time and his procedure requires two RDs. Kim & Warde (2005) considered a multinomial RR model which can handle untruthful responses. However, all these RR techniques rely on various RDs. As a result, they are usually criticized by their 1) inefficiency; 2) lack of reproductivity; 3) lack of confidence/trust from the respondents; and 4) dependence on the RD.

4.5.2 Nonrandomized response models

To overcome some of the aforementioned inadequacies of RR models, two *nonrandomized response* (NRR) models, namely the triangular and crosswise models, were developed recently by Yu *et al.* (2008b) for a single sensitive dichotomous question. Tian *et al.* (2007) proposed a nonrandomized *hidden sensitivity* (HS) model for analyzing the association between two sensitive dichotomous questions. Unlike traditional RR models, the NRR models utilize an independent (or unrelated) nonsensitive question (e.g., season of birth) in the survey to indirectly obtain a respondent's answer to a sensitive question. In general, the triangular design (which is NRR) is more efficient than the Warner's randomized design (Tan, Tian & Tang, 2009).

4.5.3 The nonrandomized hidden sensitivity model

Consider two binary sensitive variates X and Y. Let $X = 1$ denote the sensitive answer (or outcome) that a respondent may not want to reveal (e.g., take drug), and $X = 0$ the nonsensitive answer (e.g., not to take drug). Similarly, let $Y = 1$ be the sensitive answer (e.g., HIV+) and $Y = 0$ the nonsensitive one (e.g., HIV−). Let $\theta_x = \Pr(X = 1)$, $\theta_y = \Pr(Y = 1)$,

$$\begin{aligned} \theta_1 &= \Pr(X = 0, Y = 0), \\ \theta_2 &= \Pr(X = 0, Y = 1), \\ \theta_3 &= \Pr(X = 1, Y = 0), \quad \text{and} \\ \theta_4 &= \Pr(X = 1, Y = 1). \end{aligned}$$

Hence, $\theta_x = \theta_3 + \theta_4$ and $\theta_y = \theta_2 + \theta_4$. A commonly used measure of association is the odds ratio defined by $\psi = \theta_1\theta_4/(\theta_2\theta_3)$. The objective is to estimate θ_x, θ_y, θ_is and ψ.

(a) Survey design for two sensitive questions

To obtain reliable responses from respondents, Tian *et al.* (2007) introduce a nonsensitive variate W, which is independent of (X, Y). Let $\omega_i = \Pr(W = i)$ for $i = 1, \ldots, 4$. Like the triangular and crosswise models, the variate W should be chosen in such a way that all ω_is are known or can be estimated easily. Therefore, we assume that ω_is are given. For example, let $\{W = i\}$ denote that a respondent was born in the i-th quarter and we can thus assume that ω_is are approximately all equal to 1/4.

Instead of directly answering the sensitive question, each respondent is asked to answer a new question as shown in Table 4.6. Since $\{X = 0, Y = 0\}$ represents an nonsensitive subclass, we have reason to believe that a respondent will put a tick in Block i ($i = 1, \ldots, 4$) according to his/her truthful status if (s)he belongs to this category. The other categories (i.e., Blocks II to IV), however, are sensitive to the respondent. If the respondent belongs to Block II (III or IV), (s)he is asked to put a tick in Block 2 (3 or 4), where the sensitive answers are mixed with nonsensitive ones so that his/her privacy is protected. This technique is simply called the HS model in the sense that the sensitive attribute of a respondent is being hidden. Table 4.7 shows the cell probabilities θ_is and the observed frequencies n_is. Let n_1 denote the observed frequency of respondents putting a tick in Block 1. Note that n_2 represents the sum of the frequencies of respondents belonging to Block 2 and Block Ⅱ. We can interpret n_3 and n_4 similarly.

Table 4.6 *Questionnaire for the HS model*

Categories	$W=1$	$W=2$	$W=3$	$W=4$
I: $\{X=0, Y=0\}$	Block 1:_	Block 2:_	Block 3:_	Block 4:_
Ⅱ: $\{X=0, Y=1\}$	Category Ⅱ: please put a tick in Block 2			
Ⅲ: $\{X=1, Y=0\}$	Category Ⅲ: please put a tick in Block 3			
Ⅳ: $\{X=1, Y=1\}$	Category Ⅳ: please put a tick in Block 4			

Source: Tian *et al.* (2007).

Table 4.7 *Cell probabilities, observed and unobservable frequencies for the HS model*

Categories	$W=1$	$W=2$	$W=3$	$W=4$	Total
I: $\{X=0, Y=0\}$	$\omega_1\theta_1$	$\omega_2\theta_1$	$\omega_3\theta_1$	$\omega_4\theta_1$	θ_1 (Z_1)
Ⅱ: $\{X=0, Y=1\}$					θ_2 (Z_2)
Ⅲ: $\{X=1, Y=0\}$					θ_3 (Z_3)
Ⅳ: $\{X=1, Y=1\}$					θ_4 (Z_4)
Total	ω_1 (n_1)	ω_2 (n_2)	ω_3 (n_3)	ω_4 (n_4)	1 $(n.)$

Source: Tian *et al.* (2007). NOTE: $n. = \sum_{i=1}^{4} n_i$, $Z_1 = n. - (Z_2 + Z_3 + Z_4)$, where (Z_2, Z_3, Z_4) are unobservable.

Unlike the classic RR models, it is noteworthy that all the aforementioned NRR models have the following advantages: (i) they do not require any RDs and the study is thus less costly; (ii) the results can be reproducible; (iii) they can be easily operated for both interviewers and interviewees; and (iv) they can be applied to both face-to-face personal interviews and mail questionnaires.

(b) Posterior moments in closed-form

Assume that there are a total of $n. = \Sigma_{i=1}^{4} n_i$ respondents with n_i ticks put in Block i for $i = 1, \ldots, 4$ (see Table 4.7). Let $Y_{\text{obs}} = \{n_1, \ldots, n_4\}$ denote the observed frequencies and $\theta = (\theta_1, \ldots, \theta_4)^{\top}$. The observed-data likelihood function for θ is then (Tian *et al.*, 2009)

$$L(\theta|Y_{\text{obs}}) = \theta_1^{n_1} \prod_{i=2}^{4} (\omega_i \theta_1 + \theta_i)^{n_i}, \quad \theta \in \mathbb{T}_4,$$

where $\omega_i = \Pr(W = i)$, $i = 1, \dots, 4$, are assumed to be known constants. A natural prior for θ is the Dirichlet(a) with $a = (a_1, \dots, a_4)^\top$. Thus, the posterior of θ has the following explicit expression:

$$f(\theta|Y_{\text{obs}}) = c^{-1}(a, n) \times \prod_{i=1}^{4} \theta_k^{a_i - 1} \times L(\theta|Y_{\text{obs}}), \quad \theta \in \mathbb{T}_4,$$

where $n \hat{=} (n_1, \dots, n_4)^\top$, $c(a, n) = c^*(a, n)/\Gamma(\sum_{i=1}^4 a_i + n)$ and

$$\begin{aligned} c^*(a, n) &= \sum_{j_2=0}^{n_2} \sum_{j_3=0}^{n_3} \sum_{j_4=0}^{n_4} \Big\{ \Gamma(a_1 + n_1 + j_2 + j_3 + j_4) \\ &\quad \times \prod_{\ell=2}^{4} \binom{n_\ell}{j_\ell} \Gamma(a_\ell + n_\ell - j_\ell) p_\ell^{j_\ell} \Big\}. \end{aligned}$$

Let $t = (t_1, \dots, t_4)^\top$, then the posterior moment of θ is given by

$$E\Big(\theta_1^{t_1} \theta_2^{t_2} \theta_3^{t_3} \theta_4^{t_4} \Big| Y_{\text{obs}}\Big) = \frac{c^*(a + t, n)}{c^*(a, n)} \times \frac{\Gamma(\sum_{i=1}^4 a_i + n)}{\Gamma(\sum_{i=1}^4 (a_i + t_i) + n)}.$$

Hence, the posterior moments of θ_x, θ_y and ψ can be expressed as

$$\begin{aligned} E(\theta_x|Y_{\text{obs}}) &= E(\theta_3|Y_{\text{obs}}) + E(\theta_4|Y_{\text{obs}}), \\ E(\theta_x^2|Y_{\text{obs}}) &= E(\theta_3^2|Y_{\text{obs}}) + 2E(\theta_3\theta_4|Y_{\text{obs}}) + E(\theta_4^2|Y_{\text{obs}}), \\ E(\theta_y|Y_{\text{obs}}) &= E(\theta_2|Y_{\text{obs}}) + E(\theta_4|Y_{\text{obs}}), \\ E(\theta_y^2|Y_{\text{obs}}) &= E(\theta_2^2|Y_{\text{obs}}) + 2E(\theta_2\theta_4|Y_{\text{obs}}) + E(\theta_4^2|Y_{\text{obs}}), \\ E(\psi|Y_{\text{obs}}) &= E(\theta_1\theta_2^{-1}\theta_3^{-1}\theta_4|Y_{\text{obs}}), \\ E(\psi^2|Y_{\text{obs}}) &= E(\theta_1^2\theta_2^{-2}\theta_3^{-2}\theta_4^2|Y_{\text{obs}}). \end{aligned}$$

(c) The posterior mode via the EM algorithm

To derive the posterior mode of θ, we treat the observed frequencies n_2, n_3 and n_4 as incomplete data and the frequencies Z_2, Z_3 and Z_4 as missing data (see Table 4.7). Let $Z = (Z_2, Z_3, Z_4)^\top$ with $Z_1 = n. - Z_2 - Z_3 - Z_4$. Thus, the complete-data posterior distribution and the conditional predictive distribution are given by

$$f(\theta|Y_{\text{obs}}, Z) = \text{Dirichlet}(\theta|a_1 + Z_1, \dots, a_4 + Z_4), \qquad (4.13)$$

$$f(Z|Y_{\text{obs}}, \theta) = \prod_{i=2}^{4} \text{Binomial}(Z_i|n_i,\ \theta_i/(\omega_i\theta_1 + \theta_i)). \qquad (4.14)$$

The M-step of the EM algorithm calculates the complete-data posterior mode

$$\tilde{\theta}_i = \frac{a_i + Z_i - 1}{\Sigma_{\ell=1}^4 a_\ell + n - 4}, \quad i = 2, 3, 4, \quad \tilde{\theta}_1 = 1 - \sum_{i=2}^4 \tilde{\theta}_i, \tag{4.15}$$

and the E-step is to replace $\{Z_i\}$ by their conditional expectations

$$E(Z_i | Y_{\rm obs}, \theta) = \frac{n_i \theta_i}{\omega_i \theta_1 + \theta_i}, \qquad i = 2, 3, 4. \tag{4.16}$$

(d) Generation of i.i.d. posterior samples

To apply the exact IBF sampling to the current model, we simply need to identify the support of $Z|Y_{\rm obs}$. From (4.14), we have $\mathcal{S}_{(Z|Y_{\rm obs})} = \{z_1, \dots, z_K\}$ with $K = (n_2+1)(n_3+1)(n_4+1)$. For the

Table 4.8 *The values of* $\{q_k(\theta_0)\}$ *and* $\{p_k\}$

k	z_k	$q_k(\theta_0)$	p_k	k	z_k	$q_k(\theta_0)$	p_k
1	(0,0,0)	0.0008473	0.0125290	19	(0,0,2)	0.0014525	0.0214784
2	(1,0,0)	0.0008473	0.0125290	20	(1,0,2)	0.0019367	0.0286379
3	(2,0,0)	0.0004841	0.0071594	21	(2,0,2)	0.0015494	0.0229103
4	(0,1,0)	0.0008473	0.0125290	22	(0,1,2)	0.0019367	0.0286379
5	(1,1,0)	0.0009683	0.0143189	23	(1,1,2)	0.0030988	0.0458206
6	(2,1,0)	0.0006455	0.0095459	24	(2,1,2)	0.0030988	0.0458206
7	(0,2,0)	0.0004841	0.0071594	25	(0,2,2)	0.0015494	0.0229103
8	(1,2,0)	0.0006455	0.0095459	26	(1,2,2)	0.0030988	0.0458206
9	(2,2,0)	0.0005164	0.0076367	27	(2,2,2)	0.0041317	0.0610942
10	(0,0,1)	0.0012710	0.0187936	28	(0,0,3)	0.0009683	0.0143189
11	(1,0,1)	0.0014525	0.0214784	29	(1,0,3)	0.0015494	0.0229103
12	(2,0,1)	0.0009683	0.0143189	30	(2,0,3)	0.0015494	0.0229103
13	(0,1,1)	0.0014525	0.0214784	31	(0,1,3)	0.0015494	0.0229103
14	(1,1,1)	0.0019367	0.0286379	32	(1,1,3)	0.0030988	0.0458206
15	(2,1,1)	0.0015494	0.0229103	33	(2,1,3)	0.0041317	0.0610942
16	(0,2,1)	0.0009683	0.0143189	34	(0,2,3)	0.0015494	0.0229103
17	(1,2,1)	0.0015494	0.0229103	35	(1,2,3)	0.0041317	0.0610942
18	(2,2,1)	0.0015494	0.0229103	36	(2,2,3)	0.0082635	0.1221884

Note: $\theta_0 = (0.25, 0.25, 0.25, 0.25)^{\top}$.

purpose of illustration, in Table 4.7 we let $Y_{\text{obs}} = \{n_1, \dots, n_4\} = \{1, 2, 2, 3\}$, and $\omega_1 = \cdots = \omega_4 = 0.25$. Then, the corresponding $\{z_k\}_{k=1}^K$ are given in the second and sixth columns of Table 4.8. Furthermore, in (4.13) let $a_1 = \cdots = a_4 = 1$. With $\theta_0 = \mathbf{1}_4/4$, $q_k(\theta_0)$ and $\{p_k\}_{k=1}^K$ are calculated by (4.2) and (4.3). The results are shown in Table 4.8.

4.6 Zero-Inflated Poisson Model

Count data with excessive zeros relative to a Poisson distribution are common in applications of public health, biomedicine, epidemiology, sociology, psychology and engineering. Failure to account for the extra zeros in the modeling process may result in biased estimates and misleading inferences (Lambert, 1992). A variety of examples of count data (e.g., number of heart attacks, number of epileptic seizures, length of stay in a hospital, number of defects in a manufacturing process and so on) from different disciplines are available (Böhning, 1998; Ridout *et al.*, 1998). Such count data are often over-dispersed and exhibit greater variability than predicted by a Poisson model.

To model the over-dispersion of such non-Poisson data, one of the useful approaches is by a *zero-inflated Poisson* (ZIP) model (Hinde & Demetrio, 1998). From a likelihood-based point of view, Yip (1988) used the ZIP distribution to model the number of insect per leaf. Heilbron (1989) proposed ZIP and negative binomial regression models and applied them to study high-risk human behavior. Lambert (1992) used the ZIP to model covariate effects in an experiment on soldering defects on printed wiring boards. Gupta *et al.* (1996) proposed zero-adjusted discrete models including the zero-inflated modified power series distributions. From a Bayesian perspective, Rodrigues (2003), Ghosh *et al.* (2006) and Angers & Biswas (2003) analyzed the ZIP data by using MCMC methods or/and Monte Carlo integration to obtain the posterior distributions, respectively.

A discrete r.v. Y is said to follow a ZIP distribution if its pmf is

$$f(y|\phi, \lambda) = [\phi + (1-\phi)e^{-\lambda}]I_{(y=0)} + \left[(1-\phi)\frac{e^{-\lambda}\lambda^y}{y!}\right]I_{(y>0)}, \quad (4.17)$$

where $0 \le \phi < 1$. The ZIP distribution may be viewed as a mixture of a degenerate distribution with all mass at zero and a Poisson (λ) distribution. Note that ϕ is used to incorporate more zeros than those permitted by the original Poisson model ($\phi = 0$). From (4.17), it is easy to verify that

$$\begin{aligned} E(Y|\phi,\lambda) &= (1-\phi)\lambda, \quad \text{and} \\ \text{Var}(Y|\phi,\lambda) &= E(Y|\lambda,\phi) + E(Y|\lambda,\phi)\{\lambda - E(Y|\lambda,\phi)\}. \end{aligned}$$

Clearly, $\text{Var}(Y|\phi,\lambda)$ suggests that the ZIP distribution incorporates extra variation that is unaccounted for by the Poisson distribution.

Let $Y_{\text{obs}} = \{y_i\}_{i=1}^n$ denote n independent observations from the ZIP model (4.17), $\mathbb{O} \hat{=} \{y_i\colon y_i = 0,\ i = 1,\dots,n\}$, and m denote the number of elements in $\mathbb{O}$. Then the likelihood for (ϕ,λ) is

$$L(\phi,\lambda|Y_{\text{obs}}) = [\phi + (1-\phi)e^{-\lambda}]^m \times (1-\phi)^{n-m} \prod_{y_i \notin \mathbb{O}} \frac{e^{-\lambda}\lambda^{y_i}}{y_i!}.$$

We augment Y_{obs} with a latent r.v. Z by splitting the observed m into Z and $(m-Z)$ so that the conditional predictive distribution is

$$f(Z|Y_{\text{obs}},\phi,\lambda) = \text{Binomial}(Z|m,\ \phi/[\phi + (1-\phi)e^{-\lambda}]). \tag{4.18}$$

Note that the complete-data likelihood for (ϕ,λ) is given by

$$\begin{aligned} L(\phi,\lambda|Y_{\text{obs}},Z) &\propto \phi^Z[(1-\phi)e^{-\lambda}]^{m-z} \times (1-\phi)^{n-m} \prod_{y_i \notin \mathbb{O}} \frac{e^{-\lambda}\lambda^{y_i}}{y_i!} \\ &\propto \phi^Z(1-\phi)^{n-Z} e^{-(n-Z)\lambda} \lambda^{\sum_{y_i \notin \mathbb{O}} y_i}. \end{aligned}$$

Suppose that $\phi \sim \text{Beta}(a,b)$, $\lambda \sim \text{Gamma}(c,d)$ and they are independent, then, the complete-data posterior distribution is

$$f(\phi,\lambda|Y_{\text{obs}},Z) = f(\phi|Y_{\text{obs}},Z) \times f(\lambda|Y_{\text{obs}},Z), \tag{4.19}$$

where

$$\begin{aligned} f(\phi|Y_{\text{obs}},Z) &= \text{Beta}(\phi|Z+a,\ n-Z+b), \quad \text{and} \\ f(\lambda|Y_{\text{obs}},Z) &= \text{Gamma}\Big(\lambda\Big|\ {\textstyle\sum_{y_i \notin \mathbb{O}}} y_i + c,\ n-Z+d\Big). \end{aligned}$$

The exact IBF sampling in §4.1 then applies.

4.7 Changepoint Problems

Changepoint problems (CPs) are often encountered in medicine and other fields, e.g., economics, finance, psychology, signal processing, industrial system control and geology. Typically, a sequence of data is collected over a period of time, we wish to make inference about the location of one or more points of the sequence at which there is a change in the model. The literature on CPs is extensive. For binomial CPs, Smith (1975) presented a conventional Bayesian approach for a finite sequence of independent observations with details on binomial single-changepoint model. Smith (1980) studied binomial multiple-changepoint model which is investigated further by Stephens (1994) using the Gibbs sampler. For Poisson process CPs, a well-known example concerns British coal-mining disasters from 1851–1962.[3] Frequentist investigations appear in Worsley (1986) and Siegmund (1988), while traditional Bayesian analysis and MCMC hierarchical Bayesian analysis are presented in Raftery & Akman (1986) and Carlin *et al.* (1992), respectively. Arnold (1993) considered the application of the Gibbs sampler to a Poisson distribution with a changepoint. For binary CPs, Halpern (1999) applied a novel changepoint statistic based on the minimum value, over possible changepoint locations of Fisher's exact test to assessing recombination in genetic sequences of HIV. Three comprehensive reviews on CPs are provided by Brodsky & Darkhovsky (1993), Chen & Gupta (2000) and more recently by Wu (2005). This section is partly based on Tian *et al.* (2009).

4.7.1 Bayesian formulation

(a) The single-changepoint problem

Let $Y_{\text{obs}} = \{y_i\}_{i=1}^n$ denote a realization of the sequence of independent r.v.'s $\{Y_i\}_{i=1}^n$ of length n. The r.v.'s $\{Y_i\}_{i=1}^n$ are said to have a changepoint at r $(1 \le r \le n)$ if

$$\begin{aligned} Y_i &\sim f(y|\theta_1), \quad i = 1, \dots, r, \quad \text{and} \\ Y_i &\sim f(y|\theta_2), \quad i = r+1, \dots, n, \end{aligned}$$

where θ_1 and θ_2 could be vector-valued and $\theta_1 \neq \theta_2$. In particular, the point $r = n$ represents "no change." Thus, the likelihood function becomes

$$L(r, \theta_1, \theta_2 | Y_{\text{obs}}) = \prod_{i=1}^{r} f(y_i|\theta_1) \times \prod_{i=r+1}^{n} f(y_i|\theta_2). \tag{4.20}$$

[3]The original data were gathered by Maguire *et al.* (1952) and then the data were corrected by Jarrett (1979).

Using $\pi(r, \theta_1, \theta_2)$ as a joint prior distribution for r, θ_1 and θ_2, the joint posterior distribution is then given by

$$f(r, \theta_1, \theta_2 | Y_{\text{obs}}) \propto L(r, \theta_1, \theta_2 | Y_{\text{obs}}) \times \pi(r, \theta_1, \theta_2). \tag{4.21}$$

(b) The multiple-changepoint problem

The above method for single-changepoint can be easily generalized to multiple-changepoint in the sequence. The Bayesian formulation for the multiple-changepoint problem is almost identical with that for the single-changepoint problem. Let M_s represent a model with s changepoints denoted by $\mathbf{r} = (r_1, \dots, r_s)^\top$. Similar to (4.21), under M_s (s is given), we have

$$\begin{aligned} f(\mathbf{r}, \theta | Y_{\text{obs}}) &\propto L(\mathbf{r}, \theta | Y_{\text{obs}}) \cdot \pi(\mathbf{r}, \theta) \\ &= \left\{ \prod_{j=1}^{s+1} \prod_{i=r_{j-1}+1}^{r_j} f(y_i | \theta_j) \right\} \times \pi(\mathbf{r}, \theta), \end{aligned} \tag{4.22}$$

where $\theta = (\theta_1, \dots, \theta_{s+1})^\top$, $r_0 \hat{=} 0$, $r_{s+1} \hat{=} n$, and the changepoints $\mathbf{r}$ take values in the domain

$$\mathcal{S}_{(\mathbf{r}|Y_{\text{obs}})} = \{\mathbf{r}\colon 1 \le r_1 < \cdots < r_s \le n,\ r_j \text{ is an integer}\}. \tag{4.23}$$

(c) Bayesian analysis via noniterative computation

The primary objective is to make inferences on the unknown changepoints $\mathbf{r}$ and the associated parameters θ. We present an exact sampling approach that is more straightforward than the MCMC. We first treat the changepoint r (or the changepoints $\mathbf{r}$) as a latent variable Z, and then derive both the complete-data posterior distribution $f(\theta | Y_{\text{obs}}, Z)$ and the conditional predictive distribution $f(Z | Y_{\text{obs}}, \theta)$. Finally, we apply the exact IBF sampling to obtain i.i.d. posterior samples $\{Z^{(\ell)}, \theta^{(\ell)}\}_{\ell=1}^L$.

(d) Exact calculation of marginal likelihood

In practice, the number of changepoints is generally uncertain. Thus, model determination is the first task in changepoint analysis. Let M_s represent a model with s changepoints. A classical approach of selecting the most appropriate model is the likelihood ratio test by comparing M_s with M_{s+1} (e.g., Henderson & Matthews, 1993). Gelfand & Dey (1994) reviewed the behavior of the likelihood ratio statistic and some well-known adjustments to it. In Bayesian analysis, Bayes factor is a useful tool for model choice (cf. §1.4.4). However, the calculation of Bayes factor itself has proved extremely challenging (Kass & Raftery, 1995). Approximate computation of Bayes factor can be implemented by using the Gibbs output (Chib, 1995) or the more general MCMC output (Chen, 2005). In this subsection, two alternative formulae are developed to exactly calculate marginal likelihood (or Bayes factor) by using the exact IBF output and the point-wise IBF, respectively.

Denote the marginal density of Y_{obs} by $m(Y_{\text{obs}})$.[4] Let $\{Z^{(\ell)}, \theta^{(\ell)}\}_1^L$ be the output of the exact IBF sampling. From the Bayes formula:

$$m(Y_{\text{obs}}) = L(\theta|Y_{\text{obs}})\pi(\theta)/f(\theta|Y_{\text{obs}}),$$

which holds for any θ, we obtain

$$\log m(Y_{\text{obs}}) = \log L(\theta_0|Y_{\text{obs}}) + \log \pi(\theta_0) - \log f(\theta_0|Y_{\text{obs}}), \tag{4.24}$$

for an arbitrary $\theta_0 \in \mathcal{S}_{(\theta|Y_{\text{obs}})}$. For estimation efficiency, θ_0 is generally taken to be a high-density point in the support of the posterior (e.g., the posterior mode/mean as suggested by Chib, 1995). Since the observed posterior density can be written as

$$f(\theta|Y_{\text{obs}}) = \int_{\mathcal{S}_{(Z|Y_{\text{obs}})}} f(\theta|Y_{\text{obs}}, z) f(z|Y_{\text{obs}})\, dz,$$

we obtain a Monte Carlo estimate of $f(\theta|Y_{\text{obs}})$ at θ_0:[5]

$$\hat{f}(\theta_0|Y_{\text{obs}}) = \frac{1}{L}\sum_{\ell=1}^{L} f(\theta_0|Y_{\text{obs}}, Z^{(\ell)}), \tag{4.25}$$

where $\{Z^{(\ell)}\}$ are i.i.d. samples from $f(Z|Y_{\text{obs}})$. Note that this estimate is consistent, i.e., $\hat{f}(\theta_0|Y_{\text{obs}}) \to f(\theta_0|Y_{\text{obs}})$ as $L \to \infty$. Combining (4.24) with (4.25), we have an approximate formula to calculate $m(Y_{\text{obs}})$.

On the other hand, when Z is a discrete r.v. taking values on $\{z_k\}_1^K$, using the point-wise IBF (1.36), we explicitly obtain

$$f(\theta_0|Y_{\text{obs}}) = \left\{ \sum_{k=1}^{K} q_k(\theta_0) \right\}^{-1} = p_1/q_1(\theta_0), \tag{4.26}$$

where p_k and $q_k(\theta_0)$ are defined in (4.3) and (4.2), respectively. Substituting (4.26) into (4.24) yields an exact formula to calculate $m(Y_{\text{obs}})$.

---

[4]Usually, it is called marginal likelihood, cf. §1.4.5 for more details.

[5]Comparing (1.30) with (4.25).

4.7.2 Binomial changepoint models

Consider binomial model with two changepoints. Suppose that

$$\begin{aligned} Y_i &\overset{\text{ind}}{\sim} \text{Binomial}(N_i, \theta_1), \quad i = 1, \dots, r_1, \\ Y_i &\overset{\text{ind}}{\sim} \text{Binomial}(N_i, \theta_2), \quad i = r_1 + 1, \dots, r_2, \\ Y_i &\overset{\text{ind}}{\sim} \text{Binomial}(N_i, \theta_3), \quad i = r_2 + 1, \dots, n, \end{aligned}$$

where (r_1, r_2) denote two changepoints taking integer values on

$$\mathcal{S}_{(r_1, r_2|Y_{\text{obs}})} = \{(r_1, r_2)\colon\ 1 \le r_1 < r_2 < n\}.$$

If independent priors are chosen, where $(r_1, r_2) \sim U(\mathcal{S}_{(r_1,r_2|Y_{\text{obs}})})$ and $\theta_j \sim \text{Beta}(a_j, b_j)$ for $j = 1, 2, 3$, then the joint posterior distribution is given by

$$f(r_1, r_2, \theta|Y_{\text{obs}}) \propto \prod_{j=1}^{3} \theta_j^{a_j + S_j(r_{j-1}, r_j) - 1}(1 - \theta_j)^{b_j + T_j(r_{j-1}, r_j) - 1}, \quad (4.27)$$

where $\theta = (\theta_1, \theta_2, \theta_3)^{\top}$, $S_j(r_{j-1}, r_j) = \sum_{i=r_{j-1}+1}^{r_j} y_i$, $T_j(r_{j-1}, r_j) = \sum_{i=r_{j-1}+1}^{r_j} (N_i - y_i)$, $r_0 \hat{=} 0$ and $r_3 \hat{=} n$. From (4.27), we obtain the following conditional distributions

$$\begin{aligned} f(\theta|Y_{\text{obs}}, r_1, r_2) &= \prod_{j=1}^{3} \text{Beta}\Big(\theta_j | a_j + S_j(r_{j-1}, r_j), \\ &\qquad\qquad b_j + T_j(r_{j-1}, r_j)\Big), \quad (4.28) \\ f(r_1, r_2|Y_{\text{obs}}, \theta) &\propto \prod_{j=1}^{3} \theta_j^{S_j(r_{j-1}, r_j)}(1 - \theta_j)^{T_j(r_{j-1}, r_j)}. \end{aligned}$$

Treating changepoints (r_1, r_2) as latent variable Z, from (4.1), we have

$$f(r_1, r_2|Y_{\text{obs}}) \propto \prod_{j=1}^{3} \frac{\Gamma(a_j + S_j(r_{j-1}, r_j))\Gamma(b_j + T_j(r_{j-1}, r_j))}{\Gamma(a_j + b_j + S_j(r_{j-1}, r_j) + T_j(r_{j-1}, r_j))}, \quad (4.29)$$

where $1 \le r_1 < r_2 < n$. Therefore, we can obtain i.i.d. posterior samples of (r_1, r_2) and θ from (4.29) and (4.28), respectively.

Example 4.1 (*Lindisfarne scribe data*). Table 1 of Stephens (1994) gives the number of occurrences of two types of pronoun endings observed in 13 chronologically ordered medieval manuscripts (Smith, 1980). Since the proportion of each ending in individual documents

Table 4.9 *Exact joint pmf $f(r_1, r_2|Y_{\text{obs}})$ defined in (4.29)*

r_2	r_1 = 1	2	3	4	5
2	5.20×10^{-4}	–	–	–	–
3	6.09×10^{-4}	2.52×10^{-4}	–	–	–
4	3.62×10^{-4}	1.35×10^{-4}	2.05×10^{-4}	–	–
5	6.52×10^{-2}	2.93×10^{-2}	3.47×10^{-2}	0.3279	–
6	6.11×10^{-2}	2.26×10^{-2}	1.91×10^{-2}	3.63×10^{-2}	4.76×10^{-2}
7	1.37×10^{-2}	4.53×10^{-3}	3.49×10^{-3}	2.97×10^{-3}	2.95×10^{-2}
8	5.57×10^{-3}	1.80×10^{-3}	1.47×10^{-3}	8.86×10^{-4}	2.94×10^{-2}
9	1.08×10^{-3}	3.66×10^{-4}	3.51×10^{-4}	1.70×10^{-4}	2.15×10^{-2}
10	5.93×10^{-4}	2.08×10^{-4}	2.18×10^{-4}	9.96×10^{-5}	2.18×10^{-2}
11	4.66×10^{-4}	1.68×10^{-4}	1.89×10^{-4}	8.33×10^{-5}	2.62×10^{-2}
12	5.57×10^{-4}	2.05×10^{-4}	2.39×10^{-4}	1.03×10^{-4}	3.59×10^{-2}

r_2	r_1 = 6	7	8	9	10	11
2	–	–	–	–	–	–
3	–	–	–	–	–	–
4	–	–	–	–	–	–
5	–	–	–	–	–	–
6	–	–	–	–	–	–
7	0.0199	–	–	–	–	–
8	0.0184	0.0037	–	–	–	–
9	0.0159	0.0029	1.13×10^{-3}	–	–	–
10	0.0176	0.0032	1.24×10^{-3}	2.33×10^{-4}	–	–
11	0.0222	0.0040	1.52×10^{-3}	2.36×10^{-4}	1.25×10^{-4}	–
12	0.0294	0.0052	1.75×10^{-3}	2.57×10^{-4}	1.25×10^{-4}	9.92×10^{-5}

appears to change over the sequence, it is believed that the 13 documents are work of more than one author. Thus, assuming that the documents can be categorized into temporally contiguous phases, with each phase having a distinctive underlying proportion of ending one, say, and corresponding to a different author, it is clear that a binomial model with multiple changepoints is appropriate for these data.

Smith found evidence for the presence of at least two changepoints by using traditional Bayesian approach. Thus we focus our attention on model M_2. Table 4.9 contains the joint posterior probabilities $f(r_1, r_2|Y_{\text{obs}})$ defined in (4.29) for all possible pairs of changepoints for this data set using the uniform priors (i.e., $a_j = b_j = 1$).

The maximum joint posterior probability occurs at $r_1 = 4$ and $r_2 = 5$. ‖

4.7.3 Poisson changepoint models

(a) The single-changepoint model

By setting $f_j(y|\theta_j) = \text{Poisson}(y|\theta_j)$ in (4.20), $j = 1, 2$, we first consider the Poisson single-changepoint model M_1. We use independent prior distributions: r is assumed to follow a discrete uniform prior distribution on $\{1, \dots, n\}$, $\theta_j \sim \text{Gamma}(a_j, b_j)$, $j = 1, 2$. Then, the joint posterior distribution (4.21) becomes

$$f(r, \theta_1, \theta_2|Y_{\text{obs}}) \propto \theta_1^{a_1+S_r-1} e^{-(b_1+r)\theta_1} \times \theta_2^{a_2+S_n-S_r-1} e^{-(b_2+n-r)\theta_2},$$

where $S_r \triangleq \sum_{i=1}^r y_i$. Direct calculation yields

$$\begin{aligned} f(\theta_1, \theta_2|Y_{\text{obs}}, r) &= \text{Gamma}(\theta_1|a_1 + S_r,\ b_1 + r) \qquad (4.30) \\ &\quad \times \text{Gamma}(\theta_2|a_2 + S_n - S_r,\ b_2 + n - r), \\ f(r|Y_{\text{obs}}, \theta_1, \theta_2) &= \frac{(\theta_1/\theta_2)^{S_r} \exp\{(\theta_2 - \theta_1)r\}}{\sum_{i=1}^n (\theta_1/\theta_2)^{S_i} \exp\{(\theta_2 - \theta_1)i\}}. \end{aligned}$$

If the changepoint r is viewed as a latent variable Z, by (4.1), then

$$f(r|Y_{\text{obs}}) \propto \frac{\Gamma(a_1 + S_r)\Gamma(a_2 + S_n - S_r)}{(b_1 + r)^{a_1+S_r}(b_2 + n - r)^{a_2+S_n-S_r}}, \qquad (4.31)$$

where $1 \le r \le n$. Therefore, i.i.d. posterior samples of r and (θ_1, θ_2) from (4.31) and (4.30), respectively, can be obtained readily.

(b) The multiple-changepoint model

Now we consider the multiple-changepoint model M_s. In (4.22), let $f_j(y|\theta_j) = \text{Poisson}(y|\theta_j)$ for $j = 1, \dots, s+1$, where $\theta = (\theta_1, \dots, \theta_{s+1})^\top$ is the mean vector and $\mathbf{r} = (r_1, \dots, r_s)^\top$ denote the s changepoints taking integer values on the domain $\mathcal{S}_{(\mathbf{r}|Y_{\text{obs}})}$ defined in (4.23). We use independent priors: $\mathbf{r} \sim U(\mathcal{S}_{(\mathbf{r}|Y_{\text{obs}})})$ and

$$\theta_j \sim \text{Gamma}(a_j, b_j), \qquad j = 1, \dots, s + 1. \qquad (4.32)$$

Hence, the joint posterior (4.22) becomes

$$f(\mathbf{r}, \theta|Y_{\text{obs}}) \propto \prod_{j=1}^{s+1} \theta_j^{a_j+S_{r_j}-S_{r_{j-1}}-1} e^{-(b_j+r_j-r_{j-1})\theta_j},$$

where $S_r \hat{=} \Sigma_{i=1}^r y_i$, $r_0 \hat{=} 0$ and $r_{s+1} \hat{=} n$. It is easy to obtain

$$\begin{aligned} f(\theta|Y_{\text{obs}}, \mathbf{r}) &= \prod_{j=1}^{s+1} \text{Gamma}(\theta_j | a_j + S_{r_j} - S_{r_{j-1}}, \\ &\qquad\qquad b_j + r_j - r_{j-1}), \qquad (4.33) \\ f(\mathbf{r}|Y_{\text{obs}}, \theta) &\propto \prod_{j=1}^{s} (\theta_j/\theta_{j+1})^{S_{r_j}} e^{(\theta_{j+1}-\theta_j)r_j}. \end{aligned}$$

By using (4.1), we have

$$f(\mathbf{r}|Y_{\text{obs}}) \propto \prod_{j=1}^{s+1} \frac{\Gamma(a_j + S_{r_j} - S_{r_{j-1}})}{(b_j + r_j - r_{j-1})^{a_j + S_{r_j} - S_{r_{j-1}}}}, \qquad (4.34)$$

where $\mathbf{r} \in \mathcal{S}_{(\mathbf{r}|Y_{\text{obs}})}$. Therefore, we can obtain i.i.d. posterior samples of $\mathbf{r}$ and θ from (4.34) and (4.33), respectively.

(c) Determining the number of changepoints via Bayes factor

Let M_s represent a Poisson model with s changepoints denoted by $\mathbf{r} = (r_1, \dots, r_s)^\top$, and $\theta = (\theta_1, \dots, \theta_{s+1})^\top$ be its mean vector. Furthermore, let $\Theta = (\mathbf{r}, \theta)$ and $\hat{\Theta} = (\hat{\mathbf{r}}, \hat{\theta})$ denote the posterior means obtained via the exact IBF output. Under model M_s, from (4.24), the log-marginal likelihood is given by

$$\begin{aligned} \log m(Y_{\text{obs}}|M_s) &= \log L(\hat{\Theta}|Y_{\text{obs}}, M_s) + \log \pi(\hat{\Theta}|M_s) \\ &\quad - \log f(\hat{\Theta}|Y_{\text{obs}}, M_s), \qquad (4.35) \end{aligned}$$

where

$$f(\hat{\Theta}|Y_{\text{obs}}, M_s) = f(\hat{\mathbf{r}}|Y_{\text{obs}}, M_s) \times f(\hat{\theta}|Y_{\text{obs}}, \hat{\mathbf{r}}, M_s).$$

We choose the model with the largest log-marginal likelihood. Essentially, the marginal likelihood approach is the same as the Bayes factor approach (cf. §1.4.4). The Bayes factor for model M_s versus model M_{s+1} is defined by

$$B_{s,s+1} = \frac{m(Y_{\text{obs}}|M_s)}{m(Y_{\text{obs}}|M_{s+1})}. \qquad (4.36)$$

Example 4.2 (*The HUS data*). Diarrhoea-associated *hemolytic uremic syndrome* (HUS) is a disease that affects the kidneys and other organs. It poses a substantial threat to infants and young children as

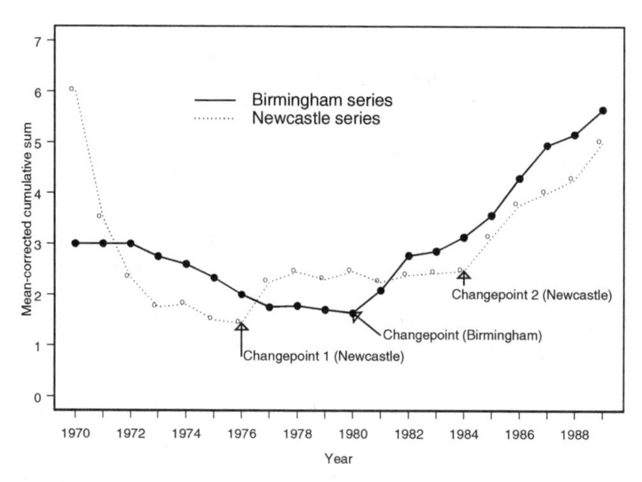

Figure 4.2 Mean-corrected cumulative sum plot for the number of cases at Birmingham and Newcastle.

one of the leading causes of both acute and chronic kidney failures. HUS is most common in the warmer months of the year, following a gastrointestinal illness caused primarily by a particular strain of bacterium, Escherichia Coli O157:H7 (Milford *et al.*, 1990). These bacteria (E. Coli O157:H7) produce extremely potent toxins which are the main cause of the symptoms related to the gastrointestinal illness. Table 1 of Henderson & Matthews (1993) displays the annual number of cases of HUS collected in Birmingham and Newcastle of England, respectively, from 1970 to 1989 (Tarr *et al.*, 1989). The primary concern is the incidence of HUS and when the frequency of cases increases sharply.

Figure 4.2 plots the mean-corrected cumulative sum. The annual totals appear to increase abruptly at about 1980 for the Birmingham series and 1976, 1984 for the Newcastle series. Therefore, a changepoint analysis with Poisson models seems to be appropriate.

The number of cases of HUS at Birmingham in Year i is denoted by y_i ($i = 1, \ldots, n$ with $n = 20$, and $i = 1$ denotes Year 1970). To determine the number of changepoints via Bayes factor, noninformative priors are not used because they are improper. We investigate models M_0, M_1 and M_2 and choose standard exponential priors, specified by setting all $a_j = b_j = 1$ in (4.32). Based on (4.35), we calculate log-marginal likelihoods for the three models, and we obtain $\log m(Y_{\text{obs}}|M_0) = -86.14$, $\log m(Y_{\text{obs}}|M_1) = -57.56$ and $\log m(Y_{\text{obs}}|M_2) = -57.00$. Therefore, M_2 seems to be the most appropriate choice. From (4.36), the Bayes factor for M_1 versus M_0

Table 4.10 *Exact posterior probabilities of the changepoint r for Birmingham data under Model M_1*

r	1	2	3	4
$f(r\|Y_{\text{obs}})$	2.249×10^{-13}	1.499×10^{-14}	2.651×10^{-14}	1.365×10^{-13}
r	5	6	7	8
$f(r\|Y_{\text{obs}})$	8.493×10^{-13}	1.994×10^{-11}	2.669×10^{-09}	7.541×10^{-07}
r	9	10	11	12
$f(r\|Y_{\text{obs}})$	1.656×10^{-05}	2.899×10^{-03}	9.795×10^{-01}	1.753×10^{-02}
r	13	14	15	16
$f(r\|Y_{\text{obs}})$	3.628×10^{-06}	3.020×10^{-05}	7.756×10^{-06}	8.459×10^{-08}
r	17	18	19	20
$f(r\|Y_{\text{obs}})$	4.596×10^{-12}	4.673×10^{-15}	1.404×10^{-15}	1.952×10^{-14}

is 2.583×10^{12}, while the Bayes factor for M_2 versus M_1 is 1.751. That is, the difference between M_2 and M_1 is not worth mentioning. Therefore, we select M_1, which is consistent with the pattern indicated in Figure 4.2.

Under M_1, we assume that

$$y_1, \dots, y_r \overset{\text{iid}}{\sim} \text{Poisson}(\theta_1) \quad \text{and} \quad y_{r+1}, \dots, y_n \overset{\text{iid}}{\sim} \text{Poisson}(\theta_2),$$

where r is the unknown changepoint and $\theta_1 \neq \theta_2$. Table 4.10 contains the exact posterior probabilities for the changepoint r using (4.31). The changepoint occurs at $r = 11$ (i.e., Year 1980) with posterior probability 0.9795. Based on (4.31) and (4.30), we generate 20,000 i.i.d. posterior samples by using the exact IBF sampling, and the Bayes estimates of r, θ_1 and θ_2 are given by 11.013, 1.593 and 9.609, respectively. The corresponding standard deviations are 0.143, 0.370 and 0.985. The 95% Bayes CIs for θ_1 and θ_2 are $[0.952, 2.393]$ and $[7.800, 11.621]$, respectively. Figure 4.3(a) and 4.3(b) show the histogram of the changepoint r and the posterior densities of θ_1 and θ_2, which are estimated by a kernel density smoother based on i.i.d. posterior samples. Figure 4.3(c) depicts the annual numbers of HUS for Birmingham series, the identified changepoint position, and the average number of cases before and after the changepoint.

Next, we analyze the Newcastle data set. Similarly, we obtain

$$\log m(Y_{\text{obs}}|M_0) = -85.24,$$

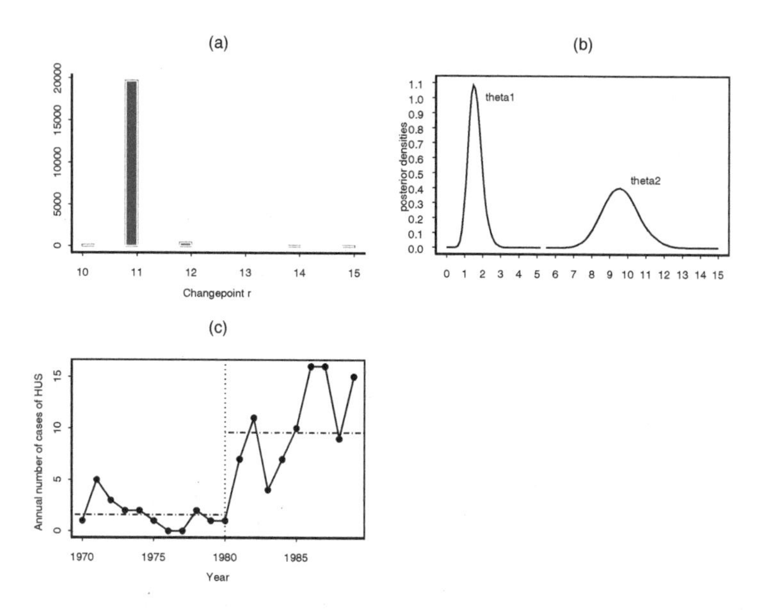

Figure 4.3 Birmingham data set. (a) Histogram of the changepoint r. (b) The posterior densities of θ_1 and θ_2 estimated by a kernel density smoother based on 20,000 i.i.d. samples generated via the exact IBF sampling. (c) The annual numbers of cases of HUS from 1970 to 1989. The dotted vertical line denotes the identified changepoint position, the lower horizontal line the average number (1.593) of cases during 1970–1980, and the upper horizontal line the average number (9.609) of cases during 1980–1989.

Table 4.11 *Posterior estimates of parameters for Birmingham data under Model M_2*

Parameters	Bayesian mean	Bayesian std	95% Bayesian CI
r_1	7.638	3.6637	[1.0000, 15.00]
r_2	15.47	1.5449	[14.000, 20.00]
θ_1	1.805	0.7723	[0.7461, 3.620]
θ_2	3.591	2.4996	[1.5085, 11.50]
θ_3	9.643	3.1975	[0.2806, 13.32]

$$\begin{aligned}\log m(Y_{\text{obs}}|M_1) &= -64.13, \quad \text{and} \\ \log m(Y_{\text{obs}}|M_2) &= -64.10.\end{aligned}$$

From (4.36), the Bayes factor for M_2 versus M_0 is 1.5169×10^9, and the Bayes factor for M_2 versus M_1 is 1.03. Therefore, we select M_2, which is also consistent with the pattern indicated in Figure 4.2.

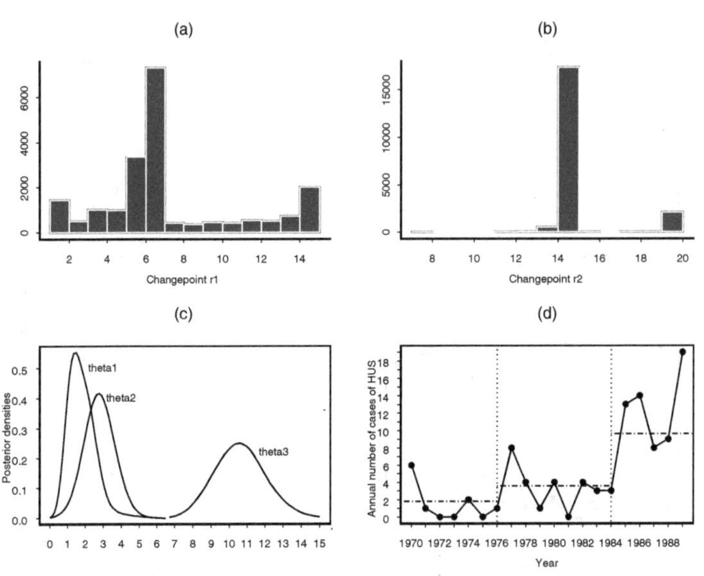

Figure 4.4 Newcastle data set. (a) Histogram of the changepoint r_1. (b) Histogram of the changepoint r_2. (c) The posterior densities of θ_1, θ_2 and θ_3 estimated by a kernel density smoother based on 20,000 i.i.d. samples generated via the exact IBF sampling. (d) The annual numbers of cases of HUS at Newcastle from 1970 to 1989. The two vertical lines denote two identified changepoint positions (1976, 1984), the three horizontal lines the average numbers (1.805, 3.591, 9.643) of cases during 1970–1976, 1976–1984 and 1984–1989, respectively.

Under M_2, we assume that

$$\begin{aligned} y_1, \dots, y_{r_1} &\overset{\text{iid}}{\sim} \text{Poisson}(\theta_1), \\ y_{r_1+1}, \dots, y_{r_2} &\overset{\text{iid}}{\sim} \text{Poisson}(\theta_2), \quad \text{and} \\ y_{r_2+1}, \dots, y_n &\overset{\text{iid}}{\sim} \text{Poisson}(\theta_3), \end{aligned}$$

where (r_1, r_2) are two changepoints and $\theta_1 \neq \theta_2 \neq \theta_3$. Using the standard exponential prior distributions, specified by letting $a_j = b_j = 1$ $(j = 1, 2, 3)$ in (4.32), we obtained exact joint posterior probabilities for the changepoint pair (r_1, r_2) from (4.34). Two changepoints occur at $r_1 = 7$ and $r_2 = 15$ (i.e., Year 1976 and Year 1984) with the joint posterior probability being 0.3589. Based on (4.34) and (4.33), we generated 20,000 i.i.d. posterior samples. The resulting Bayes estimates of parameters are given in Table 4.11. Figure 4.4(a) and 4.4(b) display the histograms of r_1 and r_2. Figure 4.4(c) shows the posterior densities of θ_j $(j = 1, 2, 3)$. Figure 4.4(d) depicts the annual numbers of HUS, two identified changepoints, and the average number of cases before and after the two changepoints. $\|$

4.8 Capture-Recapture Model

The capture-recapture models are widely used in the estimation of population sizes and related parameters such as survival rates, birth rates and migration rates (George & Robert, 1992). The models are generally classified as either closed or open (Chao, 1998). In a closed model, the size of a population is assumed to be constant during the time of the investigation. Thus, the closed model can be applied to epidemiology and health science such as birth defects, cancers, drug use, infectious diseases, injures and diabetes.

Let N be the unknown size of the population of interest and s be the number of samples taken. The probability that an individual animal is captured in sample i is θ_i $(i = 1, \dots, s)$ and $\theta = (\theta_1, \dots, \theta_s)^\top$. We denote n_i for the number of animals in sample i, m_i for the number of marked animals in sample i and M_i for the number of marked animals in the population just before the i-th sample. Then, $M_{i+1} = M_i + n_i - m_i$. Suppose that

(i) the population remains constant throughout the experiment;

(ii) there are initially no marked animals, $M_1 = 0$ and $m_1 = n_1$;

(iii) in a given sample, all animals have the same probability of being caught, regardless of their previous history of being caught.

Let $Y_{\text{obs}} = \{n_i, m_i\}_{i=1}^s$ denote the observed data, then, the likelihood function is (Castledine, 1981)

$$\begin{aligned} L(N, \theta|Y_{\text{obs}}) &= f(m_1, \dots, m_s|n_1, \dots, n_s, N, \theta) f(n_1, \dots, n_s|N, \theta) \\ &= \prod_{i=1}^s \binom{N - M_i}{n_i - m_i} \binom{M_i}{m_i} \theta_i^{n_i} (1 - \theta_i)^{N - n_i} \\ &\propto \frac{N!}{(N - r)!} \prod_{i=1}^s \theta_i^{n_i} (1 - \theta_i)^{N - n_i}, \end{aligned}$$

where

$$r = \sum_{i=1}^s (n_i - m_i) \hat{=} n. - m.$$

is the total number of different captured animals. We note that sufficient statistics for the problem are $\{n_1, \dots, n_s, m.\}$.

The independent priors of the form $\pi(N) \times \pi(\theta)$ lead to the following full conditional distributions:

$$f(N|Y_{\text{obs}}, \theta) \quad \propto \quad \pi(N) \times \frac{N!}{(N-r)!} \prod_{i=1}^{s} (1-\theta_i)^N, \tag{4.37}$$

$$f(\theta|Y_{\text{obs}}, N) \quad \propto \quad \pi(\theta) \times \prod_{i=1}^{s} \theta_i^{n_i}(1-\theta_i)^{N-n_i}. \tag{4.38}$$

In the special case where the θ_i's are **a priori** independent,

$$\pi(\theta) = \prod_{i=1}^{s} \text{Beta}(\theta_i|a, b),$$

it is easy to see that (4.38) becomes

$$f(\theta|Y_{\text{obs}}, N) = \prod_{i=1}^{s} \text{Beta}(\theta_i|n_i + a, N - n_i + b). \tag{4.39}$$

By using (4.1) with $\theta_0 = (0.5, \ldots, 0.5)^{\top}$, we have

$$f(N|Y_{\text{obs}}) = c^{-1} \times \pi(N) \frac{N!}{(N-r)!} \prod_{i=1}^{s} \frac{\Gamma(N - n_i + b)}{\Gamma(N + a + b)}, \tag{4.40}$$

where $N = r, r+1, \ldots$ and the normalizing constant c does not depend on N. Thus, (4.40) can be computed by the following recursion:

$$\frac{f(N+1|Y_{\text{obs}})}{f(N|Y_{\text{obs}})} = \frac{\pi(N+1)}{\pi(N)} \times \frac{N+1}{N+1-r} \prod_{i=1}^{s} \frac{N - n_i + b}{N + a + b}.$$

Using Jeffreys' prior: $\pi(N) \propto 1/N$, we obtain

$$\begin{aligned} f(N = r|Y_{\text{obs}}) &= c^{-1} \times (r-1)! \frac{\prod_{i=1}^{s} \Gamma(r - n_i + b)}{[\Gamma(r + a + b)]^s}, \\ \frac{f(N+1|Y_{\text{obs}})}{f(N|Y_{\text{obs}})} &= \frac{N}{N+1-r} \times \frac{\prod_{i=1}^{s}(N - n_i + b)}{(N + a + b)^s}. \end{aligned} \tag{4.41}$$

Therefore, based on (4.41) and (4.39), the implementation of the exact IBF sampling is straightforward.

Example 4.3 (*Gordy Lake sunfish data*). Table 4.12 consists of $s = 14$ capture occasions from a population of sunfish. At the i-th capture, n_i fish are captured out of which m_i have been previously captured. Therefore, $r = \Sigma(n_i - m_i) = 138$ is the total number of different fish captured.

Table 4.12 *Capture-recapture counts of Gordy Lake sunfish data*

i	1	2	3	4	5	6	7	8	9	10	11	12	13	14
n_i	10	27	17	7	1	5	6	15	9	18	16	5	7	19
m_i	0	0	0	0	0	0	2	1	5	5	4	2	2	3

Source: Castledine (1981).

We analyze this data by using the prior formulation

$$\pi(N) \times \prod_{i=1}^{s} \pi(\theta_i|a, b)$$

with Jeffreys' prior

$$\pi(N) \propto 1/N \quad \text{and} \quad \pi(\theta_i|a, b) = \text{Beta}(\theta_i|a, b)$$

for four different pairs (a, b). Note that $(a, b) = (1, 1)$ is corresponding to the uniform prior, $(a, b) = (0, 0)$ is the noninformative prior,

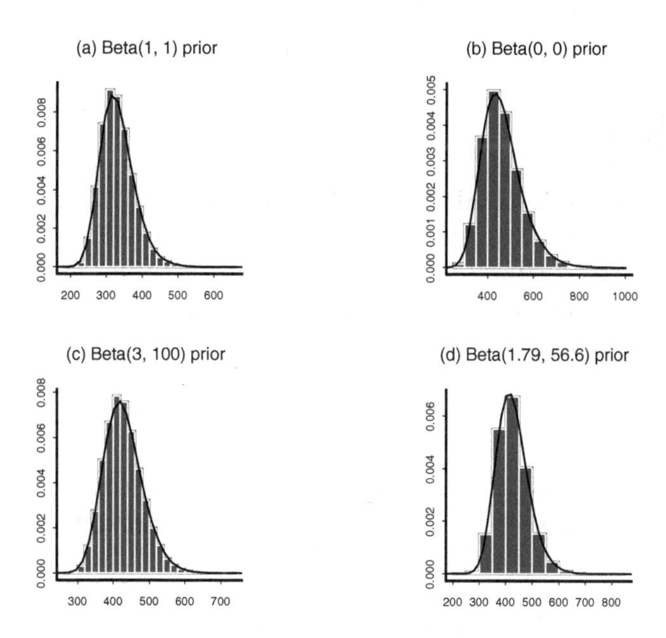

Figure 4.5 Histograms of the population size N for the Gordy Lake sunfish data using the prior formulation $\pi(N) \times \Pi_{i=1}^{14} \pi(\theta_i|a, b)$ with Jeffreys' prior $\pi(N) \propto 1/N$ and $\pi(\theta_i|a, b) = \text{Beta}(\theta_i|a, b)$ for four different (a, b). (a) Uniform prior $a = b = 1$; (b) Noninformative prior $a = b = 0$; (c) Informative prior $a = 3$ and $b = 100$; (d) Empirical Bayes prior $a = 1.79$ and $b = 56.6$.

$(a,b) = (3, 100)$ can be viewed as an informative prior, and $(a,b) = (1.79, 56.6)$, which maximizes the likelihood, is motivated as the empirical Bayes prior.

Table 4.13 *Posterior estimates of N for various a and b*

a	b	Bayesian mean	Bayesian std	95% Bayesian CI
1	1	330.879	45.247	[256, 433]
0	0	462.159	86.175	[328, 663]
3	100	428.007	52.900	[337, 544]
1.79	56.6	426.407	58.264	[329, 556]

For each prior, we first compute $f(N|Y_{\text{obs}})$ based on (4.41) for $N = r, r+1, \dots, N_{\max}$ (say, $N_{\max} = 1{,}000$). Then we generate $L = 50{,}000$ i.i.d. posterior samples of N from $f(N|Y_{\text{obs}})$. Table 4.13 lists posterior mean, standard deviation and a 95% credible interval for N obtained from the 2.5% and 97.5% quantiles. Figure 4.5 shows the four corresponding histograms of N. ‖

Problems

4.1 Grouped Dirichlet distribution (Tang *et al.*, 2007; Ng *et al.*, 2008). An n-vector $x \in \mathbb{T}_n$ is said to follow a *grouped Dirichlet distribution* (GDD) with two partitions, if the density of $x_{-n} \hat{=} (x_1, \dots, x_{n-1})^\top \in \mathbb{V}_{n-1}$ is

$$\begin{aligned} \text{GD}_{n,2,s}(x_{-n}|a,b) &= c_{\text{GD}}^{-1} \times \left(\textstyle\sum_{i=1}^{n} x_i^{a_i-1}\right) \\ &\quad \times \left(\textstyle\sum_{i=1}^{s} x_i\right)^{b_1} \left(\textstyle\sum_{i=s+1}^{n} x_i\right)^{b_2}, \quad (4.42) \end{aligned}$$

where $a = (a_1, \dots, a_n)^\top$ and $b = (b_1, b_2)^\top$ are two nonnegative parameter vectors, s is a known positive integer less than n and the normalizing constant is given by

$$\begin{aligned} c_{\text{GD}} &= B(a_1, \dots, a_s) \times B(a_{s+1}, \dots, a_n) \\ &\quad \times B\left(\textstyle\sum_{i=1}^{s} a_i + b_1,\ \sum_{i=s+1}^{n} a_i + b_2\right). \end{aligned}$$

We write $x \sim \text{GD}_{n,2,s}(a,b)$ on $\mathbb{T}_n$ or $x_{-n} \sim \text{GD}_{n,2,s}(a,b)$ on $\mathbb{V}_{n-1}$ accordingly. Especially, when $b_1 = b_2 = 0$ the GDD (4.42) reduces to $\text{Dirichlet}_n(a)$. Show that

(a) Let $x^{(1)} = (x_1, \ldots, x_s)^\top$. An n-vector $x = (x^{(1)\top}, x^{(2)\top})^\top \sim \mathrm{GD}_{n,2,s}(a, b)$ on $\mathbb{T}_n$ iff

$$x = \begin{pmatrix} x^{(1)} \\ x^{(2)} \end{pmatrix} \stackrel{d}{=} \begin{pmatrix} R \cdot y^{(1)} \\ (1-R) \cdot y^{(2)} \end{pmatrix} \tag{4.43}$$

where $y^{(1)}$, $y^{(2)}$ and R are mutually independent,

$$\begin{aligned} y^{(1)} &\sim \text{Dirichlet}(a_1, \ldots, a_s) \text{ on } \mathbb{T}_s, \\ y^{(2)} &\sim \text{Dirichlet}(a_{s+1}, \ldots, a_n) \text{ on } \mathbb{T}_{n-s}, \\ R &\sim \text{Beta}(\textstyle\sum_{i=1}^s a_i + b_1,\ \sum_{i=s+1}^n a_i + b_2). \end{aligned}$$

(b) The mode of the grouped Dirichlet density (4.42) is

$$\begin{cases} \hat{x}_i = \dfrac{a_i - 1}{\Delta} \cdot \dfrac{\Delta_1}{\sum_{i=1}^s a_i - s}, & 1 \le i \le s, \\ \hat{x}_i = \dfrac{a_i - 1}{\Delta} \cdot \dfrac{\Delta - \Delta_1}{\sum_{i=s+1}^n a_i - (n-s)}, & s+1 \le i \le n, \end{cases}$$

where $\Delta = \sum_{i=1}^n a_i + b_1 + b_2 - n$ and $\Delta_1 = \sum_{i=1}^s a_i + b_1 - s$.

4.2 Multiplying the likelihood (4.4) by the prior (4.11) results in a grouped Dirichlet posterior distribution. Use (4.43) to generate this posterior and to calculate the corresponding Bayes estimates. Compare them with the results in Table 4.3.

4.3 **Nested Dirichlet distribution** (Tian *et al.*, 2003; Ng *et al.*, 2009). An n-vector $x \in \mathbb{T}_n$ is said to follow a *nested Dirichlet distribution* (NDD), if the density of $x_{-n} \hat{=} (x_1, \ldots, x_{n-1})^\top \in \mathbb{V}_{n-1}$ is

$$\mathrm{ND}_{n,n-1}(x_{-n}|a, b) = c_{\mathrm{ND}}^{-1} \times \prod_{i=1}^n x_i^{a_i - 1} \prod_{j=1}^{n-1} (\textstyle\sum_{k=1}^j x_k)^{b_j}, \tag{4.44}$$

where $a = (a_1, \ldots, a_n)^\top$ are positive parameters, $b = (b_1, \ldots, b_{n-1})^\top$ are nonnegative parameters, and

$$c_{\mathrm{ND}} = \textstyle\prod_{j=1}^{n-1} B(d_j,\ a_{j+1}), \quad d_j \hat{=} \sum_{k=1}^j (a_k + b_k).$$

We will write $x \sim \mathrm{ND}_{n,n-1}(a, b)$ on $\mathbb{T}_n$ or $x_{-n} \sim \mathrm{ND}_{n,n-1}(a, b)$ on $\mathbb{V}_{n-1}$ accordingly. In particular, when all $b_j = 0$ the NDD (4.44) reduces to $\text{Dirichlet}_n(a)$. Verify the following facts:

(a) An n-vector $x \sim \mathrm{ND}_{n,n-1}(a, b)$ on $\mathbb{T}_n$ iff[6]

$$\begin{cases} x_i \stackrel{d}{=} (1 - y_{i-1}) \prod_{j=i}^{n-1} y_j, \ 1 \le i \le n-1, \\ x_n \stackrel{d}{=} 1 - y_{n-1}, \end{cases} \tag{4.45}$$

where $y_0 \hat{=} 0$, $y_j \sim \mathrm{Beta}(d_j, \ a_{j+1})$ and $y_1, \ldots, y_{n-1}$ are mutually independent.

(b) The mode of the nested Dirichlet density (4.44) is[7]

$$\begin{cases} \hat{x}_n = (a_n - 1)/(d_{n-1} + a_n - n), \\ \hat{x}_i = \dfrac{(a_i - 1)(1 - \Sigma_{j=i+1}^n \hat{x}_j)}{d_{i-1} + a_i - i}, \ 2 \le i \le n-1, \\ \hat{x}_1 = 1 - \hat{x}_2 - \cdots - \hat{x}_n. \end{cases} \tag{4.46}$$

4.4 Dental caries data (Paulino & Pereira, 1995). To determine the degree of sensitivity to dental caries, dentists often consider three risk levels: low, medium and high. Each subject will be assigned a risk level based on the spittle color obtained using a coloration technique. However, some subjects may not be fully categorized due to the inability to distinguish adjacent categories. Of 97 subjects, only 51 were fully categorized with $n_1 = 14$, $n_2 = 17$ and $n_3 = 20$ subjects being classified as low, medium and high, respectively. A total of $n_{12} = 28$ subjects were only classified as low or medium risk, and $n_{23} = 18$ as medium or high risk. The primary objective of this study is to estimate the cell probability vector $\theta = (\theta_1, \theta_2, \theta_3)^\top \in \mathbb{T}_3$. Let $Y_{\text{obs}} = \{(n_1, n_2, n_3); (n_{12}, n_{23})\}$ denote the observed counts. Under MAR assumption, the observed-data likelihood is

$$L(\theta|Y_{\text{obs}}) \propto \left\{ \left(\prod_{i=1}^3 \theta_i^{n_i}\right) \theta_1^0 (\theta_1 + \theta_2)^{n_{12}} \right\} \times (\theta_2 + \theta_3)^{n_{23}}.$$

Note that the first term in $L(\theta|Y_{\text{obs}})$ follows the $\mathrm{ND}_{3,2}(a, b)$ with $a = (n_1, n_2, n_3)^\top$ and $b = (0, n_{12})^\top$ up to a normalizing

[6]The SR (4.45) provides a simple procedure for generating i.i.d. samples from NDD, which in turn plays a crucial role in Bayesian analysis for incomplete categorical data. The result indicates that the NDD can be stochastically represented by a sequence of mutually independent beta variates.

[7]Eq.(4.46) gives a closed-form expression for the mode of an NDD density, implying that explicit MLEs of cell probabilities are available in the frequentist analysis of incomplete categorical data.

constant. The problem is to (i) develop an EM algorithm to estimate θ; (ii) use the exact IBF sampling in §4.1 to generate i.i.d. posterior samples of θ.
(*Hint*: Introduce a latent r.v. Z to split $(\theta_2+\theta_3)^{n_{23}}$ and utilize (4.46) to obtain complete-data MLEs.)

4.5 **The triangular model for sensitive surveys** (Yu *et al.*, 2008b). Let $Y = 1$ denote the class of people with a sensitive characteristic (e.g., drug-taking) and $Y = 0$ the complementary class. Let W be a binary and nonsensitive r.v. and be independent of Y. For example, $W = 1$ may represent the class of people who were born between July and December. Without loss of generality, let p be known. The aim is to estimate the proportion $\pi = \Pr(Y = 1)$.

For a face-to-face personal interview, investigators may replace the sensitive question by the tabular form presented in Table 4.14 and ask the respondent to put a tick in the circle or in the triangle formed by the three dots according to his/her truthful status. It is noteworthy that $\{Y = 0, W = 0\}$ represents a nonsensitive subclass. On the other hand, a tick in the triangle indicates the respondent can be either a drug user or a non-drug user born between July and December. Thus, $\{Y = 1\} \cup \{Y = 0, W = 1\}$ can be regarded as a nonsensitive subclass as well. Such mix of sensitive and nonsensitive classes would presumably encourage respondents to not only participate in the survey but also provide truthful responses. This is called **triangular model** by Yu *et al.* (2008b).

Table 4.14 *The triangular model*

Categories	$W = 0$	$W = 1$
$Y = 0$	○	•
$Y = 1$	•	•

Let $Y_{\text{obs}} = \{n, s\}$ denote the observed data for n respondents with s ticks in the triangle. Prove that

(a) The likelihood function is given by

$$L(\pi|Y_{\text{obs}}) \propto [\pi + (1-\pi)p]^s[(1-\pi)(1-p)]^{n-s}.$$

(b) If Beta(a, b) is chosen to be the prior, then the posterior of π takes the following closed-form expression:

$$f(\pi|Y_{\text{obs}}) = c_{\text{T}}^{-1}\cdot\pi^{a-1}(1-\pi)^{b+n-s-1}[\pi+(1-\pi)p]^s, \quad (4.47)$$

where $c_{\mathrm{T}} = \sum_{j=0}^{s}\binom{s}{j}p^{s-j}B(a+j, b+n-j)$.

(c) Let Z be the number of respondents with the sensitive attribute, then

$$\pi|(Y_{\text{obs}}, Z) \sim \text{Beta}(a+Z, b+n-Z), \tag{4.48}$$
$$Z|(Y_{\text{obs}}, \pi) \sim \text{Binomial}(s, \pi/[\pi+(1-\pi)p]). \tag{4.49}$$

(d) Based on (4.48) and (4.49), develop an EM algorithm to compute the posterior mode of π. In addition, compare the exact posterior curve given by (4.47) with the curve estimated by a kernel density smoother based on i.i.d. posterior samples of π generated via the exact IBF sampling.

4.6 Pancreas disorder data (Lee *et al.*, 2004). Table 4.15 reports counts of pancreas disorder *length of stay* (LOS) for a group of 261 patients hospitalized from 1998 to 1999 in Western Australia. The LOS is recorded as discrete count representing the duration between admission and discharge from the hospital. The excess zeros in the data may lead to over-dispersion and hence a Poisson modeling would not suffice. Fit the data with the ZIP model presented in §4.6 and estimate posterior by generating i.i.d. posterior samples for parameters of interest via the exact IBF sampling and the DA algorithm.

Table 4.15 *Observed counts of pancreas disorder data*

LOS in days	0	1	2	3	4	5	6	7	8	9	10	11–14
Frequency	45	35	35	47	40	20	13	8	4	5	3	6

4.7 Continuous changepoint problems (Stephens, 1994). In many applications, the response Y_t is a measurement of some substance of interest at time t so that Y_t is a continuous r.v.. A sequence $\{Y_t\colon t \ge 0\}$ is said to have a continuous changepoint γ if $Y_t \sim f_1(\cdot|\theta_1)$ for $t \le \gamma$ and $Y_t \sim f_2(\cdot|\theta_2)$ for $t > \gamma$. For example, consider the switching straight line regression model:

$$\begin{aligned} Y_t &\sim N(\alpha_1 + \beta_1 t,\ \sigma^2), \quad t \le \gamma, \quad \text{and} \\ Y_t &\sim N(\alpha_2 + \beta_2 t,\ \sigma^2), \quad t > \gamma, \end{aligned} \tag{4.50}$$

where the constraint $\beta_2 = \beta_1 + (\alpha_1 - \alpha_2)/\gamma$ ensures continuity of two straight lines intersecting at the changepoint γ. Thus, the model (4.50) has five unknown parameters, denoted by $(\gamma, \Theta) \hat{=} (\gamma, \alpha_1, \beta_1, \alpha_2, \sigma^2)$. Let $Y_{\text{obs}} = \{y_t\colon 1 \le t \le n\}$ denote a realization of the sequence $\{Y_t\colon t \ge 0\}$ with length n, then the likelihood $L(\gamma, \Theta | Y_{\text{obs}})$ is proportional to

$$\sigma^{-n} \exp\left\{ -\frac{\Sigma_{t \le \gamma}(y_t - \alpha_1 - \beta_1 t)^2 + \Sigma_{t > \gamma}(y_t - \alpha_2 - \beta_2 t)^2}{2\sigma^2} \right\}.$$

Obviously, this likelihood is nonlinear in γ so that the analytic approximation might be inappropriate. In Bayesian settings, using $\pi(\gamma, \Theta)$ as the prior will result in the following posterior

$$f(\gamma, \Theta | Y_{\text{obs}}) \propto L(\gamma, \Theta | Y_{\text{obs}}) \times \pi(\gamma, \Theta). \tag{4.51}$$

Interest centers on the derivation of the marginal posterior distribution of γ as well as that of other parameters.

In general, from (4.51) we can easily obtain $f(\gamma | Y_{\text{obs}}, \Theta)$ known up to a normalizing constant and $f(\Theta | Y_{\text{obs}}, \gamma)$ in closed-form. By applying (4.1), we have an unnormalized density $f(\gamma | Y_{\text{obs}})$. Note that the changepoint γ varies on the interval

$$\Big[\min\{y_1, \ldots, y_n\},\ \max\{y_1, \ldots, y_n\} \Big]. \tag{4.52}$$

The most straightforward procedure for drawing from the continuous pdf $f(\gamma | Y_{\text{obs}})$ is to approximate it with a discrete distribution on a grid of points (cf. Ex.2.13). Specifically, let $\{\gamma_1, \ldots, \gamma_K\}$ denote a set of uniformly spaced values on the interval (4.52). When these points are closely spaced enough (theoretically speaking, $K \to \infty$) and nothing important beyond their boundaries, this method is expected to work well. Implement the procedure and evaluate its performance in general and in conjunction with the next Problem 4.8.

4.8 Renal transplant data (Smith & Cook, 1980). Table 4.16 contains data from two patients who have each undergone a failed kidney transplant, where the observed response Y_t is the level of a substance reflecting the healthy or otherwise functioning of the transplanted kidney. The changepoint denotes the point in time at which the kidney is rejected. The data model is presumed to be that in Eq.(4.50), the model is assumed to be continuous in time and all the parameters are unknown. Use the method introduced in Problem 4.7 to generate posterior densities for the changepoint positions and other parameters for both patients.

Table 4.16 *Renal transplant data*

t	1	2	3	4	5	6	7	8	9	10
Patient A	48.6	58.0	62.3	71.9	80.6	54.8	49.3	43.4	–	–
Patient B	36.8	46.5	50.8	66.2	75.0	71.5	68.5	60.5	31.5	19

4.9 Capture-recapture model with complex priors (George & Robert, 1992). Recall (4.37) and (4.38). In some situations, more complicated priors such as a truncated Poisson prior on N and a logit prior on the θ_i's may be more appropriate, i.e.,

$$\begin{aligned} \pi(N) &\propto \lambda_0^N e^{-\lambda_0}/N!, \quad N = r,\ r+1, \dots, \\ \alpha_i = \text{logit}(\theta_i) &\sim N(\mu_i, \sigma_0^2), \quad i = 1, \dots, s, \end{aligned}$$

where λ_0 and σ_0^2 are known. Let $\alpha = (\alpha_1, \dots, \alpha_s)^\top$. Prove that (4.37) and (4.38) become

$$N - r|(Y_{\text{obs}}, \alpha) \sim \text{Poisson}(\lambda_0 \textstyle\prod_{i=1}^s (1+e^{\alpha_i})^{-1}), \tag{4.53}$$

$$f(\alpha|Y_{\text{obs}}, N) = \prod_{i=1}^s f(\alpha_i|Y_{\text{obs}}, N), \tag{4.54}$$

$$f(\alpha_i|Y_{\text{obs}}, N) \propto \frac{\exp[\alpha_i n_i - (\alpha_i - \mu_i)^2/(2\sigma_0^2)]}{(1+e^{\alpha_i})^N}. \tag{4.55}$$

Note that (4.55) is log concave in α_i, then these α_i's can be simulated by the rejection method (cf. §2.2.2(c)). Therefore, the Gibbs sampler applies to (4.53) and (4.54). Since (4.55) is known up to a normalizing constant, the exact IBF sampling is not available for the current situation. However, the IBF sampler introduced in the next chapter is a possibility.

CHAPTER 5

Computing Posteriors in the EM-Type Structures

In the previous chapter, we introduced a noniterative sampling procedure (i.e., the exact IBF sampling) to obtain i.i.d. samples **exactly** from an observed posterior distribution for discrete MDPs. Generally, the exact IBF sampling is feasible only when the discrete latent vector (or missing data) Z is of low dimension. For more general cases (e.g., Problem 4.9, or when Z is discrete but of high dimension, or when Z is continuous and so on), the noniterative sampling method may need to be modified.

The purpose of this chapter is to develop such a noniterative sampling method (called IBF sampler), as opposed to the iterative sampling in an MCMC, for computing posteriors based on IBF and SIR to obtain i.i.d. samples **approximately** from the observed posterior distribution while utilizing the posterior mode and structure from an EM-type algorithm. The idea of the IBF sampler in the EM framework is to use EM algorithm to obtain an optimal importance sampling density and the sampling IBF to get i.i.d. samples from the posterior. Specifically,

- First, we augment the observed data with latent data and obtain the structure of augmented posterior/conditional predictive distributions as in the EM or the DA algorithm;

- Then, in the class of built-in *importance sampling densities* (ISDs) provided by the sampling IBF, we choose the best ISD by using preliminary estimates from the EM algorithm so that the overlap area under the target density and the ISD is large;

- Finally the sampling IBF and SIR are combined to generate i.i.d. samples approximately from the observed posterior distribution.

The synergy of IBF, EM and SIR creates an attractive sampling approach for Bayesian computation. Since the sampling IBF and the EM share the DA structure, the IBF sampler via the EM does not require extra derivations, and can be applied to problems where the EM is applicable while obtaining the whole posterior.

In §5.1, we present the IBF sampler in the DA-type structure and theoretically justify an optimal choice of ISD. In §5.2–§5.7, we illustrate the noniterative algorithm with incomplete pre-post test problems, the right censored regression model, linear mixed models for longitudinal data, the probit regression model, the probit-normal GLMM, hierarchical models for correlated binary data and several related real datasets. In §5.8, we propose a hybrid algorithm by combining the IBF sampler with the Gibbs sampler. As another application of the IBF sampler, two monitoring approaches for assessing the convergence of an MCMC are introduced in §5.9 after the introduction of the well-known Gelman–Rubin statistic. Some remarks are presented in §5.10.

5.1 The IBF Method

In this section, we first develop an IBF sampling approach in the EM structure. Then, we extend it to more complicated situations — the ECM structure and the Monte Carlo EM structure.

5.1.1 The IBF sampling in the EM structure

Again let $Y_{\rm obs}$ denote the observed data and θ the parameter vector of interest. The observed data $Y_{\rm obs}$ are augmented with latent variables (or missing data) Z to build augmented (or complete-data) posterior distribution $f(\theta|Y_{\rm obs}, Z)$ and conditional predictive distribution $f(Z|Y_{\rm obs}, \theta)$. Let $\tilde{\theta}$ denote the mode of the observed posterior density $f(\theta|Y_{\rm obs})$ and $\mathcal{S}_{(\theta,Z|Y_{\rm obs})}$, $\mathcal{S}_{(\theta|Y_{\rm obs})}$ and $\mathcal{S}_{(Z|Y_{\rm obs})}$ denote the supports of $(\theta, Z)|Y_{\rm obs}$, $\theta|Y_{\rm obs}$ and $Z|Y_{\rm obs}$, respectively. In this subsection, we make the following three basic assumptions:

- Both $f(\theta|Y_{\rm obs}, Z)$ and $f(Z|Y_{\rm obs}, \theta)$ are available;[1]

- The posterior mode $\tilde{\theta}$ is already obtained via an EM algorithm;

- The joint support is a product space, i.e.,

$$\mathcal{S}_{(\theta,Z|Y_{\rm obs})} = \mathcal{S}_{(\theta|Y_{\rm obs})} \times \mathcal{S}_{(Z|Y_{\rm obs})}.$$

[1]With "available," we mean that both densities have closed-form expressions or they can easily be evaluated or sampled.

The goal is to obtain i.i.d. posterior samples from $f(\theta|Y_{\text{obs}})$.

(a) Formulation of the IBF sampler

According to the discussion in the second paragraph of §4.1, the key is to be able to generate independent samples from $f(Z|Y_{\text{obs}})$. This can be achieved by using the sampling IBF (4.1). For convenience, we rewrite (4.1) as follows:

$$f(Z|Y_{\text{obs}}) \propto \frac{f(Z|Y_{\text{obs}}, \theta_0)}{f(\theta_0|Y_{\text{obs}}, Z)}, \tag{5.1}$$

for some arbitrary $\theta_0 \in \mathcal{S}_{(\theta|Y_{\text{obs}})}$ and all $Z \in \mathcal{S}_{(Z|Y_{\text{obs}})}$. In general, $\mathcal{S}_{(\theta|Y_{\text{obs}})} = \mathcal{S}_\theta$, but $\mathcal{S}_{(Z|Y_{\text{obs}})} \neq \mathcal{S}_Z$.[2] Considering the conditional predictive density as an approximation to the marginal predictive density $f(Z|Y_{\text{obs}})$, the IBF sampling is realized via SIR[3] as follows.

THE IBF SAMPLER:

Calculate the posterior mode $\tilde{\theta}$ via an EM algorithm based on $f(\theta|Y_{\text{obs}}, Z)$ and $f(Z|Y_{\text{obs}}, \theta)$, and set $\theta_0 = \tilde{\theta}$;[4]

Step 1. Draw J i.i.d. samples $\{Z^{(j)}\}_{j=1}^J$ of Z from $f(Z|Y_{\text{obs}}, \theta_0)$;

Step 2. Calculate the reciprocals of the augmented posterior densities to obtain the weights

$$\omega_j = \frac{f^{-1}(\theta_0|Y_{\text{obs}}, Z^{(j)})}{\sum_{\ell=1}^J f^{-1}(\theta_0|Y_{\text{obs}}, Z^{(\ell)})}, \quad j = 1, \dots, J; \tag{5.2}$$

Step 3. Choose a subset from $\{Z^{(j)}\}_1^J$ via resampling **without replacement** from the discrete distribution on $\{Z^{(j)}\}$ with probabilities $\{\omega_j\}_1^J$ to obtain an i.i.d. sample of size I ($< J$) approximately from $f(Z|Y_{\text{obs}})$, denoted them by $\{Z^{(k_i)}\}_1^I$;

Step 4. Generate $\theta^{(i)} \sim f(\theta|Y_{\text{obs}}, Z^{(k_i)})$ for $i = 1, \dots, I$, then $\{\theta^{(i)}\}_1^I$ are i.i.d. samples from $f(\theta|Y_{\text{obs}})$.

---

[2]For example, in §5.3, we have $\mathcal{S}_{(Z|Y_{\text{obs}})} = \prod_{i=r+1}^m (c_i, +\infty) \neq \mathbb{R}^{m-r} = \mathcal{S}_Z$.

[3]See §2.2.3 for more details on Rubin's *sampling/importance resampling* (SIR) method.

[4]A theoretical justification is given in Theorem 5.1.

Remark 5.1 Since a subset of independent r.v.'s is still independent, in the IBF sampler, $\{Z^{(k_i)}\}_1^I$ is an independent sample. However, resampling **with replacement** would result in dependent samples. The second part of Step 3, i.e., "resampling from the discrete distribution on $\{Z^{(j)}\}$ with probabilities $\{\omega_j\}_1^J$," implies $\{Z^{(k_i)}\}_1^I$ are approximately from $f(Z|Y_{\text{obs}})$ with the approximation "improving" as J increases (Smith & Gelfand, 1992). ¶

Remark 5.2 The weights $\{\omega_j\}$ defined in (5.2) differ fundamentally from those associated with the harmonic mean estimate of Newton & Raftery (1994) which, as pointed out by Gelfand & Dey (1994), is likely to suffer from numeric instability since the reciprocals of augmented posterior densities may approach infinity. However, in the IBF sampler, the weights $\{\omega_j\}$ are **ratios** that are free from this kind of numeric instability. In fact, for any j_0 $(1 \le j_0 \le J)$, if $f^{-1}(\theta_0|Y_{\text{obs}}, Z^{(j_0)}) \to \infty$, we have

$$\omega_{j_0} = \left\{ 1 + \sum_{\ell=1,\, \ell \ne j_0}^{J} \frac{f^{-1}(\theta_0|Y_{\text{obs}}, Z^{(\ell)})}{f^{-1}(\theta_0|Y_{\text{obs}}, Z^{(j_0)})} \right\}^{-1} \to 1.$$

When J is very large, say $J = 10^5$, some weights will be extremely small. Empirically, the use of the exponent of the logarithm of the ratio in calculating weights $\{\omega_j\}$ increases numeric accuracy. ¶

(b) Theoretical justification for choosing $\theta_0 = \tilde{\theta}$

It is worth noting that only one pre-specified θ_0 is needed for the whole IBF sampling process although the sampling IBF (5.1) holds for any θ_0 in the support of $\theta|Y_{\text{obs}}$. Clearly, the sampling IBF (5.1) provides a natural class of ISDs:

$$\Big\{ f(Z|Y_{\text{obs}}, \theta) \colon \ \theta \in \mathcal{S}_{(\theta|Y_{\text{obs}})} \Big\},$$

which are available from the model specification. However, the efficiency of the IBF sampler depends on how well the ISD approximates the target function $f(Z|Y_{\text{obs}})$. Since (5.1) holds for any given $\theta_0 \in \mathcal{S}_{(\theta|Y_{\text{obs}})}$, it suffices to select a θ_0 such that $f(Z|Y_{\text{obs}}, \theta_0)$ best approximates $f(Z|Y_{\text{obs}})$. Heuristically, if θ_0 is chosen to be the observed posterior mode $\tilde{\theta}$, the overlap area under the two functions would be substantial since the approximation is accurate to the order of $O(1/n)$, as shown in the following theorem.

Theorem 5.1 (Tan, Tian & Ng, 2003). Let the observed posterior density $f(\theta|Y_{\rm obs})$ be unimodal with mode $\tilde{\theta}$ and n be the sample size of the observed data $Y_{\rm obs}$. Then

$$f(Z|Y_{\rm obs}) = f(Z|Y_{\rm obs}, \tilde{\theta})\{1 + O(1/n)\}. \qquad ¶ \quad (5.3)$$

PROOF. Let $g(\theta)$ be an arbitrarily smooth, positive function for $\theta \in \mathcal{S}_{(\theta|Y_{\rm obs})} \subseteq \mathbb{R}^d$, $L(\theta|Y_{\rm obs})$ be the likelihood function and $\pi(\theta)$ be the prior. The posterior mean of $g(\theta)$ is given by

$$\begin{aligned} E\{g(\theta)|Y_{\rm obs}\} &= \int_{\mathcal{S}_{(\theta|Y_{\rm obs})}} g(\theta) f(\theta|Y_{\rm obs})\, d\theta \\ &= \frac{\int g(\theta) \exp\{n\,\ell(\theta)\}\, d\theta}{\int \exp\{n\,\ell(\theta)\}\, d\theta}, \end{aligned} \qquad (5.4)$$

where

$$n\,\ell(\theta) = \log\{L(\theta|Y_{\rm obs})\pi(\theta)\} \propto \log\{f(\theta|Y_{\rm obs})\}.$$

Thus $\ell(\theta)$ has the same mode as $f(\theta|Y_{\rm obs})$, i.e., $\ell'(\tilde{\theta}) = 0$. Applying Laplace's method to the numerator in (5.4) gives

$$\int g(\theta) \exp\{n\,\ell(\theta)\}\, d\theta \doteq g(\tilde{\theta}) \exp\{n\,\ell(\tilde{\theta})\} \Big(\frac{2\pi}{n}\Big)^{d/2} |\Sigma|^{1/2},$$

where

$$\Sigma_{d\times d} = -\left(\frac{\partial^2 \ell(\tilde{\theta})}{\partial\theta\,\partial\theta^{\top}}\right)^{-1}.$$

Similarly, for the denominator in (5.4), we have

$$\int \exp\{n\,\ell(\theta)\}\, d\theta \doteq \exp\{n\,\ell(\tilde{\theta})\} \Big(\frac{2\pi}{n}\Big)^{d/2} |\Sigma|^{1/2}.$$

The resulting ratio is $g(\tilde{\theta})$ up to error $O(1/n)$ as shown in Tierney & Kadane (1986). Thus,

$$E\{g(\theta)|Y_{\rm obs}\} = g(\tilde{\theta})\{1 + O(1/n)\}.$$

Since $f(Z|Y_{\rm obs}) = \int f(Z|Y_{\rm obs}, \theta) f(\theta|Y_{\rm obs})\, d\theta = E\{f(Z|Y_{\rm obs}, \theta)|Y_{\rm obs}\}$, (5.3) follows immediately. ||END||

Example 5.1 (*The genetic linkage model revisited*). To illustrate the IBF sampler, we revisit the genetic linkage model introduced in §3.3 with observed data specified by $Y_{\rm obs} = (y_1, y_2, y_3, y_4)^{\top} = (125, 18, 20, 34)^{\top}$. We first use the EM algorithm to compute the posterior mode $\tilde{\theta}$. Based on (3.2) and (3.3), both E-step and M-step have following closed-form expressions:

$$z^{(t)} = \frac{y_1\theta^{(t)}}{\theta^{(t)}+2}, \quad \theta^{(t+1)} = \frac{a+y_4+z^{(t)}-1}{(a+y_4+z^{(t)}-1)+(b+y_2+y_3-1)}.$$

Setting $\theta^{(0)} = 0.5$ and $a = b = 1$ corresponding to the uniform prior, the EM converged to $\tilde{\theta} = 0.6268$ after four iterations.

We implement the IBF sampler based on (5.1) by generating

$$Z^{(j)} \overset{\text{iid}}{\sim} \text{Binomial}(y_1, \tilde{\theta}/(\tilde{\theta}+2)), \quad j = 1, \dots, J,$$

with $J = 30{,}000$ and computing the weights $\{\omega_j\}$ according to (5.2). Then resample without replacement from the discrete distribution on $\{Z^{(j)}\}$ with probabilities $\{\omega_j\}$ to obtain an i.i.d. sample of size $I = 10{,}000$ approximately from $f(Z|Y_{\text{obs}})$, denoted by $\{Z^{(k_i)}\}_{i=1}^{I}$. Finally, we generate

$$\theta^{(i)} \overset{\text{ind}}{\sim} \text{Beta}(1+y_4+Z^{(k_i)},\ 1+y_2+y_3), \quad i = 1, \dots, I,$$

then $\{\theta^{(i)}\}_1^I$ are i.i.d. posterior samples from $f(\theta|Y_{\text{obs}})$.

The accuracy of the IBF sampler is remarkable as shown in Figure 5.1(a), where the solid curve is given exactly by (3.4) while the

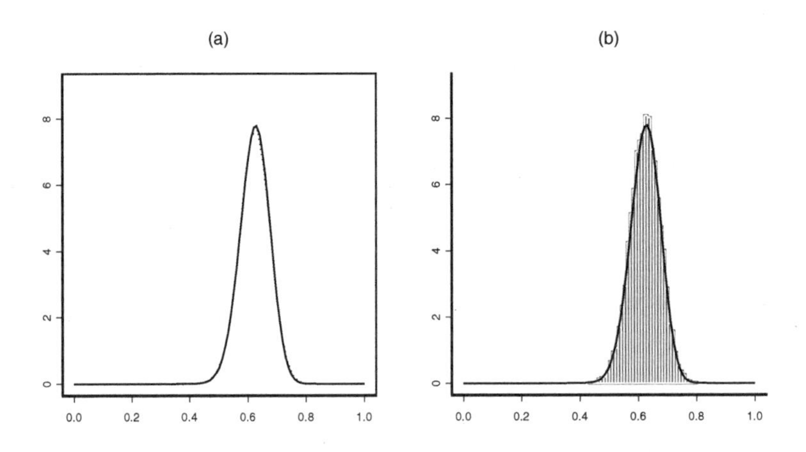

Figure 5.1 (a) The comparison between the observed posterior density of θ (solid curve) given exactly by (3.4) with the dotted curve estimated by a kernel density smoother based on i.i.d. samples obtained via the IBF sampler ($J = 30{,}000$, $I = 10{,}000$, without replacement). (b) The histogram of θ based on $I = 10{,}000$ i.i.d. samples generated via the IBF sampler.

dotted curve is estimated by a kernel density smoother based on these i.i.d. IBF output. In addition, the histogram based on these samples is plotted in Figure 5.1(b), which shows that the IBF sampler has recovered the density completely. ||

(c) IBF sampling: An alternative

An alternative sampling method can be derived by exchanging the role of θ and Z in sampling IBF (5.1). The observed posterior is then given by

$$f(\theta|Y_{\text{obs}}) \propto \frac{f(\theta|Y_{\text{obs}}, Z_0)}{f(Z_0|Y_{\text{obs}}, \theta)}, \tag{5.5}$$

for some arbitrary $Z_0 \in \mathcal{S}_{(Z|Y_{\text{obs}})}$ and all $\theta \in \mathcal{S}_{(\theta|Y_{\text{obs}})}$. Similarly, the sampling IBF (5.5) can always be combined with SIR using $f(\theta|Y_{\text{obs}}, Z_0)$ as the ISD to generate i.i.d. samples approximately from the observed posterior.

Now the key is to be able to find a Z_0 such that $f(\theta|Y_{\text{obs}}, Z_0)$ approximates $f(\theta|Y_{\text{obs}})$ well. The idea is to simply take the Z_0 at which the EM algorithm for finding the observed mode $\tilde{\theta}$ converges. When Z is a continuous random variable (or vector), we choose

$$Z_0 = E(Z|Y_{\text{obs}}, \tilde{\theta}), \quad Z_0 \in \mathcal{S}_{(Z|Y_{\text{obs}})}. \tag{5.6}$$

A real example based on right censored regression model will be presented in §5.3 to illustrate this approach.

When Z is discrete, Z_0 obtained from (5.6) may not belong to $\mathcal{S}_{(Z|Y_{\text{obs}})}$. Let $\tilde{\theta}_{\text{aug}}(Z)$ denote the mode of the augmented posterior density $f(\theta|Y_{\text{obs}}, Z)$, then, we choose the $Z_0 \in \mathcal{S}_{(Z|Y_{\text{obs}})}$ such that the distance between $\tilde{\theta}_{\text{aug}}(Z)$ and $\tilde{\theta}$ is minimized, i.e.,

$$Z_0 = \arg \min_{z \in \mathcal{S}_{(Z|Y_{\text{obs}})}} ||\tilde{\theta}_{\text{aug}}(Z) - \tilde{\theta}||. \tag{5.7}$$

Note that both $f(\theta|Y_{\text{obs}})$ and $f(\theta|Y_{\text{obs}}, Z_0)$ with Z_0 given by (5.6) or (5.7) share the mode $\tilde{\theta}$, thus there is substantial overlap in the areas under the target density curve and the ISD.

Example 5.2 (*The triangular model revisited*). To illustrate this alternative IBF sampler with discrete latent variable Z, we revisit the triangular model introduced in Problem 4.5 with observed data $Y_{\text{obs}} = \{n, s\} = \{346, 258\}$. We first use the EM algorithm to find the best Z_0. Based on (4.49) and (4.48), both E-step and M-step have following explicit expressions:

$$z^{(t)} = \frac{s\pi^{(t)}}{\pi^{(t)} + (1 - \pi^{(t)})p}, \qquad \pi^{(t+1)} = \frac{a + z^{(t)} - 1}{a + b + n - 2}.$$

Setting $\pi^{(0)} = 0.5$, $p = 0.5$ and $a = b = 1$ corresponding to the uniform prior, the EM algorithm converges in 28 iterations. The resultant posterior mode of π is $\tilde{\pi} = 0.49133$. Therefore, from (5.6), we have

$$Z_0 = \frac{s\tilde{\pi}}{\tilde{\pi} + (1 - \tilde{\pi})p} = 170.01.$$

Since Z is a discrete variable, Z_0 should be an integer belonging to $\mathcal{S}_{(Z|Y_{\text{obs}})} = \{0, 1, \ldots, s\}$. From (5.7), we have

$$\tilde{\pi}_{\text{aug}}(Z) - \tilde{\pi} = \frac{a + Z - 1}{a + b + n - 2} - 0.49133.$$

Note that $||\tilde{\pi}_{\text{aug}}(170) - \tilde{\pi}|| = 5.3 \times 10^{-6} \le 0.00289 = ||\tilde{\pi}_{\text{aug}}(171) - \tilde{\pi}||$, we choose $Z_0 = 170$.

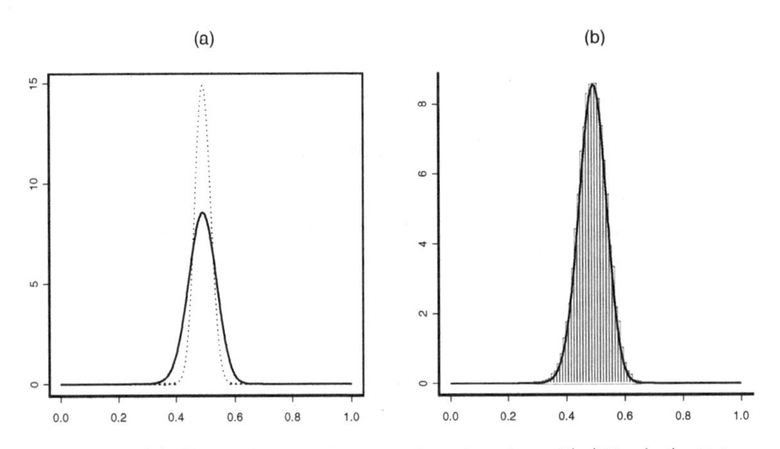

Figure 5.2 (a) The observed posterior density $f(\pi|Y_{\text{obs}})$ (solid curve) given exactly by (4.47) and the augmented posterior density $f(\pi|Y_{\text{obs}}, Z_0) = \text{Beta}(\pi|a + Z_0, b + n - Z_0)$ with $Z_0 = 170$ (dotted curve) share the mode $\tilde{\pi} = 0.49133$. (b) The histogram of π based on i.i.d. samples obtained via the alternative IBF sampler ($J = 30{,}000$, $I = 10{,}000$, without replacement) entirely recovers the $f(\pi|Y_{\text{obs}})$ (solid curve) given exactly by (4.47).

Figure 5.2(a) shows that as the best ISD, the augmented posterior $f(\pi|Y_{\text{obs}}, 170) = \text{Beta}(\pi|a + 170, b + n - 170)$ and the observed posterior $f(\pi|Y_{\text{obs}})$ given exactly by (4.47) overlap most in the class of ISDs

$$\Big\{\text{Beta}(\pi|a+Z, b+n-Z)\colon\ Z=0,1,\ldots,s\Big\}$$

since both curves share the mode $\tilde{\pi} = 0.49133$.

We implement the alternative IBF sampling based on (5.5) by first drawing $J = 30{,}000$ i.i.d. samples $\{\pi^{(j)}\}_{j=1}^{J}$ from $f(\pi|Y_{\text{obs}}, 170)$ so that the weights are given by

$$\omega_j \propto f^{-1}(170|Y_{\text{obs}}, \pi^{(j)}), \quad j = 1, \ldots, J.$$

Then, we resample without replacement from the discrete distribution on $\{\pi^{(j)}\}$ with probabilities $\{\omega_j\}$ to obtain an i.i.d. sample of size $I = 10{,}000$ from $f(\pi|Y_{\text{obs}})$. Based on these samples, the histogram is plotted in Figure 5.2(b), which shows that this alternative IBF sampling entirely recovers the $f(\pi|Y_{\text{obs}})$ (solid curve in Figure 5.2(b)) given exactly by (4.47). ||

5.1.2 The IBF sampling in the ECM structure

In the beginning of §5.1.1, we assumed that the complete-data posterior $f(\theta|Y_{\text{obs}}, Z)$ and the conditional predictive density $f(Z|Y_{\text{obs}}, \theta)$ have closed-form expressions so that the EM algorithm can be applied. However, we often encounter the situation where only one has explicit expression while the other does not. In this subsection, we present an IBF sampling in ECM (Meng & Rubin, 1993) structure where the E-step is simple but the M-step is complicated. This means that there are closed-form expectations with respect to $f(Z|Y_{\text{obs}}, \theta)$ and the complete-data posterior mode associated to $f(\theta|Y_{\text{obs}}, Z)$ does not have closed-form expression. In such cases, one may partition θ into θ_1 and θ_2 so that both $f(\theta_1|Y_{\text{obs}}, Z, \theta_2)$ and $f(\theta_2|Y_{\text{obs}}, Z, \theta_1)$ are available. Therefore, we can first use ECM algorithm to obtain the posterior mode $\tilde{\theta} = (\tilde{\theta}_1, \tilde{\theta}_2)$ and the corresponding

$$Z_0 = E(Z|Y_{\text{obs}}, \tilde{\theta}),$$

then apply (5.5) twice, namely,

$$f(\theta_2|Y_{\text{obs}}, Z_0) \propto \frac{f(\theta_2|Y_{\text{obs}}, Z_0, \tilde{\theta}_1)}{f(\tilde{\theta}_1|Y_{\text{obs}}, Z_0, \theta_2)}, \tag{5.8}$$

$$f(\theta_1, \theta_2|Y_{\text{obs}}, Z_0) = f(\theta_1|Y_{\text{obs}}, Z_0, \theta_2) \cdot f(\theta_2|Y_{\text{obs}}, Z_0), \tag{5.9}$$

$$f(\theta_1, \theta_2|Y_{\text{obs}}) \propto \frac{f(\theta_1, \theta_2|Y_{\text{obs}}, Z_0)}{f(Z_0|Y_{\text{obs}}, \theta_1, \theta_2)}, \tag{5.10}$$

to obtain i.i.d. samples approximately from $f(\theta|Y_{\text{obs}})$, where we still need the assumption of the product measurable space that

$$\mathcal{S}_{(\theta_1,\theta_2,Z|Y_{\text{obs}})} = \mathcal{S}_{(\theta_1|Y_{\text{obs}})} \times \mathcal{S}_{(\theta_2|Y_{\text{obs}})} \times \mathcal{S}_{(Z|Y_{\text{obs}})}.$$

In §6.2, we present a real study in tumor xenograft experiments by using the ECM algorithm and the IBF sampling.

5.1.3 The IBF sampling in the MCEM structure

Now, we develop an IBF sampler in the structure of the Monte Carlo EM algorithm (Wei & Tanner, 1990) where sampling from $f(\theta|Y_{\text{obs}}, Z)$ is straightforward and the complete-data posterior mode has closed-form expression, while there are no closed-form expectations with respect to the conditional predictive density $f(Z|Y_{\text{obs}}, \theta)$. We further augment the latent vector Z by another latent vector b such that all $f(\theta|Y_{\text{obs}}, Z, b)$, $f(Z|Y_{\text{obs}}, b, \theta)$ and $f(b|Y_{\text{obs}}, Z, \theta)$ are available. Let the joint support be a product measurable space, i.e.,

$$\mathcal{S}_{(\theta,Z,b|Y_{\text{obs}})} = \mathcal{S}_{(\theta|Y_{\text{obs}})} \times \mathcal{S}_{(Z|Y_{\text{obs}})} \times \mathcal{S}_{(b|Y_{\text{obs}})}.$$

Applying (5.1) twice, we have,

$$\begin{aligned} f(Z|Y_{\text{obs}}, \tilde{\theta}) &\propto \frac{f(Z|Y_{\text{obs}}, b_0, \tilde{\theta})}{f(b_0|Y_{\text{obs}}, Z, \tilde{\theta})}, & (5.11)\\ f(Z, b|Y_{\text{obs}}, \tilde{\theta}) &= f(b|Y_{\text{obs}}, Z, \tilde{\theta}) \cdot f(Z|Y_{\text{obs}}, \tilde{\theta}), & (5.12)\\ f(Z, b|Y_{\text{obs}}) &\propto \frac{f(Z, b|Y_{\text{obs}}, \tilde{\theta})}{f(\tilde{\theta}|Y_{\text{obs}}, Z, b)}, & (5.13) \end{aligned}$$

where $b_0 = E\{b|Y_{\text{obs}}, \tilde{\theta}\}$ and $\tilde{\theta}$ is the observed posterior mode. We have the following noniterative algorithm.

THE IBF SAMPLER IN THE MCEM STRUCTURE:

Step 1. Based on (5.11), independently generate $\{Z^{(j)}\}_1^J$ approximately from $f(Z|Y_{\text{obs}}, \tilde{\theta})$ with the IBF sampler;

Step 2. Based on (5.12), generate J independent samples $b^{(j)} \sim f(b|Y_{\text{obs}}, Z^{(j)}, \tilde{\theta})$, then $\{Z^{(j)}, b^{(j)}\}_1^J \overset{\text{iid}}{\sim} f(Z, b|Y_{\text{obs}}, \tilde{\theta})$;

Step 3. Based on (5.13), generate $I\,(< J)$ independent samples $\{Z^{(k_i)}, b^{(k_i)}\}_{i=1}^I$ approximately from $f(Z, b|Y_{\text{obs}})$ with the IBF sampler;

Step 4. Generate $\theta^{(i)} \sim f(\theta|Y_{\text{obs}}, Z^{(k_i)}, b^{(k_i)})$ for $i = 1, \dots, I$. Then $\{\theta^{(i)}\}_1^I \stackrel{\text{iid}}{\sim} f(\theta|Y_{\text{obs}})$.

Therefore, the key for this noniterative algorithm is to find the $\tilde{\theta}$ and $b_0 = E\{b|Y_{\text{obs}}, \tilde{\theta}\}$. On one hand, the posterior mode can be determined using any methods such as the NR algorithm, the scoring algorithm, the Laplace method and so on. On the other hand, the posterior mode can be determined using the MCEM algorithm. For more details, see §5.6 and §5.7.

5.2 Incomplete Pre-Post Test Problems

Pre-post test design is one of the commonly used designs in clinical trials where patients serve as their own control and the differential effect of a treatment is assessed. Because this design avoids within patient variability and reduces sample size, it is often used in drug development and clinical studies (Bonate, 1998). The same scenario also arises in comparing pre-post changes in either physiological variables or molecular or genetic targets in more complex design or observational studies. Statistically, this is an incomplete data problem with underlying binormal distribution. In the growing literature on dealing with incomplete data problems, three main approaches emerge:

- The likelihood-based approach using EM algorithm (Dempster *et al.*, 1977; Liu, 1999);
- The Bayesian approach using DA algorithm (Tanner & Wong, 1987); and
- The Gibbs sampler (Gelfand & Smith, 1990).

No closed-form solutions have been obtained with these approaches and most recent solutions focus on the MCMC or iterative sampling. In §3.6, we obtained an explicit Bayesian solution to the covariance matrix Σ when the mean vector μ is known for a binormal model with missing data. In this section, for two cases that Σ is known and unknown (Tan *et al.*, 2001), we further show that closed-form solutions can be derived by the function-wise IBF or i.i.d. posterior samples can be generated by the IBF sampler.

5.2.1 Motivating example: Sickle cell disease study

Sickle cell disease (SCD) is the most common hemoglobinopathy seen in the United States, affecting approximately 30,000 children. Children with SCD have decreased height and weight when compared to their healthy peers. Patients with SCD had *resting energy expenditure* (REE) measurements that were 18%–22% higher than healthy controls (Singhal *et al.*, 1993). It is believed that REE ratios (the ratio of actual REE to predicted REE) may decrease after a glutamine supplementation (Williams *et al.*, 2002). St. Jude Children's Research Hospital conducted such a study, where the SCD patients were treated by glutamine. To demonstrate such a decrease, patients receive glutamine supplementation for 24 weeks. REE is measured at Day 1 and the end of Week 24 using a breath by breath analyzer while the patient is in a supine position for 15–20 minutes after a steady state has been achieved. The predicted REE is defined by the Harris–Benedict equations. The ratio of actual REE to predicted REE is obtained for each patient. REE is considered to be fairly normally distributed based on previous data. The REE ratios of patients at Day 1 and Week 24 are listed in Table 5.1.

Table 5.1 *REE ratios of patients at Day 1 and Week 24*

i	1	2	3	4	5	6	7	8	9	10	11
x_{1i}	1.092	1.213	1.021	1.304	1.003	1.504	1.463	1.082	1.280	1.333	1.131
x_{2i}	0.985	1.219	1.123	1.165	1.108	1.393	1.283	1.180	1.194	1.160	1.143
i	12	13	14	15	16	17	18	19	20	21	22
x_{1i}	1.178	1.249	1.457	1.023	1.150	1.065	1.414	1.043	1.214	*	*
x_{2i}	1.288	1.052	1.177	*	*	*	*	*	*	0.982	1.273

Source: Tan *et al.* (2001). NOTE: x_{1i} and x_{2i} denote the corresponding REE ratio at Day 1 and Week 24 for patient i. * Value not observed (missing at random).

Let x_{1i} and x_{2i} denote the corresponding REE ratio at Day 1 and Week 24 for patient i. A total of $n = 22$ patients are enrolled in the SCD study. There are $n_1 = 14$ patients with complete observed data, $n_2 = 6$ patients with the observations of the REE ratios at Week 24 missing, and $n_3 = n - n_1 - n_2 = 2$ patients with the observations of the REE ratios at Day 1 missing. Suppose that

$$x_i = (x_{1i}, x_{2i})^\top \stackrel{\text{iid}}{\sim} N_2(\mu, \Sigma), \qquad i = 1, \ldots, n,$$

where

$$\mu = \begin{pmatrix} \mu_1 \\ \mu_2 \end{pmatrix} \quad \text{and} \quad \Sigma = \begin{pmatrix} \sigma_1^2 & \rho\sigma_1\sigma_2 \\ \rho\sigma_1\sigma_2 & \sigma_2^2 \end{pmatrix}.$$

The observed data and the missing data are denoted by

$$\begin{aligned} Y_{\text{obs}} &= \{x_i\}_{i=1}^{n_1} \cup \{x_{1i}\}_{n_1+1}^{n_1+n_2} \cup \{x_{2i}\}_{n_1+n_2+1}^{n} \quad \text{and} \\ Z &= \{x_{2i}\}_{n_1+1}^{n_1+n_2} \cup \{x_{1i}\}_{n_1+n_2+1}^{n}, \end{aligned}$$

respectively.

5.2.2 Binormal model with missing data and known variance

When the covariance matrix Σ is known, we adopt $N_2(\mu_0, \Sigma_0)$ as the prior of μ, where μ_0 and Σ_0 are assumed to be known. This prior becomes the noninformative or flat prior if $\Sigma_0^{-1} \to 0$. It is easy to show that (Gelman *et al.*, 1995, p.79)

$$f(\mu|Y_{\text{obs}}, Z) = N_2(\mu|\omega, \Omega), \tag{5.14}$$

where $\Omega^{-1} = n\Sigma^{-1} + \Sigma_0^{-1}$,

$$\omega = \Omega\left\{\Sigma^{-1}\begin{pmatrix} n_1\bar{x}_1 + n_2\bar{x}_3 + n_3\bar{x}_4^* \\ n_1\bar{x}_2 + n_2\bar{x}_3^* + n_3\bar{x}_4 \end{pmatrix} + \Sigma_0^{-1}\mu_0\right\}, \tag{5.15}$$

$$\begin{aligned} \bar{x}_1 &= \frac{1}{n_1}\sum_{i=1}^{n_1} x_{1i}, & \bar{x}_2 &= \frac{1}{n_1}\sum_{i=1}^{n_1} x_{2i}, \\ \bar{x}_3 &= \frac{1}{n_2}\sum_{i=n_1+1}^{n_1+n_2} x_{1i}, & \bar{x}_3^* &= \frac{1}{n_2}\sum_{i=n_1+1}^{n_1+n_2} x_{2i}, \\ \bar{x}_4^* &= \frac{1}{n_3}\sum_{i=n_1+n_2+1}^{n} x_{1i}, & \bar{x}_4 &= \frac{1}{n_3}\sum_{i=n_1+n_2+1}^{n} x_{2i}. \end{aligned} \tag{5.16}$$

On the other hand, the conditional predictive distribution is

$$\begin{aligned} f(Z|Y_{\text{obs}}, \mu) &= \prod_{i=n_1+1}^{n_1+n_2} N\left(x_{2i}\middle|\mu_2 + (x_{1i} - \mu_1)\frac{\rho\sigma_2}{\sigma_1},\ \sigma_2^2(1-\rho^2)\right) \\ &\quad \times \prod_{i=n_1+n_2+1}^{n} N\left(x_{1i}\middle|\mu_1 + (x_{2i} - \mu_2)\frac{\rho\sigma_1}{\sigma_2},\ \sigma_1^2(1-\rho^2)\right). \end{aligned} \tag{5.17}$$

With the sampling IBF (1.37), from (5.14) and (5.17), we have

$$f(\mu|Y_{\text{obs}}) = N_2(\mu|q, Q), \tag{5.18}$$

where

$$\begin{aligned}
Q^{-1} &= n_1\Sigma^{-1} + n_2\begin{pmatrix} \sigma_1^{-2} & 0 \\ 0 & 0 \end{pmatrix} + n_3\begin{pmatrix} 0 & 0 \\ 0 & \sigma_2^{-2} \end{pmatrix} + \Sigma_0^{-1} \\
&= n_1\Sigma^{-1} + \text{diag}(n_2/\sigma_1^2, n_3/\sigma_2^2) + \Sigma_0^{-1} \qquad (5.19) \\
q &= Q\Big\{ n_1\Sigma^{-1}\begin{pmatrix} \bar{x}_1 \\ \bar{x}_2 \end{pmatrix} + n_2\begin{pmatrix} \sigma_1^{-2} & 0 \\ 0 & 0 \end{pmatrix}\begin{pmatrix} \bar{x}_3 \\ 0 \end{pmatrix} \\
&\quad + n_3\begin{pmatrix} 0 & 0 \\ 0 & \sigma_2^{-2} \end{pmatrix}\begin{pmatrix} 0 \\ \bar{x}_4 \end{pmatrix} + \Sigma_0^{-1}\mu_0 \Big\} \\
&= Q\Big\{ \Sigma^{-1}\begin{pmatrix} n_1\bar{x}_1 + n_2\bar{x}_3 + \rho\sigma_1\sigma_2^{-1}n_3\bar{x}_4 \\ n_1\bar{x}_2 + \rho\sigma_2\sigma_1^{-1}n_2\bar{x}_3 + n_3\bar{x}_4 \end{pmatrix} + \Sigma_0^{-1}\mu_0 \Big\}. \qquad (5.20)
\end{aligned}$$

Thus, routine Bayesian inferences such as the Bayesian point and interval estimates, hypothesis testing and predictive inference can be carried out based upon (5.18), (5.19) and (5.20).

Interestingly, the above explicit results also give a clear picture of the relative effect of observed and missing data on inference. For example, Q^{-1} consists of four parts which are the corresponding inverse covariance matrices of $(\bar{x}_1, \bar{x}_2)^\top$, $(\bar{x}_3, 0)^\top$, $(0, \bar{x}_4)^\top$ and μ_0. On the other hand, the q specified by (5.20) has quite a similar structure to ω given by (5.15). Filling the missing parts of ω with their conditional expectations evaluating at $\mu = (0, 0)^\top$ yields the value of q.

5.2.3 Binormal model with missing data and unknown mean and variance

When both μ and Σ are unknown, the likelihood function for the complete data $(Y_{\text{obs}}, Z) = \{x_i\}_1^n$ is given by

$$L(\mu, \Sigma|Y_{\text{obs}}, Z) \propto |\Sigma|^{-n/2} \exp\left(-\frac{1}{2}\sum_{i=1}^{n}(x_i - \mu)^\top\Sigma^{-1}(x_i - \mu) \right).$$

We again use a noninformative prior for (μ, Σ), which is the multivariate Jeffreys' prior density (Box & Tiao, 1973, p.426),

$$\pi(\mu, \Sigma) \propto |\Sigma|^{-(d+1)/2} = (\sigma_1\sigma_2\sqrt{1-\rho^2}\,)^{-(d+1)}, \qquad (5.21)$$

where d is the dimension of the multivariate normal distribution (for the current situation, $d = 2$). Here we chose Jeffreys' prior is for its scale invariant property. The prior (5.21) indicates that $\pi(\mu) \propto 1$ and $\pi(\Sigma) \propto |\Sigma|^{-(d+1)/2}$.

(a) Sampling via the IBF sampler

The complete-data posterior distribution can be written as

$$\begin{aligned} f(\mu, \Sigma|Y_{\text{obs}}, Z) &= f(\mu|Y_{\text{obs}}, Z, \Sigma) \cdot f(\Sigma|Y_{\text{obs}}, Z) \\ &= N_2(\mu|\bar{x}, \Sigma/n) \cdot \text{IWishart}_d(\Sigma|S^{-1}, n-1), \end{aligned} \tag{5.22}$$

where

$$\bar{x} = \frac{1}{n}\sum_{i=1}^{n} x_i \quad \text{and} \quad S = \sum_{i=1}^{n}(x_i - \bar{x})(x_i - \bar{x})^{\top}. \tag{5.23}$$

The conditional predictive distribution $f(Z|Y_{\text{obs}}, \mu, \Sigma)$ is the same as (5.17).

To implement the IBF sampler presented in §5.2, we first need to find the observed posterior mode $(\tilde{\mu}, \tilde{\Sigma})$ using the EM algorithm. Based on (5.17), the E-step calculates the following first- and second-order conditional moments:

$$\begin{aligned} &E(x_{2i}|Y_{\text{obs}}, \mu, \Sigma),\ E(x_{2i}x_{2i'}|Y_{\text{obs}}, \mu, \Sigma),\ i, i' = n_1+1, \dots, n_1+n_2, \\ &E(x_{1i}|Y_{\text{obs}}, \mu, \Sigma),\ E(x_{1i}x_{1i'}|Y_{\text{obs}}, \mu, \Sigma),\ i, i' = n_1+n_2+1, \dots, n. \end{aligned}$$

The M-step is to find the complete-data posterior mode:

$$\tilde{\mu} = \bar{x} \quad \text{and} \quad \tilde{\Sigma} = S/(n+d+1).$$

(b) An alternative strategy without using posterior mode

All inferences on (μ, Σ) are based on the observed posterior distribution $f(\mu, \Sigma|Y_{\text{obs}})$, from which an i.i.d. sample can be obtained by a two-step sampling process. By using the SIR technique in the first step, we can draw an i.i.d. sample from $f(\Sigma|Y_{\text{obs}})$, which is given by (5.26). The second step draws an independent sample from the conditional density $f(\mu|Y_{\text{obs}}, \Sigma)$ (cf. (5.24)), which is rather straightforward. A main advantage for this strategy over the IBF sampler is that it avoids computing the posterior mode $(\tilde{\mu}, \tilde{\Sigma})$. In what follows, we first derive $f(\mu|Y_{\text{obs}}, \Sigma)$ and $f(\mu, \Sigma|Y_{\text{obs}})$, and then present an SIR algorithm.

Theorem 5.2 (Tan *et al.*, 2001). The conditional pdf of $\mu|(Y_{\text{obs}}, \Sigma)$ is given by

$$f(\mu|Y_{\text{obs}}, \Sigma) = N_2(\mu|\delta, \Delta), \tag{5.24}$$

where

$$\begin{aligned} \Delta^{-1} &= n_1\Sigma^{-1} + \text{diag}(n_2/\sigma_1^2, n_3/\sigma_2^2), \\ \delta &= \Delta\left(n_1\Sigma^1\binom{\bar{x}_1}{\bar{x}_2} + \text{diag}(n_2/\sigma_1^2, n_3/\sigma_2^2)\binom{\bar{x}_3}{\bar{x}_4}\right), \end{aligned} \tag{5.25}$$

and $\{\bar{x}_i\}_{i=1}^4$ are specified by (5.16). In addition, we have

$$\begin{aligned} f(\Sigma|Y_{\text{obs}}) &\propto c_1^{-1}(\Sigma)\cdot|\Delta|^{1/2}\exp\{\delta^{\top}\Delta^{-1}\delta/2\} \\ &\quad\times\exp\left\{-\frac{1}{2}\,\text{tr}\,\Sigma^{-1}((1-\rho^2)\text{diag}(t_3,t_4)+T)\right\}, \end{aligned} \tag{5.26}$$

$$\begin{aligned} f(\Sigma^{-1}|Y_{\text{obs}}) &\propto c_2^{-1}(\Sigma^{-1})\cdot|\Delta|^{1/2}\exp\{\delta^{\top}\Delta^{-1}\delta/2\} \\ &\quad\times\exp\left\{-\frac{1}{2}\,\text{tr}\,\Sigma^{-1}((1-\rho^2)\text{diag}(t_3,t_4)+T)\right\}, \end{aligned} \tag{5.27}$$

where

$$\begin{aligned} c_1(\Sigma) &= \sigma_1^{n+d+1-n_3}\sigma_2^{n+d+1-n_2}(1-\rho^2)^{(n_1+d+1)/2}, \\ c_2(\Sigma^{-1}) &= \sigma_1^{n-d-1-n_3}\sigma_2^{n-d-1-n_2}(1-\rho^2)^{(n_1-d-1)/2}, \\ t_3 &= \sum_{i=n_1+1}^{n_1+n_2} x_{1i}^2, \quad t_4 = \sum_{i=n_1+n_2+1}^{n} x_{2i}^2, \end{aligned} \tag{5.28}$$

and $T = \sum_{i=1}^{n_1} x_i x_i^{\top}$. ¶

PROOF. Applying the point-wise IBF (1.36) to (5.17) and (5.22), we obtain

$$f(\mu,\Sigma|Y_{\text{obs}}) \propto \frac{\exp\{-\frac{1}{2}\,\text{tr}\,\Sigma^{-1}((1-\rho^2)\text{diag}(a_3,a_4)+A)\}}{c_1(\Sigma)}, \tag{5.29}$$

where

$$\begin{aligned} A &= \sum_{i=1}^{n_1}(x_i-\mu)(x_i-\mu)^{\top}, \\ a_3 &= \sum_{i=n_1+1}^{n_1+n_2}(x_{1i}-\mu_1)^2 \quad\text{and}\quad a_4 = \sum_{i=n_1+n_2+1}^{n}(x_{2i}-\mu_2)^2. \end{aligned}$$

Since $f(\mu|Y_{\text{obs}},\Sigma) \propto$ (5.29), we have

$$f(\mu|Y_{\text{obs}},\Sigma) \propto \exp\left\{-\frac{1}{2}\,\text{tr}\,\Sigma^{-1}\Big((1-\rho^2)\text{diag}(a_3,a_4)+A\Big)\right\}. \tag{5.30}$$

Note that the matrix A, the vectors a_3 and a_4 can be rewritten as

$$\begin{aligned} A &= \sum_{i=1}^{n_1}(x_i - \bar{x}_{12})(x_i - \bar{x}_{12})^{\top} + n_1(\bar{x}_{12} - \mu)(\bar{x}_{12} - \mu)^{\top}, \\ a_3 &= \sum_{i=n_1+1}^{n_1+n_2} (x_{1i} - \bar{x}_3)^2 + n_2(\mu_1 - \bar{x}_3)^2, \\ a_4 &= \sum_{i=n_1+n_2+1}^{n} (x_{2i} - \bar{x}_4)^2 + n_3(\mu_2 - \bar{x}_4)^2, \end{aligned}$$

where $\bar{x}_{12} = (\bar{x}_1, \bar{x}_2)^{\top}$, $\bar{x}_{34} = (\bar{x}_3, \bar{x}_4)^{\top}$ with $\{\bar{x}_k\}_{k=1}^4$ being specified by (5.16), we obtain

$$\operatorname{tr} \Sigma^{-1} A \;\propto\; (\mu - \bar{x}_{12})^{\top}\Lambda_1^{-1}(\mu - \bar{x}_{12}), \quad (5.31)$$

$$\operatorname{tr}\left(\Sigma^{-1}(1-\rho^2)\operatorname{diag}(a_3, a_4)\right) \;\propto\; (\mu - \bar{x}_{34})^{\top}\Lambda_2^{-1}(\mu - \bar{x}_{34}), \quad (5.32)$$

where $\Lambda_1 = \Sigma/n_1$ and $\Lambda_2 = \operatorname{diag}(\sigma_1^2/n_2,\ \sigma_2^2/n_3)$. Since both (5.31) and (5.32) are of quadratic forms in μ, the summation is still of quadratic form in μ. From the formula (3.18) of Gelman *et al.* (1995, p.79) and combining (5.31) with (5.32), the right-hand side of (5.30) is proportional to

$$\exp\left\{ -\frac{1}{2}(\mu - \delta)^{\top}\Delta^{-1}(\mu - \delta)\right\}$$

with δ given by (5.25). Hence, (5.24) follows immediately.

The definition of conditional probability indicates that

$$f(\Sigma|Y_{\text{obs}}) = \frac{f(\mu, \Sigma|Y_{\text{obs}})}{f(\mu|Y_{\text{obs}}, \Sigma)}$$

for an arbitrary choice of μ. In particular, we may let $\mu = (0,0)^{\top}$. The formula (5.26) follows immediately from (5.29) and (5.24). Since the Jacobian determinant of the transformation from Σ to Σ^{-1} is $|\Sigma|^3$ (cf. Box & Tiao, 1973, p.475), the posterior density of Σ^{-1} is

$$f(\Sigma^{-1}|Y_{\text{obs}}) = f(\Sigma|Y_{\text{obs}}) \cdot |\Sigma|^3,$$

which gives (5.27). ||END||

Now, we present the SIR algorithm (cf. §2.2.3) to draw from $f(\Sigma|Y_{\text{obs}})$. A random matrix Σ from $f(\Sigma|Y_{\text{obs}})$ can be obtained by drawing a matrix W from $f(W|Y_{\text{obs}})$ and inverting it, where $W \hat{=} \Sigma^{-1}$. From (5.27), the posterior density of W can be written as $f(W|Y_{\text{obs}}) = c \cdot g(W) \cdot h(W)$, where c is the normalizing constant,

$$g(W) = \frac{\exp\{\delta^{\top}\Delta^{-1}\delta/2\} \exp\left\{ -\frac{t_3}{2\sigma_1^2} - \frac{t_4}{2\sigma_2^2} \right\}}{\sigma_1^{n_2}\sigma_2^{n_3}(n_1 n + n_2 n_3(1-\rho^2))^{1/2}}, \tag{5.33}$$

and $h(W) = \text{Wishart}_2(W|T^{-1}, n_1 - 1)$ denotes the pdf of a Wishart pdf with $n_1 - 1$ degrees of freedom and expectation $(n_1 - 1)T^{-1}$ and takes the role of a proposal density. Assuming that $\{W^{(j)}\}_1^J \overset{\text{iid}}{\sim} h(W)$, we can construct the weights

$$\omega_j = \frac{g(W^{(j)})}{\sum_{\ell=1}^J g(W^{(\ell)})}, \quad j = 1, \ldots, J.$$

A second sample of size I is drawn from the discrete distribution on $\{W^{(j)}\}$ with probabilities $\{\omega_j\}$. The resulting sample has approximate pdf $f(W|Y_{\text{obs}})$.

(c) Bayesian inference via importance sampling

In certain applications, our interest centers on some function of μ, say $f(\mu) = b^{\top}\mu$. For instance, to determine the posterior mean of $b^{\top}\mu$ by (5.24), we know that the distribution of $b^{\top}\mu|(Y_{\text{obs}}, \Sigma)$ is uninormal with mean $b^{\top}\delta$. This allows us to obtain the posterior mean of $b^{\top}\mu$ directly by importance sampling, which is much easier than to draw from $f(\mu, \Sigma|Y_{\text{obs}})$ first, then make the inference. For example, we have

$$\begin{aligned}
E(b^{\top}\mu|Y_{\text{obs}}) &= E\{E(b^{\top}\mu|Y_{\text{obs}}, \Sigma)|Y_{\text{obs}}\} = E(b^{\top}\delta|Y_{\text{obs}}) \\
&= \int b^{\top}\delta \cdot f(\Sigma^{-1}|Y_{\text{obs}})\, d\Sigma^{-1} \\
&= c \int b^{\top}\delta \cdot g(W) \cdot h(W)\, dW \\
&\doteq \frac{\sum_{j=1}^J b^{\top}\delta^{(j)} \cdot g(W^{(j)})}{\sum_{j=1}^J g(W^{(j)})},
\end{aligned} \tag{5.34}$$

where $g(W)$ is given by (5.33) and $\{W^{(j)}\} \overset{\text{iid}}{\sim} \text{Wishart}_2(T^{-1}, n_1 - 1)$.

Furthermore, the posterior probability of the null hypothesis H_0: $a^{\top}\mu \le a_0$ with specific constant vector a and scalar a_0 is

$$\Pr\{H_0|Y_{\text{obs}}\} = \Pr\{a^{\top}\mu \le a_0|Y_{\text{obs}}\}$$

$$
\begin{aligned}
&= \int \Pr\left\{\frac{a^\top\mu - a^\top\delta}{\sqrt{a^\top\Delta a}} \le \frac{a_0 - a^\top\delta}{\sqrt{a^\top\Delta a}}\Big|Y_{\rm obs}, \Sigma^{-1}\right\} \\
&\quad \times f(\Sigma^{-1}|Y_{\rm obs})\, d\Sigma^{-1} \\
&\doteq \frac{\sum_{j=1}^J \Phi\left(\frac{a_0 - a^\top\delta^{(j)}}{\sqrt{a^\top\Delta^{(j)}a}}\right)\cdot g(W^{(j)})}{\sum_{j=1}^J g(W^{(j)})}, \qquad (5.35)
\end{aligned}
$$

where $\Phi(\cdot)$ denotes the cdf of $N(0,1)$.

Example 5.3 (*The SCD data*). To compute the posterior mean of $b^\top\mu$ given by (5.34), we first calculate the values of t_3, t_4 and T. Using the SCD data in Table 5.1, from (5.28), we obtain $t_3 = 8.0643$, $t_4 = 2.5849$,

$$
T = \begin{pmatrix} 21.7508 & 20.4936 \\ 20.4936 & 19.5098 \end{pmatrix} \quad \text{and} \quad T^{-1} = \begin{pmatrix} 4.4685 & -4.6938 \\ -4.6938 & 4.9817 \end{pmatrix}.
$$

In (5.34), let $b = (1,0)^\top$ and $b = (0,1)^\top$, respectively. Then, the Bayesian estimates of μ_1 and μ_2 are given by

$$
E(\mu_1|Y_{\rm obs}) = 1.2086 \quad \text{and} \quad E(\mu_2|Y_{\rm obs}) = 1.1511.
$$

Therefore, the reduction in REE is

$$
E(\mu_1|Y_{\rm obs}) - E(\mu_2|Y_{\rm obs}) = 0.0575.
$$

To obtain a 95% Bayesian CI for $\mu_1 - \mu_2$, we first draw a sample of size $I = 10{,}000$ from $f(\Sigma^{-1}|Y_{\rm obs})$ by using the SIR method described in §5.2.3(b), then conditionally draw a sample of size $I = 10{,}000$ from $f(\mu|Y_{\rm obs}, \Sigma)$ according to (5.24). Therefore, we obtain a sample of $\mu_1 - \mu_2$ with size $I = 10{,}000$. A 95% Bayesian CI for $\mu_1 - \mu_2$ is

$$
[-0.0102,\ 0.1206].
$$

In addition, in (5.35), let $a = (1,-1)^\top$ and $a_0 = 0.10$, i.e., H_0: $\mu_1 - \mu_2 \le 10\%$, we obtain $\Pr\{H_0|Y_{\rm obs}\} = 0.8501$. That is, with 0.85 probability, the reduction in REE is less than 10%. ||

5.3 Right Censored Regression Model

In Ex.2.4, we considered a right censored regression model. The complete-data likelihood function and the conditional predictive density are given by (2.14) and (2.15), respectively. Consider the following independent prior distributions:

$$
\begin{aligned}
\beta &\sim N_d(a_0, A_0^{-1}), \quad A_0 \to 0, \quad \text{and} \\
\sigma^2 &\sim \text{IGamma}(\sigma^2|q_0/2, \lambda_0/2), \quad q_0 = \lambda_0 = 0.
\end{aligned}
$$

Then, the augmented posterior is given by

$$\begin{aligned}
f(\beta, \sigma^2 | Y_{\text{obs}}, Z) &\propto \frac{\exp\{-\frac{1}{2\sigma^2}(y - X\beta)^\top (y - X\beta)\}}{\sigma^{m+2}} \qquad (5.36) \\
&= f(\beta | Y_{\text{obs}}, Z, \sigma^2) \times f(\sigma^2 | Y_{\text{obs}}, Z) \\
&= N_d(\beta | \tilde{\beta},\, \sigma^2 (X^\top X)^{-1}) \\
&\quad \times \text{IGamma}\Big(\sigma^2 \Big| \frac{m-d}{2},\, \frac{(m+2)\tilde{\sigma}^2}{2}\Big), \qquad (5.37)
\end{aligned}$$

where

$$\tilde{\beta} = (X^\top X)^{-1} X^\top y \quad \text{and} \quad \tilde{\sigma}^2 = \frac{(y - X\tilde{\beta})^\top (y - X\tilde{\beta})}{m+2} \qquad (5.38)$$

denote the complete-data posterior modes of β and σ^2. The goal here is to obtain an i.i.d. sample from $f(\beta, \sigma^2 | Y_{\text{obs}})$. With the sampling IBF (5.5), we have

$$f(\beta, \sigma^2 | Y_{\text{obs}}) \propto \frac{f(\beta, \sigma^2 | Y_{\text{obs}}, Z_0)}{f(Z_0 | Y_{\text{obs}}, \beta, \sigma^2)}$$

for some arbitrary $Z_0 \in \mathcal{S}_{(Z|Y_{\text{obs}})} = \prod_{i=r+1}^{m} (c_i, +\infty)$. It is quite important to distinguish $\mathcal{S}_{(Z|Y_{\text{obs}})}$ from $\mathcal{S}_Z = \mathbb{R}^{m-r}$.

The best Z_0 can be obtained by using the EM algorithm. The E-step requires calculating

$$\begin{aligned}
E\{Z_i | Y_{\text{obs}}, \beta, \sigma^2\} &= x_{(i)}^\top \beta + \sigma \Psi\Big(\frac{c_i - x_{(i)}^\top \beta}{\sigma}\Big) \quad \text{and} \\
E\{Z_i^2 | Y_{\text{obs}}, \beta, \sigma^2\} &= (x_{(i)}^\top \beta)^2 + \sigma^2 + \sigma(c_i + x_{(i)}^\top \beta) \Psi\Big(\frac{c_i - x_{(i)}^\top \beta}{\sigma}\Big),
\end{aligned}$$

for $i = r+1, \ldots, m$, where $\Psi(\cdot)$ was defined by (2.16). The M-step is to update (5.38) by replacing Z_i and Z_i^2 by $E\{Z_i | Y_{\text{obs}}, \beta, \sigma^2\}$ and $E\{Z_i^2 | Y_{\text{obs}}, \beta, \sigma^2\}$, respectively. Let the EM converge at $(\tilde{\beta}, \tilde{\sigma})$, then we choose

$$Z_0 = (Z_{0,r+1}, \ldots, Z_{0,m})^\top, \qquad (5.39)$$

where

$$Z_{0,i} = x_{(i)}^\top \tilde{\beta} + \tilde{\sigma} \Psi\Big(\frac{c_i - x_{(i)}^\top \tilde{\beta}}{\tilde{\sigma}}\Big), \quad i = r+1, \ldots, m.$$

Example 5.4 (*The insulation life data revisited*). We revisit the insulation life data with censoring time in Table 2.3. Starting from $(\beta_0^{(0)}, \beta_1^{(0)}, \sigma^{(0)}) = (1, 1, 1)$, the EM algorithm converged to $\tilde{\beta}_0 = -5.9612$, $\tilde{\beta}_1 = 4.2803$ and $\tilde{\sigma} = 0.2433$ after 40 iterations with precision 10^{-5}. By (5.39), we obtain

$$\begin{aligned} Z_0 &= (Z_{0,18}, \dots, Z_{0,40})^{\top} = (4.22, 4.22, 4.22, 4.22, 4.22, \\ &\quad 4.22, 4.22, 4.22, 4.22, 4.22, 3.92, 3.92, 3.92, 3.44, \\ &\quad 3.44, 3.44, 3.44, 3.44, 2.91, 2.91, 2.91, 2.91, 2.91)^{\top}. \end{aligned} \tag{5.40}$$

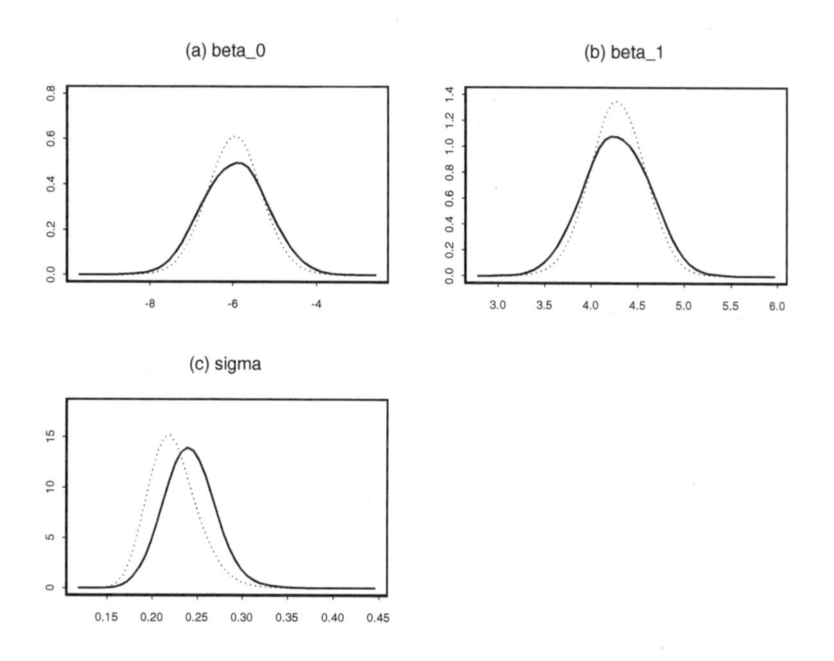

Figure 5.3 The observed posterior density (solid curve) estimated by a kernel density smoother based on i.i.d. samples obtained via the alternative IBF sampler (J = 30,000, I = 10,000, without replacement) and the best augmented posterior density (dotted curve) with Z_0 given by (5.40). (a) β_0; (b) β_1; (c) σ.

Table 5.2 *Posterior estimates of* β_0, β_1 *and* σ

Parameter	Posterior mode†	Posterior mean	Posterior std	95% Posterior CI
β_0	−5.9612	−5.9520	0.7569	[−7.4010, −4.4780]
β_1	4.2803	4.2744	0.3449	[3.6048, 4.9375]
σ	0.2433	0.2417	0.0278	[0.1901, 0.2994]

The IBF sampler is implemented by first generating an i.i.d. sample of size $J = 30{,}000$ of $\beta = (\beta_0, \beta_1)^{\top}$ and σ^2 from (5.37) with $Z = Z_0$. Then we resample without replacement from the discrete distribution with corresponding weights to obtain the desired i.i.d. posterior samples of (β, σ^2) with size $I = 10{,}000$. The observed and augmented posterior densities of β_0, β_1 and σ are plotted in Figure 5.3. As shown in Figure 5.3(a) and 5.3(b), the modes of both curves are the same. However, for the shape parameter σ, none of the curves peaks at the same location because the EM finds the global mode. In fact, from (5.36) and (5.37), the global mode of σ^2 for the augmented posterior $f(\beta, \sigma^2|Y_{\text{obs}}, Z)$ is $\tilde{\sigma}^2$ given by (5.38), but the marginal mode of σ^2 for the augmented posterior $f(\sigma^2|Y_{\text{obs}}, Z)$ is given by

$$\tilde{\sigma}^2_{\text{marg}} = \frac{(y - X\tilde{\beta})^{\top}(y - X\tilde{\beta})}{m}.$$

When the EM converged, $(y - X\tilde{\beta})^{\top}(y - X\tilde{\beta}) = 2.4862$, thereby,

$$\tilde{\sigma}^2 = 0.2433^2 < 0.2493^2 = \tilde{\sigma}^2_{\text{marg}}.$$

Corresponding Bayesian estimates of parameters are given in Table 5.2. ‖

5.4 Linear Mixed Models for Longitudinal Data

This is perhaps one of most widely used statistical models and the likelihood-based analysis is implemented in PROC MIXED of SAS. Let Y_{ij} be the j-th response for subject i, where $j = 1, \ldots, n_i$ and $i = 1, \ldots, N$. The normal linear mixed-effects model (Laird & Ware, 1982; Liu & Rubin, 1994) is

$$\begin{aligned} Y_i &= X_i^{\top}\beta + W_i^{\top}b_i + \varepsilon_i, \quad 1 \le i \le N, \\ b_i &\sim N_q(\mathbf{0},\ D), \\ \varepsilon_i &\sim N_{n_i}(\mathbf{0},\ \sigma^2 R_i), \end{aligned} \tag{5.41}$$

where Y_i are $n_i \times 1$ vectors of responses for subject i, $X_i\,(p \times n_i)$ and $W_i\,(q \times n_i)$ are known design matrices relating to the covariates, β are the $p \times 1$ fixed effects, b_i are $q \times 1$ random effects, D is an unknown $q \times q$ positive definite matrix relating to the correlation structure of Y_i, σ^2 is an unknown variance parameter, the $R_i > 0$

are known $n_i \times n_i$ correlation matrices, and b_i is independent of ε_i. The model (5.41) can be rewritten in a hierarchical form:

$$\begin{aligned} Y_i|b_i &\sim N_{n_i}(X_i^\top\beta + W_i^\top b_i,\ \sigma^2 R_i), \quad 1 \le i \le N, \\ b_i &\sim N_q(\mathbf{0},\ D). \end{aligned}$$

Let $Y_{\text{obs}} = \{Y_i, X_i, W_i, R_i\}_{i=1}^N$ denote the observed data. For convenience, we define $\xi \mathrel{\hat{=}} (\sigma^2, D)$, $\theta \mathrel{\hat{=}} (\beta, \sigma^2, D)$ and treat $b = \{b_1, \ldots, b_N\}$ as missing data. Then, the likelihood function for the complete-data $\{Y_{\text{obs}}, b\}$ is

$$L(\theta|Y_{\text{obs}}, b) = \prod_{i=1}^N \Big\{N_q(b_i|\mathbf{0},\ D) \cdot N_{n_i}(Y_i|X_i^\top\beta + W_i^\top b_i,\ \sigma^2 R_i)\Big\}.$$

Consider independent prior distributions:

$$\begin{aligned} \beta &\sim N_p(\mu_0,\ \Sigma_0) \quad \text{with} \quad \Sigma_0^{-1} \to 0, \\ \sigma^2 &\sim \text{IGamma}(q_0/2,\ \lambda_0/2), \quad \text{and} \\ D &\sim \text{IWishart}_q(\Lambda_0^{-1},\ \nu_0). \end{aligned}$$

Then the complete-data posterior distribution of θ is

$$\begin{aligned} f(\theta|Y_{\text{obs}}, b) &= f(\beta|Y_{\text{obs}}, b, \sigma^2) \times f(\sigma^2|Y_{\text{obs}}, b) \times f(D|Y_{\text{obs}}, b) \\ &= N_p(\beta|\hat{\beta},\ \sigma^2\hat{\Sigma}) \\ &\quad \times \text{IGamma}\Big(\sigma^2\Big|\frac{q_0 + n - p}{2}, \frac{\lambda_0 + s}{2}\Big) \\ &\quad \times \text{IWishart}_q(D|\Lambda^{-1}, \nu_0 + N), \end{aligned} \tag{5.42}$$

where

$$\begin{aligned} \hat{\beta} &= \hat{\Sigma} \cdot \Sigma_{i=1}^N X_i R_i^{-1}(Y_i - W_i^\top b_i), \\ \hat{\Sigma} &= (\Sigma_{i=1}^N X_i R_i^{-1} X_i^\top)^{-1}, \\ n &= \Sigma_{i=1}^N n_i, \\ s &= \Sigma_{i=1}^N (Y_i - X_i^\top\hat{\beta} - W_i^\top b_i)^\top R_i^{-1}(Y_i - X_i^\top\hat{\beta} - W_i^\top b_i), \quad \text{and} \\ \Lambda &= \Lambda_0 + \Sigma_{i=1}^N b_i b_i^\top. \end{aligned}$$

The conditional predictive density is

$$f(b|Y_{\text{obs}}, \theta) = \prod_{i=1}^N N_q(b_i|\hat{b}_i(\theta),\ \Omega_i(\xi)), \tag{5.43}$$

where the mean vector $\hat{b}_i(\theta)$ and the covariance matrix $\Omega_i(\xi)$ have two alternative expressions:

$$\begin{aligned}
\hat{b}_i(\theta) &= DW_i\Delta_i(\xi)(Y_i - X_i^\top\beta) \\
&= (\sigma^2 D^{-1} + W_i R_i^{-1} W_i^\top)^{-1} W_i R_i^{-1}(Y_i - X_i^\top\beta), \\
\Omega_i(\xi) &= D - DW_i\Delta_i(\xi)W_i^\top D \\
&= \sigma^2(\sigma^2 D^{-1} + W_i R_i^{-1} W_i^\top)^{-1}
\end{aligned}$$

with $\Delta_i(\xi) \hat{=} (\sigma^2 R_i + W_i^\top D W_i)^{-1}$. The objective is to obtain i.i.d. samples from $f(\theta|Y_{\text{obs}})$. According to the IBF sampler, we only need to obtain i.i.d. samples from $f(b|Y_{\text{obs}})$.

To implement the IBF sampler, we need to find the observed posterior mode $\tilde{\theta} = (\tilde{\beta}, \tilde{\sigma}^2, \tilde{D})$. The MLE of θ was considered in Liu & Rubin (1994). The posterior mode $\tilde{\theta}$ can be derived similarly. In fact, using the current estimates $\theta^{(t)} = (\beta^{(t)}, \xi^{(t)}) = (\beta^{(t)}, \sigma^{2(t)}, D^{(t)})$, the E-step calculates

$$\begin{aligned}
E(b_i|Y_{\text{obs}}, \theta^{(t)}) &= \hat{b}_i(\theta^{(t)}) \quad \text{and} \\
E(b_i b_i^\top|Y_{\text{obs}}, \theta^{(t)}) &= \Omega_i(\xi^{(t)}) + \hat{b}_i(\theta^{(t)})\hat{b}_i(\theta^{(t)})^\top
\end{aligned}$$

for $i = 1, \ldots, N$. The M-step is to find the posterior modes based on the complete-data. We have

$$\begin{aligned}
\beta^{(t+1)} &= \hat{\Sigma} \cdot \sum_{i=1}^{N} X_i R_i^{-1}\{Y_i - W_i^\top \hat{b}_i(\theta^{(t)})\}, \\
\sigma^{2(t+1)} &= \frac{1}{q_0 + 2 + n}\bigg\{\lambda_0 + \sum_{i=1}^{N}\Big[r_i^{(t+1)\top} R_i^{-1} r_i^{(t+1)} \\
&\quad + \sigma^{2(t)}\,\mathrm{tr}\left(\mathbf{I}_q - \sigma^{2(t)}\Delta_i(\xi^{(t)})R_i\right)\Big]\bigg\}, \\
D^{(t+1)} &= \frac{1}{\nu_0 + q + 1 + N}\left\{\Lambda_0 + \sum_{i=1}^{N} E\left(b_i b_i^\top|Y_{\text{obs}}, \theta^{(t)}\right)\right\},
\end{aligned}$$

where $r_i^{(t+1)} \hat{=} Y_i - X_i^\top\beta^{(t+1)} - W_i^\top\hat{b}_i(\theta^{(t)})$, $i = 1, \ldots, N$.

Example 5.5 (*The orthodontic growth data*). Table 5.3 displays the orthodontic growth data introduced by Pothoff & Roy (1964). These data consist of growth measurements for 16 boys and 11 girls. For each subject, the distance from the center of the pituitary to the maxillary fissure was recorded at ages 8, 10, 12 and 14. The data were used by Jennrich & Schluchter (1986) to illustrate estimation methods for unbalanced longitudinal data. It is also used in SAS PROC MIXED to illustrate the SAS procedure.

A regression model is fitted where the response is a linear function of age, with separate regressions for boys and girls. If $Y_{(s)ij}$ is the measurement for subject i in sex group s ($s = 1$ for boys and $s = -1$ for girls) at age x_j, then

$$Y_{(s)ij} = \alpha^*_{si} + \gamma^*_{si} x_j + \varepsilon_{(s)ij}, \quad i = 1, \dots, 27, \quad j = 1, \dots, 4,$$

where α^*_{si} and γ^*_{si} are random intercept and slope for subject i in group s, $\mathbf{x} = (x_1, x_2, x_3, x_4)^\top = (8, 10, 12, 14)^\top$, and $\varepsilon_{(s)ij}$ are errors. Furthermore, we assume that

$$(\alpha^*_{si}, \gamma^*_{si})^\top \sim N_2((\alpha_s, \gamma_s)^\top,\ D).$$

Using matrix notation, we have two models:

$$Y_{(s)i} = (\mathbf{1}_4, \mathbf{x})\begin{pmatrix} \alpha_s \\ \gamma_s \end{pmatrix} + (\mathbf{1}_4, \mathbf{x})b_i + \varepsilon_{(s)i}, \qquad s = 1,\ -1.$$

The original goal is to estimate α_1, γ_1, α_{-1}, γ_{-1}, σ^2 and D. A unified model can be written as

$$\begin{aligned} Y_{(s)i} &= (\mathbf{1}_4, s\mathbf{1}_4, \mathbf{x}, s\mathbf{x})\beta + (\mathbf{1}_4, \mathbf{x})b_i + \varepsilon_{(s)i}, \\ b_i &\sim N_2(\mathbf{0}, D), \qquad \varepsilon_{(s)i} \sim N_4(\mathbf{0}, \sigma^2 \mathbf{I}_4), \end{aligned}$$

where $\beta = (\beta_1, \beta_2, \beta_3, \beta_4)^\top$. The relationship between (α_s, γ_s) and β is given by

$$\begin{aligned} \alpha_1 &= \beta_1 + \beta_2, \qquad \gamma_1 = \beta_3 + \beta_4, \\ \alpha_{-1} &= \beta_1 - \beta_2, \quad \gamma_{-1} = \beta_3 - \beta_4. \end{aligned}$$

Therefore, we only need to estimate β, σ^2 and D. We take noninformative priors, i.e., $q_0 = \lambda_0 = \nu_0 = 0$ and $\Lambda_0 = 0$. Using the MLEs $\hat{\beta} = (16.8566, -0.5160, 0.6319, 0.1524)^\top$, $\hat{\sigma}^2 = 1.7162$ and

$$\hat{D} = \begin{pmatrix} 4.5569 & -0.1983 \\ -0.1983 & 0.0238 \end{pmatrix}$$

as the initial values (Verbeke & Molenberghs, 2000, p.253), the EM algorithm converged to the posterior mode $\tilde{\theta} = (\tilde{\beta}, \tilde{\sigma}^2, \tilde{D})$, where

$$\begin{aligned} \tilde{\beta} &= (16.8578, -0.5271, 0.6331, 0.1541)^\top, \\ \tilde{\sigma}^2 &= 1.3049, \quad \text{and} \\ \tilde{D} &= \begin{pmatrix} 2.2012 & -0.0091 \\ -0.0091 & 0.0065 \end{pmatrix}. \end{aligned}$$

Table 5.3 *The orthodontic growth data for 16 boys and 11 girls*

	Age (in year)					Age (in year)			
Boy	8	10	12	14	Girl	8	10	12	14
1	26.0	25.0	29.0	31.0	1	21.0	20.0	21.5	23.0
2	21.5	22.5	23.0	26.5	2	21.0	21.5	24.0	25.5
3	23.0	22.5	24.0	27.5	3	20.5	24.0	24.5	26.0
4	25.5	27.5	26.5	27.0	4	23.5	24.5	25.0	26.5
5	20.0	23.5	22.5	26.0	5	21.5	23.0	22.5	23.5
6	24.5	25.5	27.0	28.5	6	20.0	21.0	21.0	22.5
7	22.0	22.0	24.5	26.5	7	21.5	22.5	23.0	25.0
8	24.0	21.5	24.5	25.5	8	23.0	23.0	23.5	24.0
9	23.0	20.5	31.0	26.0	9	20.0	21.0	22.0	21.5
10	27.5	28.0	31.0	31.5	10	16.5	19.0	19.0	19.5
11	23.0	23.0	23.5	25.0	11	24.5	25.0	28.0	28.0
12	21.5	23.5	24.0	28.0					
13	17.0	24.5	26.0	29.5					
14	22.5	25.5	25.5	26.0					
15	23.0	24.5	26.0	30.0					
16	22.0	21.5	23.5	25.0					

Source: Pothoff & Roy (1964).

Table 5.4 *Posterior estimates for parameters of interest for the orthodontic growth data*

	MLEs	Posterior mode	Posterior mean	Posterior std	95% Posterior CI
β_1	16.856	16.857	16.865	0.5800	[15.743, 18.017]
β_2	−.516	−.5271	−.5315	0.5839	[−1.668, 0.6167]
β_3	0.6319	0.6331	0.6315	0.0515	[0.5315, 0.7314]
β_4	0.1524	0.1541	0.1537	0.0519	[0.0508, 0.2542]
σ^2	1.7162	1.3049	1.3631	0.1744	[1.0748, 1.7742]
d_{11}	4.5569	2.2012	2.4487	0.7398	[1.3438, 4.2482]
d_{22}	0.0238	0.0065	0.0067	0.0020	[0.0037, 0.0113]
d_{12}	−.198	−.0091	−.0087	0.0266	[−0.065, 0.0413]

Based on (5.42) and (5.43), we implement IBF sampling using $J = 30{,}000$ to obtain an i.i.d. sample of size $I = 10{,}000$ approximately from $f(b|Y_{\text{obs}})$, denoted by $\{b^{(i)}\}_{i=1}^{I}$. Generating $\theta^{(i)} \sim f(\theta|Y_{\text{obs}}, b^{(i)})$ for $i = 1, \dots, I$, then $\{\theta^{(i)}\}_{i=1}^{I} \overset{\text{iid}}{\sim} f(\theta|Y_{\text{obs}})$. The corresponding posterior estimates are given in Table 5.4. ||

5.5 Probit Regression Models for Independent Binary Data

The probit regression model (Albert & Chib, 1993) for analyzing independent binary data assumes

$$\begin{aligned} Y_i &\stackrel{\text{ind}}{\sim} \text{Bernoulli}(p_i), \quad i = 1, \ldots, n, \\ p_i &= \Pr(Y_i = 1|\beta) = \Phi(x_i^\top \beta), \end{aligned} \tag{5.44}$$

where Y_i is a binary response for subject i with success probability p_i, β is a $r \times 1$ vector of unknown parameters, $x_i = (x_{i1}, \ldots, x_{ir})^\top$ is an $r \times 1$ vector of known covariates associated with subject i, and $\Phi(\cdot)$ is the standard normal cdf. Albert & Chib (1993) augment the observed data $Y_{\text{obs}} = \{Y_i\}_{i=1}^n$ with a latent vector $Z = (Z_1, \ldots, Z_n)^\top$, where $\{Z_i\} \stackrel{\text{ind}}{\sim} N(x_i^\top \beta, 1)$. Let

$$Y_i = I_{(Z_i > 0)}, \quad i = 1, \ldots, n.$$

In other words, if the latent variable crosses the threshold, then a success is observed; otherwise a failure is observed. It can be shown that

$$Z \sim N_n(X\beta, \mathbf{I}_n), \quad \text{where} \quad X_{n \times r} \mathrel{\hat{=}} (x_1, \ldots, x_n)^\top.$$

With $\pi(\beta) = N_r(\beta|a, A^{-1})$ as the prior of β, the joint posterior of β and Z given the observed data Y_{obs} is given by

$$f(\beta, Z|Y_{\text{obs}}) \propto \pi(\beta) \prod_{i=1}^n \Big\{ I_{(Z_i > 0)} I_{(Y_i = 1)} + I_{(Z_i \le 0)} I_{(Y_i = 0)} \Big\} N(Z_i | x_i^\top \beta, 1).$$

Hence, the augmented posterior distribution is

$$f(\beta|Y_{\text{obs}}, Z) = N_r(\beta|(X^\top X + A)^{-1}(X^\top Z + Aa), (X^\top X + A)^{-1}). \tag{5.45}$$

Note that the conditional predictive distribution of Z_i given Y_i and β follows a truncated normal distribution:[5]

$$Z_i|(Y_i, \beta) \sim \begin{cases} TN(x_i^\top \beta, 1; \mathbb{R}_+), & \text{if } Y_i = 1, \\ TN(x_i^\top \beta, 1; \mathbb{R}_-), & \text{if } Y_i = 0. \end{cases}$$

[5] Truncated multivariate normal distribution is defined in Problem 1.1. Please also see (2.15).

If we sort the data so that the first m observations of Y_i take value 1 and the others take value 0, then the conditional predictive distribution is given by

$$f(Z|Y_{\text{obs}}, \beta) = \prod_{i=1}^{m} TN(Z_i|x_i^{\top}\beta, 1; \mathbb{R}_+) \cdot \prod_{i=m+1}^{n} TN(Z_i|x_i^{\top}\beta, 1; \mathbb{R}_-). \quad (5.46)$$

From the sampling IBF (5.5), the observed posterior is

$$f(\beta|Y_{\text{obs}}) \propto \frac{f(\beta|Y_{\text{obs}}, Z_0)}{f(Z_0|Y_{\text{obs}}, \beta)},$$

for some arbitrary $Z_0 \in \mathbb{R}_+^m \times \mathbb{R}_-^{n-m}$. The best Z_0 can be obtained via the EM algorithm. Given the current value $\beta^{(t)}$, the E-step computes the following conditional expectations:

$$\begin{aligned} Z_i^{(t)} &= E\{Z_i|Y_{\text{obs}}, \beta^{(t)}\} = x_i^{\top}\beta^{(t)} + \Psi(-x_i^{\top}\beta^{(t)}), \quad 1 \le i \le m, \\ Z_i^{(t)} &= E\{Z_i|Y_{\text{obs}}, \beta^{(t)}\} = x_i^{\top}\beta^{(t)} - \Psi(x_i^{\top}\beta^{(t)}), \quad m+1 \le i \le n, \end{aligned}$$

where $\Psi(x)$ is defined by (2.16). The M-step computes

$$\beta^{(t+1)} = (X^{\top}X + A)^{-1}(X^{\top}Z^{(t)} + Aa),$$

where $Z^{(t)} = (Z_1^{(t)}, \ldots, Z_m^{(t)}, Z_{m+1}^{(t)}, \ldots, Z_n^{(t)})^{\top}$. If the EM algorithm converged at $\tilde{\beta}$, then we choose

$$Z_0 = (Z_{0,1}, \ldots, Z_{0,n})^{\top} \quad (5.47)$$

where

$$Z_{0,i} = \begin{cases} x_i^{\top}\tilde{\beta} + \Psi(-x_i^{\top}\tilde{\beta}), & i = 1, \ldots, m, \\ x_i^{\top}\tilde{\beta} - \Psi(x_i^{\top}\tilde{\beta}), & i = m+1, \ldots, n. \end{cases}$$

Example 5.6 (*The prostatic cancer data*). Consider the prostatic cancer data reported by Brown (1980) and re-analyzed by Chib (1995). The outcome of interest is a binary variable Y_i that takes the value unity if the i-th patient's cancer had spread to the surrounding lymph nodes and value zero otherwise. The goal was to determine if five common variables were prognostic to whether or not the cancer has spread to the lymph nodes. The five variables were: the age of patient at diagnosis (in years); the level of serum acid phosphatase (in King–Armstrong units); the result of an X-ray examination (0 = negative, 1 = positive); the size of the tumor (0 = small, 1 = large); and the pathological grade of the tumor (0 = less serious, 1 = more serious). The data in Table 5.5 are sorted so that the first m (= 20) observations of Y_i take value 1.

Table 5.5 *The prostatic cancer data*

i	Y_i	Age	AL	x3	x4	TG	Z_0	i	Y_i	Age	AL	x3	x4	TG	Z_0
1	1	50	0.56	0	0	1	0.44	28	0	60	0.62	1	0	0	-0.83
2	1	67	0.67	1	0	1	0.79	29	0	49	0.55	1	0	0	-0.90
3	1	59	0.99	0	0	1	0.59	30	0	61	0.62	0	0	0	-1.51
4	1	61	1.36	1	0	0	1.28	31	0	58	0.71	0	0	0	-1.37
5	1	56	0.82	0	0	0	0.53	32	0	51	0.65	0	0	0	-1.46
6	1	58	0.48	1	1	0	1.02	33	0	67	0.47	0	0	1	-1.81
7	1	57	0.51	1	1	1	1.07	34	0	51	0.49	0	0	0	-1.76
8	1	65	0.49	0	1	0	0.60	35	0	56	0.50	0	0	1	-1.74
9	1	65	0.84	1	1	1	1.50	36	0	60	0.78	0	0	0	-1.29
10	1	50	0.81	1	1	1	1.46	37	0	52	0.83	0	0	0	-1.23
11	1	60	0.76	1	1	1	1.40	38	0	56	0.98	0	0	0	-1.10
12	1	45	0.70	0	1	1	0.74	39	0	67	0.52	0	0	0	-1.69
13	1	56	0.78	1	1	1	1.43	40	0	63	0.75	0	0	0	-1.32
14	1	46	0.70	0	1	0	0.74	41	0	64	1.87	0	0	0	-0.72
15	1	67	0.67	0	1	0	0.72	42	0	64	0.40	0	1	0	-1.24
16	1	63	0.82	0	1	0	0.82	43	0	61	0.50	0	1	0	-1.07
17	1	57	0.67	0	1	1	0.72	44	0	64	0.50	0	1	0	-1.07
18	1	51	0.72	1	1	0	1.35	45	0	63	0.40	0	1	0	-1.24
19	1	64	0.89	1	1	0	1.56	46	0	52	0.55	0	1	0	-1.00
20	1	68	1.26	1	1	1	1.95	47	0	66	0.59	0	1	0	-0.95
21	0	66	0.48	0	0	0	-1.78	48	0	65	0.48	0	1	1	-1.10
22	0	68	0.56	0	0	0	-1.61	49	0	59	0.63	1	1	1	-0.54
23	0	66	0.50	0	0	0	-1.74	50	0	61	1.02	0	1	0	-0.67
24	0	56	0.52	0	0	0	-1.69	51	0	53	0.76	0	1	0	-0.81
25	0	58	0.50	0	0	0	-1.74	52	0	67	0.95	0	1	0	-0.70
26	0	60	0.49	0	0	0	-1.76	53	0	53	0.66	0	1	1	-0.89
27	0	65	0.46	1	0	0	-1.02								

Source: Chib (1995). NOTE: x1 = 1, x2 = log(Acid Level), x3 = X-ray result, x4 = tumor size. AL = Acid Level, TG = Tumor Grade, Z_0 are the predictive values specified by (5.47).

Collett (1991) concludes that the logistic model with x1 = 1, x2 = log(acid level), x3 = X-ray result and x4 = tumor size fits the data the best among 32 possible models without interactions using the classical deviance statistic. This is further supported by Chib (1995) who identified the same set of prognostic variables using the probit link. Hence, we adopt the probit regression model:

$$p_i = \Phi(\beta_1 + \beta_2 x_{i2} + \beta_3 x_{i3} + \beta_4 x_{i4}), \quad i = 1, \ldots, 53,$$

where $\beta = (\beta_1, \ldots, \beta_4)^\top$ and $x_i = (1, x_{i2}, x_{i3}, x_{i4})^\top$. Take the normal prior $\beta \sim N_4(a, A^{-1})$ with $a = 0.75 \times \mathbf{1}_4$ and $A^{-1} = \text{diag}(25, \ldots, 25)$. Using $\beta^{(0)} = \mathbf{0}_4$ as the initial value, the EM algorithm converged at the observed posterior mode $\tilde{\beta}$ (given in the second column of Table 5.6) after 20 iterations with precision 10^{-5}. The best Z_0 specified by (5.47) is given in Table 5.5. We implement the IBF sampling using $J = 30{,}000$ and $I = 10{,}000$. The posterior estimates of parameters are given in Table 5.6. The observed and augmented posterior densities of β_j for $j = 1, \ldots, 4$ are plotted in Figure 5.4.

Table 5.6 *Posterior estimates of parameters for probit regression model for the prostatic cancer data*

Parameter	Posterior mode†	Posterior mean	Posterior std	95% Posterior CI
β_1	−0.6619	−0.6680	0.3379	[−1.3246, −0.0005]
β_2	1.3985	1.4000	0.5310	[0.3692, 2.4213]
β_3	1.2205	1.2298	0.3676	[0.5136, 1.9401]
β_4	1.0053	1.0074	0.3323	[0.3613, 1.6390]

†The observed posterior mode $\tilde{\beta}$ was calculated by an EM algorithm converged at the 20-th iteration with precision 10^{-5}.

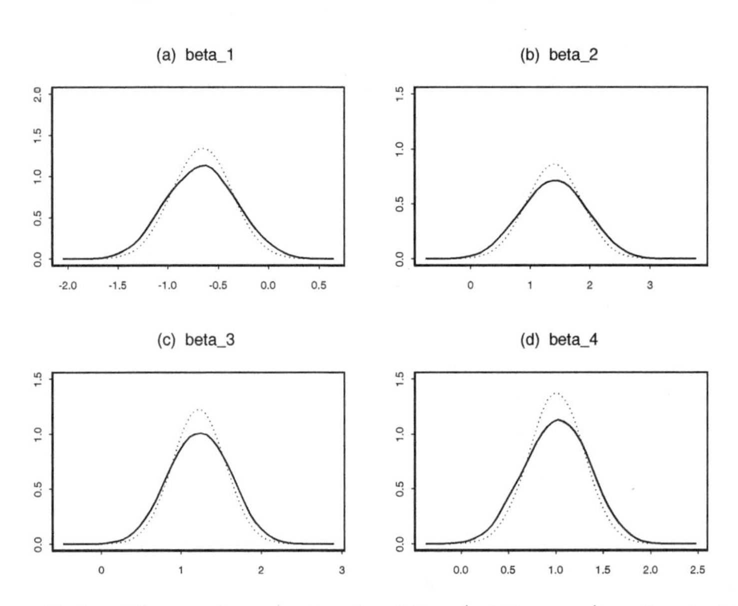

Figure 5.4 Observed posterior densities (solid curve) estimated by a kernel density smoother based on i.i.d. samples obtained via the IBF sampler ($J = 30{,}000$, $I = 10{,}000$, without replacement) and the corresponding augmented posterior densities (dotted curve) with Z_0 given in Table 5.5. (a) β_1; (b) β_2; (c) β_3; (d) β_4. ‖

5.6 A Probit-Normal GLMM for Repeated Binary Data

Generalized linear mixed models (GLMMs) are widely used in biomedical research. Although likelihood-based methods for the GLMM for Gaussian responses are well developed (Laird & Ware, 1982; Meng & van Dyk, 1998), maximum likelihood fitting of the GLMM for repeated/correlated/clustered binary data remains to be a challenge because of the complexity of the likelihood function. To tackle the complicated likelihood, Breslow & Clayton (1993) proposed approximate MLE with penalized quasi-likelihood estimates for the fixed effects parameters and restricted MLEs for the variance parameters in the random effects. However, the method is known to yield biased estimates, in particular, to underestimate the variance parameters (Jiang, 1998). To correct the bias, Lin & Breslow (1996) used a four-order Laplace approximation but it remains to be problematic for correlated binary data. Higher order approximations have been proposed but they are restricted to one random effect per cluster with a large sample size (Raudenbush *et al.*, 2000). In addition, these approximate MLEs have been shown to be inconsistent under standard (small domain) asymptotic assumptions and the asymptotic bias can be severe if the variance components are not small (Kuk, 1995; Breslow & Lin, 1995; Lin & Breslow, 1996).

Another approach is to derive the exact MLE in GLMMs by the MCEM algorithm (Wei & Tanner, 1990). While the M-step is relatively straightforward, the Monte Carlo E-step involves an intractable high-dimensional integral. To fit a probit-normal GLMM for repeated binary data, McCulloch (1994) proposed an MCEM algorithm with a Gibbs sampler at each E-step. Later, McCulloch (1997) used a Hastings–Metropolis algorithm at each E-step in the MCEM to fit more general models. Both of these two algorithms lead to problems of convergence and slow convergence. Booth & Hobert (1999) recognized that MCEM algorithms based on independent samples can be computationally more efficient than MCMC EM algorithms based on dependent samples.

In this section, an efficient MCEM algorithm is presented to find MLEs of parameters in the probit-normal GLMM. Specifically, utilizing the IBF at each E-step, an importance sampling (i.e., weighted Monte Carlo integration) is developed to numerically evaluate the first- and second-order moments of a truncated multinormal distribution, thus eliminating problems of convergence and slow convergence associated with the MCMC.

5.6.1 Model formulation

Let Y_{ij} denote the binary outcome 0 or 1 of the j-th measurement and $Y_i = (Y_{i1}, \ldots, Y_{in_i})^\top$ be the collection of responses from subject i. A probit-normal GLMM for repeated binary data (McCulloch, 1994) assumes

$$\begin{aligned} \Pr\{Y_{ij} = 1|b_i, \beta\} &= \Phi(\mu_{ij}), \quad 1 \le i \le m,\ 1 \le j \le n_i, \qquad (5.48)\\ \mu_{ij} &= x_{ij}^\top \beta + w_{ij}^\top b_i, \\ b_i|D &\overset{\text{iid}}{\sim} N_q(\mathbf{0},\ D), \end{aligned}$$

where $x_{ij}^\top = (x_{ij1}, \ldots, x_{ijp})$ and $w_{ij}^\top = (w_{ij1}, \ldots, w_{ijq})$ are covariates, β is the $p \times 1$ fixed effect, $\{b_i\}_{i=1}^m$ are the $q \times 1$ random effects, D is a $q \times q$ unknown matrix relating to the correlation structure of Y_i. Let $Y_{\text{obs}} = \{Y_i, X_i, W_i\}_1^m$ denote the observed data and $X_i = (x_{i1}, \ldots, x_{in_i})$ and $W_i = (w_{i1}, \ldots, w_{in_i})$ be two $p \times n_i$ and $q \times n_i$ matrices, then the observed-data likelihood for $\theta = (\beta, D)$ is

$$L(\theta|Y_{\text{obs}}) = \prod_{i=1}^m \int N_q(b_i|\mathbf{0}, D)\psi_i(\beta, b_i)\, db_i, \qquad (5.49)$$

where

$$\psi_i(\beta, b_i) \hat{=} \prod_{j=1}^{n_i} [\Phi(\mu_{ij})]^{y_{ij}} [1 - \Phi(\mu_{ij})]^{1-y_{ij}} \qquad (5.50)$$

and $y_i \hat{=} (y_{i1}, \ldots, y_{in_i})^\top$ denotes a realization of Y_i.

Directly maximizing $L(\theta|Y_{\text{obs}})$ is often difficult and this is particularly true when m, n_i and q are very large. Alternatively, we augment the Y_{obs} with the latent data $\{b_i,\ Z_i\}_1^m$ by defining

$$Y_{ij} = I_{(Z_{ij}>0)}, \quad i = 1, \ldots, m, \quad j = 1, \ldots, n_i,$$

where $Z_i|(b_i, \beta) \overset{\text{ind}}{\sim} N_{n_i}(\mu_i,\ \mathbf{I}_{n_i})$ with $Z_i = (Z_{i1}, \ldots, Z_{in_i})^\top$,

$$\mu_i = (\mu_{i1}, \ldots, \mu_{in_i})^\top = X_i^\top \beta + W_i^\top b_i. \qquad (5.51)$$

Thus, the model (5.48) can be rewritten as

$$\begin{aligned} \Pr\{Y_i = y_i|b_i, \beta\} &= \int_{B_i} N_{n_i}(Z_i|\mu_i,\ \mathbf{I}_{n_i})\, dZ_i, \qquad (5.52)\\ b_i|D &\overset{\text{iid}}{\sim} N_q(\mathbf{0},\ D), \end{aligned}$$

where $B_i = B_{i1} \times \cdots \times B_{in_i}$ and B_{ij} is the interval $(0, \infty)$ if $y_{ij} = 1$ and the interval $(-\infty, 0]$ if $y_{ij} = 0$. Note that B_i depends only on the value of y_i and not on the parameters. It is important to distinguish $\mathcal{S}_{(Z|Y_{\text{obs}})} = \prod_{i=1}^m B_i$ from $\mathcal{S}_Z = \prod_{i=1}^m \mathbb{R}^{n_i}$.

5.6.2 An MCEM algorithm without using the Gibbs sampler at E-step

(a) The derivation of M-step

We treat both $b \hat{=} \{b_i\}_1^m$ and $Z \hat{=} \{Z_i\}_1^m$ as missing data. From the definition of the latent data Z, we have $\{Y_{\text{obs}}, Z\} = Z$. Thus, the joint density for the complete-data $Y_{\text{com}} = \{Y_{\text{obs}}, b, Z\} = \{b, Z\}$ is

$$\begin{aligned} f(Y_{\text{com}}|\theta) &= \prod_{i=1}^m f(b_i|D) f(Z_i|b_i, \beta) \\ &= \prod_{i=1}^m N_q(b_i|\mathbf{0},\ D) N_{n_i}(Z_i|\mu_i,\ \mathbf{I}_{n_i}), \end{aligned} \tag{5.53}$$

where $\{\mu_i\}_1^m$ are defined in (5.51). The M-step of the MCEM algorithm is to find the complete-data MLE of θ. We obtain the following closed-form expressions:

$$\begin{aligned} \hat{\beta} &= \left(\sum_{i=1}^m X_i X_i^\top\right)^{-1} \sum_{i=1}^m X_i(Z_i - W_i^\top b_i), \quad \text{and} \quad (5.54) \\ \hat{D} &= \frac{1}{m}\sum_{i=1}^m b_i b_i^\top. \end{aligned}$$

(b) The derivation of E-step

The E-step computes conditional expectations of the complete-data sufficient statistics, i.e, $E(Z_i|Y_i, \theta)$, $E(b_i|Y_i, \theta)$ and $E(b_i b_i^\top|Y_i, \theta)$ for $i = 1, \ldots, m$. To calculate them, we first derive the conditional predictive distribution of the missing data, which is given by

$$\begin{aligned} f(b, Z|Y_{\text{obs}}, \theta) &= f(b|Y_{\text{obs}}, Z, \theta)\, f(Z|Y_{\text{obs}}, \theta) \quad &(5.55) \\ &= f(Z|Y_{\text{obs}}, b, \theta)\, f(b|Y_{\text{obs}}, \theta). \quad &(5.56) \end{aligned}$$

Since $f(b|Y_{\text{obs}}, Z, \theta) \propto$ (5.53), we immediately obtain

$$\begin{aligned} f(b|Y_{\text{obs}}, Z, \theta) &= \prod_{i=1}^m f(b_i|Y_i, Z_i, \theta) = \prod_{i=1}^m f(b_i|Z_i, \theta) \\ &= \prod_{i=1}^m N_q\Big(b_i\Big|\Delta_i(Z_i - X_i^\top\beta),\ \Lambda_i\Big), \end{aligned} \tag{5.57}$$

where $\Delta_i \hat{=} DW_i\Omega_i^{-1}$, $\Lambda_i \hat{=} D - DW_i\Omega_i^{-1}W_i^{\top}D$, and $\Omega_i \hat{=} W_i^{\top}DW_i + \mathbf{I}_{n_i}$, $i = 1, \ldots, m$. To derive the second term on the right-hand side of (5.55), we use the following result (Chib & Greenberg, 1998, p.350)

$$\begin{aligned}\Pr\{Y_i = y_i|b_i, Z_i, \theta\} &= I_{(Z_i \in B_i)} \\ &= \prod_{j=1}^{n_i} \Big\{ I_{(Z_{ij}>0)} I_{(Y_{ij}=1)} + I_{(Z_{ij}\le 0)} I_{(Y_{ij}=0)} \Big\}, \qquad (5.58)\end{aligned}$$

which indicates that given Z_i, the conditional probability of Y_i is independent of b_i. Hence (5.58) implies $\Pr\{Y_i = y_i|Z_i, \theta\} = I_{(Z_i \in B_i)}$. Since the joint density of (Z_i, b_i) is normally distributed, the marginal distribution of $Z_i|\theta$ follows $N_{n_i}(X_i^{\top}\beta,\ \Omega_i)$. Moreover, from

$$\begin{aligned} f(Z_i|Y_i, \theta) &\propto f(Z_i, Y_i|\theta) \\ &= f(Z_i|\theta) \cdot \Pr\{Y_i = y_i|Z_i, \theta\} \\ &= N_{n_i}(Z_i|X_i^{\top}\beta,\ \Omega_i) \cdot I_{(Z_i \in B_i)}, \end{aligned}$$

we obtain

$$f(Z|Y_{\text{obs}}, \theta) = \prod_{i=1}^{m} f(Z_i|Y_i, \theta) = \prod_{i=1}^{m} TN_{n_i}(Z_i|X_i^{\top}\beta,\ \Omega_i;\ B_i). \qquad (5.59)$$

Below an importance sampling is provided to evaluate $E(Z_i|Y_i, \theta) \hat{=} M_1^{(i)}$ and $E(Z_iZ_i^{\top}|Y_i, \theta) \hat{=} M_2^{(i)}$ based on (5.59). Once both $M_1^{(i)}$ and $M_2^{(i)}$ are available, Eq.(5.57) gives the Rao–Blackwellized estimates:

$$\begin{aligned} E(b_i|Y_i, \theta) &= E\Big\{E(b_i|Y_i, Z_i, \theta)\Big|Y_i, \theta\Big\} \\ &= \Delta_i\Big[M_1^{(i)} - X_i^{\top}\beta\Big], \qquad (5.60) \\ E(b_ib_i^{\top}|Y_i, \theta) &= E\Big\{E(b_ib_i^{\top}|Y_i, Z_i, \theta)\Big|Y_i, \theta\Big\} \qquad (5.61) \\ &= \Lambda_i + \Delta_i\Big[M_2^{(i)} + \gamma_i\gamma_i^{\top} - M_1^{(i)}\gamma_i^{\top} - (M_1^{(i)}\gamma_i^{\top})^{\top}\Big]\Delta_i^{\top}, \end{aligned}$$

where $\gamma_i \hat{=} X_i^{\top}\beta$.

(c) The use of importance sampling at each E-step

McCulloch (1994) suggested using a Gibbs sampler at each E-step to estimate $E(Z_i|Y_i, \theta)$ and $E(Z_iZ_i^{\top}|Y_i, \theta)$ from the truncated multinormal distribution (5.59). In fact, utilizing the IBF, an importance sampling procedure can be formed to evaluate the two expectations at each E-step. For this purpose, we first need to derive the first term on the right-hand side of (5.56). From (5.53) and (5.58), we have

$$\begin{aligned} f(Z_i|Y_i, b_i, \theta) &\propto f(Y_i, b_i, Z_i|\theta) \\ &= f(b_i|\theta) \cdot f(Z_i|b_i, \theta) \cdot \Pr\{Y_i = y_i|b_i, Z_i, \theta\} \\ &\propto N_{n_i}(Z_i|\mu_i,\ \mathbf{I}_{n_i}) \cdot I_{(Z_i \in B_i)}, \end{aligned}$$

so that

$$\begin{aligned} f(Z|Y_{\rm obs}, b, \theta) &= \prod_{i=1}^m f(Z_i|Y_i, b_i, \theta) \\ &= \prod_{i=1}^m TN_{n_i}(Z_i|\mu_i,\ \mathbf{I}_{n_i};\ B_i), \end{aligned} \tag{5.62}$$

where $\{\mu_i\}_1^m$ are defined in (5.51). Next, from (5.55) and (5.56), we have $f(Z_i|Y_i,\theta) \propto f(Z_i|Y_i,b_i,\theta)/f(b_i|Y_i,Z_i,\theta)$ for an arbitrary b_i. Let b_i^0 be an arbitrary point in the support of b_i, the function-wise IBF gives

$$f(Z_i|Y_i,\theta) = \left\{ \int \frac{f(Z_i|Y_i, b_i^0, \theta)}{f(b_i^0|Y_i, Z_i, \theta)}\, dZ_i \right\}^{-1} \frac{f(Z_i|Y_i, b_i^0, \theta)}{f(b_i^0|Y_i, Z_i, \theta)}, \tag{5.63}$$

where the denominator and the numerator are given by (5.57) and (5.62), respectively. Let $\{Z_i^{(k)}\}_{k=1}^K \stackrel{\rm iid}{\sim} f(Z_i|Y_i, b_i^0, \theta)$, then the moments can be estimated by the weighted means

$$\begin{aligned} E(Z_i|Y_i,\theta) &\doteq \sum_{k=1}^K \omega_i^{(k)} Z_i^{(k)}, \\ E(Z_i Z_i^\top|Y_i,\theta) &\doteq \sum_{k=1}^K \omega_i^{(k)} Z_i^{(k)} Z_i^{(k)\top}, \end{aligned} \tag{5.64}$$

and the weights are given by

$$\omega_i^{(k)} = \frac{\delta_i^{(k)}}{\delta_i^{(1)} + \cdots + \delta_i^{(K)}}, \qquad \delta_i^{(k)} \hat{=} f^{-1}(b_i^0|Y_i, Z_i^{(k)}, \theta). \tag{5.65}$$

A natural problem for efficiently computing (5.64) is how to choose b_i^0 in (5.63). It suffices to select a b_i^0 such that $f(Z_i|Y_i, b_i^0, \theta)$

best approximates $f(Z_i|Y_i, \theta)$. Theorem 5.1 has shown that the best choice of b_i^0 is the mode of $f(b_i|Y_i, Z_i, \theta)$. Since the mode and the mean for a normal distribution is identical, from (5.57), theoretically, we can choose $b_i^0 = \Delta_i(Z_i - X_i^\top \beta)$. In practice, noting that Z_i is unknown, we may replace Z_i by $E(Z_i|Y_i, \theta) \, (= M_1^{(i)})$ and choose $b_i^0 = b_i^{(t)} = E(b_i|Y_i, \theta^{(t)})$ calculated according to (5.60) since the function-wise IBF (5.63) holds for any possible values of b_i^0 in the support of b_i.

(d) Monitoring the convergence of the MCEM algorithm

To monitor the convergence of the MCEM algorithm, we again employ importance sampling to directly calculate the log-likelihood values and then to plot $\log L(\theta^{(t)}|Y_{\text{obs}})$ against the MCEM iteration t. Specifically, let

$$b_i^{(\ell)} \stackrel{\text{iid}}{\sim} N_q(\mathbf{0}, D), \quad i = 1, \ldots, m, \quad \ell = 1, \ldots, M,$$

then, from (5.49), the log-likelihood can be approximated by

$$\begin{aligned} \log L(\theta|Y_{\text{obs}}) &= \sum_{i=1}^{m} \log L(\theta|Y_i) \\ &\doteq \sum_{i=1}^{m} \log \left[\frac{1}{M} \sum_{\ell=1}^{M} \psi_i(\beta, b_i^{(\ell)}) \right], \end{aligned} \tag{5.66}$$

where $L(\theta|Y_i)$ is the observed likelihood of θ contributed from subject i, and $\psi_i(\beta, b_i)$ is defined in (5.50). Given $\theta^{(t)}$ and $\theta^{(t+1)}$, we plot

$$\log \left[\frac{L(\theta^{(t+1)}|Y_{\text{obs}})}{L(\theta^{(t)}|Y_{\text{obs}})} \right] = \sum_{i=1}^{m} \log \left[\frac{L(\theta^{(t+1)}|Y_i)}{L(\theta^{(t)}|Y_i)} \right] \tag{5.67}$$

against t. If the plot shows that the differences vanish or stabilize around zero, we consider the algorithm has achieved approximate convergence. This is probably what can be done regarding the convergence of the MCEM.

(e) The calculation of standard errors

Denote the MLE from the MCEM algorithm by $\hat{\theta} = (\hat{\beta}, \hat{D})$. Louis (1982) showed that the observed information matrix is given by

$$-E\left\{ \frac{\partial^2 \ell(\theta|Y_{\text{obs}}, b, Z)}{\partial\theta\partial\theta^\top} \right\}\bigg|_{\theta=\hat{\theta}} - \text{Var}\left\{ \frac{\partial \ell(\theta|Y_{\text{obs}}, b, Z)}{\partial\theta} \right\}\bigg|_{\theta=\hat{\theta}} \tag{5.68}$$

where the expectation and variance are with respect to $f(b,Z|Y_{\text{obs}},\hat{\theta})$. Based on (5.57) and (5.62), a DA algorithm can be used to obtain dependent samples from $f(b,Z|Y_{\text{obs}},\hat{\theta})$ so that (5.68) can be estimated by Monte Carlo methods. Standard errors are equal to the square roots of the diagonal elements of the inverse of the estimated information matrix.

Example 5.7 (*Six cities children's wheeze data*). Consider the longitudinal study on health effects of air pollution in six cities (Chib & Greenberg, 1998). The data in Table 5.7 consist of an annual binary response indicating the presence or absence of wheeze at age 7, 8, 9 and 10 years for each of 537 children from one city. Maternal smoking was categorized as 1 if the mother smoked regularly and 0 otherwise. The objective of the study is to model the probability of wheeze status as a function of the child's age and the mother's smoking habit.

Table 5.7 *Children's wheeze data in six cities*

No maternal smoking					Maternal smoking				
Age of child (year)					Age of child (year)				
7	8	9	10	Frequency	7	8	9	10	Frequency
0	0	0	0	237	0	0	0	0	118
0	0	0	1	10	0	0	0	1	6
0	0	1	0	15	0	0	1	0	8
0	0	1	1	4	0	0	1	1	2
0	1	0	0	16	0	1	0	0	11
0	1	0	1	2	0	1	0	1	1
0	1	1	0	7	0	1	1	0	6
0	1	1	1	3	0	1	1	1	4
1	0	0	0	24	1	0	0	0	7
1	0	0	1	3	1	0	0	1	3
1	0	1	0	3	1	0	1	0	3
1	0	1	1	2	1	0	1	1	1
1	1	0	0	6	1	1	0	0	4
1	1	0	1	2	1	1	0	1	2
1	1	1	0	5	1	1	1	0	4
1	1	1	1	11	1	1	1	1	7

Source: Chib & Greenberg (1998).

The probability $\Pr\{Y_{ij} = 1|b_i, \beta\}$ of wheeze status of the i-th child at the j-th observation is assumed to be equal to

$$\Phi\Big(\beta_1 + \text{age}\ \beta_2 + \text{smoking}\ \beta_3 + (\text{age} \times \text{smoking})\beta_4 + w_{ij}^{\top} b_i\Big),$$

where "age" is the age of the child centered at nine years, "smoking" $= 1$ if mother smokes, 0 otherwise, $w_{ij}^{\top} = (1, \text{age})$, implying that both intercept and the age effects are children-specific, and $b_i|D \sim N_2(\mathbf{0},\ D)$, $i = 1, \ldots, m\ (m = 537)$, $j = 1, \ldots, n_i\ (n_i = 4)$.

To find the MLEs $\hat{\beta}$ and $\hat{D}$, we use the importance sampling described in §5.6.2(c) at each E-step. Specifically, for a fixed i, we generate

$$\{Z_i^{(k)}\}_{k=1}^{K} \overset{\text{iid}}{\sim} f(Z_i|Y_i, b_i^0, \theta)$$

(see (5.63) and (5.62)) and calculate $\{\omega_i^{(k)}\}$ according to (5.65). Thus, we can estimate $E(Z_i|Y_i, \theta)$ and $E(Z_i Z_i^{\top}|Y_i, \theta)$ by (5.64) and compute $E(b_i|Y_i, \theta)$ and $E(b_i b_i^{\top}|Y_i, \theta)$ via (5.60) and (5.61). Because of the iterative nature of the EM algorithm, we also use a K that increases linearly with the number of iterations as does McCulloch (1994). Specifically, we choose $K = 50$ for iteration 1 to 20, $K = 100$ for iteration 21 to 40, $K = 200$ for iteration 41 to 60, $K = 500$ for iteration 61 to 80, and $K = 1000$ for iteration 81 and over. The M-step is straightforward since (5.54) has a closed-form expression. Using $\theta^{(0)} = (\beta^{(0)}, D^{(0)})$ with $\beta^{(0)} = \mathbf{0}_4$ and $D^{(0)} = \mathbf{I}_2$ as initial values, the MCEM algorithm converged at the 100-th iteration to the MLEs $\hat{\beta}$ and $\hat{D}$. Standard errors are calculated according to (5.68). These results are listed in the third and fourth columns of Table 5.8.

Table 5.8 *MLEs and standard errors of β and D*

Variable	Parameter	MLE*	SE*	MLE†	SE†
Intercept	β_1	−1.8245	0.0289	−1.8145	0.0295
Age	β_2	−0.1006	0.0237	−0.1145	0.0239
Smoking	β_3	0.1925	0.0490	0.2742	0.0496
Age × Smoking	β_4	0.0368	0.0405	0.1032	0.0403
Covariance	d_{11}	1.7517	0.1080	1.6251	0.1005
	d_{12}	−0.0005	0.0070	0.0005	0.0127
	d_{22}	0.0148	0.0009	0.0525	0.0032

Source: Tan, Tian & Fang (2007). *Values obtained by the MCEM algorithm with an importance sampling at each E-step, converged at the 100-th iteration. †Values obtained by the MCEM algorithm with a Gibbs sampling at each E-step (McCulloch, 1994), nearly converged at 100-th iteration.

Convergence of the MCEM was determined from Figures 5.5(a), 5.6 and 5.7(a). As Figure 5.5(a) shows, the logs of individual components of $\theta^{(t)} = (\beta^{(t)}, D^{(t)})$ appear to have stabilized after about 40 iterations. Similarly, the log-likelihood values $\log L(\theta^{(t)}|Y_{\rm obs})$ estimated by (5.66) also appear to stabilize after 40 EM cycles (Figure 5.6). Figure 5.7(a) shows that the logs of the likelihood ratios estimated from (5.67) decrease to zero after 40 iterations. The computing time for finding the MLEs is 40.82 minutes (0.68033 hour) for 40 iterations or 102.05 minutes (1.7008 hours) for 100 iterations.

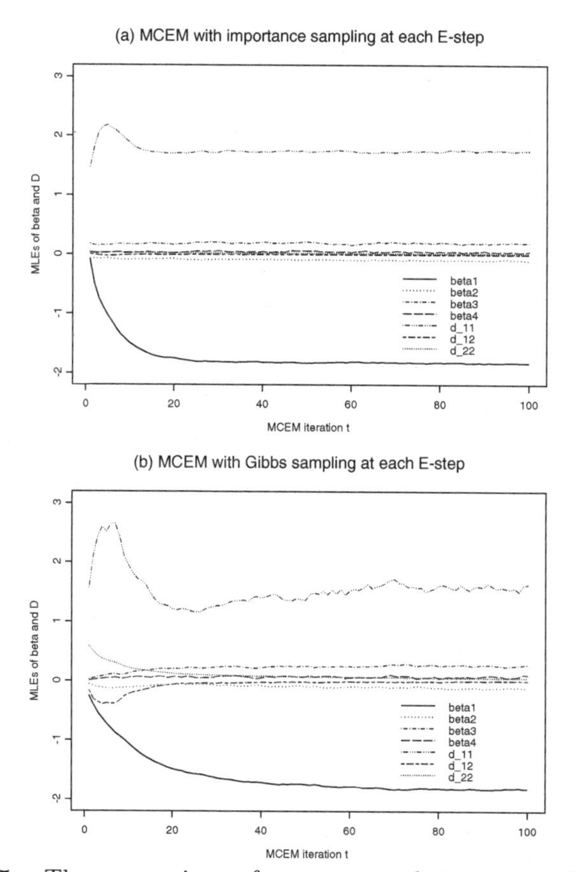

Figure 5.5 The comparison of convergence between two MCEM algorithms by plotting the MLEs of $\beta = (\beta_1, \dots, \beta_4)^\top$ and D against the MCEM iteration t for the wheeze data in six cities.

To compare the new MCEM algorithm with the MCEM of McCulloch (1994), in the E-step, for a fixed i, we run a Gibbs sampler with a single chain to obtain a dependent sample of size $2K$ from the truncated multinormal distribution $TN_{n_i}(Z_i|X_i^\top\beta,\ \Omega_i;\ B_i)$ (see

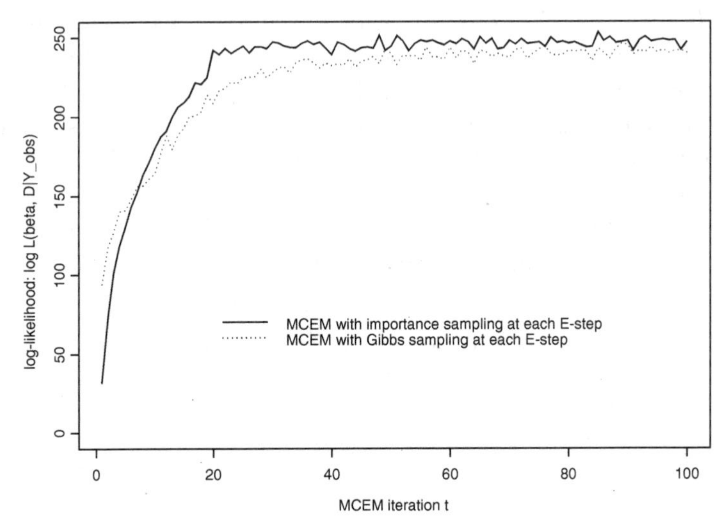

Figure 5.6 The comparison of convergence between two MCEM algorithms with importance/Gibbs sampling at each E-step by plotting the log-likelihood values against the MCEM iteration t for the children's wheeze data in six cities.

(5.59)) and no assessment of convergence of the Markov chain to its stationary distribution is made. Then, we use the second half of the sequence to estimate $E(Z_i|Y_i, \theta)$ and $E(Z_i Z_i^{\top}|Y_i, \theta)$. Note that $E(b_i|Y_i, \theta)$ and $E(b_i b_i^{\top}|Y_i, \theta)$ are still given by (5.60) and (5.61), respectively, and the M-step is also the same as (5.54). We use the same K and the same initial values $(\beta^{(0)}, D^{(0)})$ as that of the proposed MCEM above. We terminate the MCEM at the 100-th iteration. The corresponding MLEs $\hat{\beta}$ and $\hat{D}$ and their standard errors calculated according to (5.68) are listed in the fifth and sixth columns of Table 5.8. Convergence of the MCEM can be assessed based on Figures 5.5(b), 5.6 and 5.7(b). Although Figure 5.7(b) shows that the logs of the likelihood ratios estimated from (5.67) decrease to zero after 80 iterations, Figure 5.5(b) shows that the logs of d_{11} seem to have not stabilized after 100 iterations. From Figure 5.6, the log-likelihood values $\log L(\theta^{(t)}|Y_{\text{obs}})$ estimated by (5.66) do not stabilize after 80 EM cycles and the convergence is thus slower than the new MCEM. The computing time for the MLEs is 25.406 hours for 100 iterations, which is $25.406/0.68033 = 37.344$ (or at least $25.406/1.7008 = 14.938$) times slower than the new MCEM.

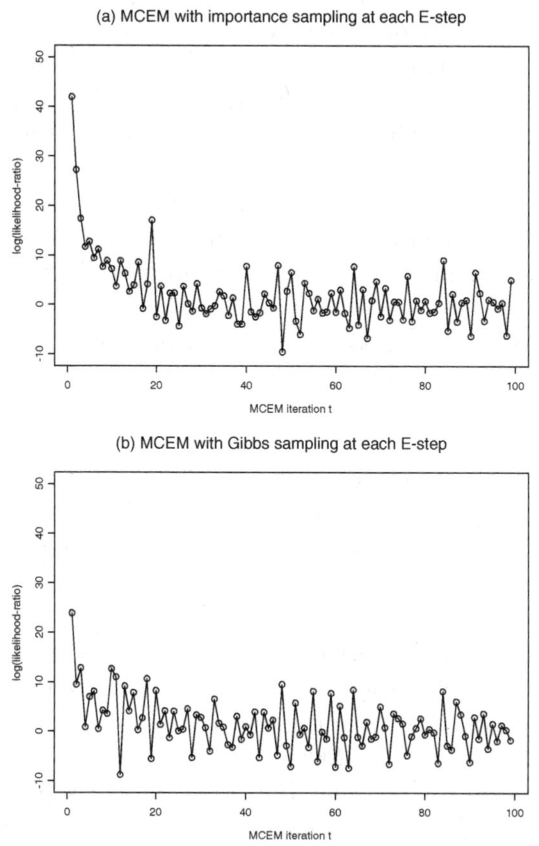

Figure 5.7 The assessment of convergence for two MCEM algorithms by plotting the difference of the consecutive log-likelihood values against the MCEM iteration t for the children's wheeze data in six cities. ||

5.7 Hierarchical Models for Correlated Binary Data

In the previous section, we introduced an MCEM algorithm without using the Gibbs sampler at the E-step to find MLEs of parameters for a probit-normal GLMM with repeated binary data. However, inference based on these results still depend on large sample size (Louis, 1982).

An alternative is to use a hierarchical model to compute the entire posterior distribution of the parameter of interest. Zeger & Karim (1991) use MCMC methods in the hierarchical logit-normal model where rejection sampling is used in each iteration to obtain samples of the fixed and random effects. Thus, each iteration involves finding the mode and curvature of a complicated likelihood. For longitudinal binary data, Chib (2000) proposes a four-block Gibbs sampler in the probit-normal model whose advantages over the logit-normal model are summarized in McCulloch (1994). Two difficulties for Chib's approach are

1) each cycle of the Gibbs sampler requires another Gibbs sampler to generate truncated multivariate normal distribution; and

2) the Gibbs sampler possibly suffers from the slow convergence owing to the introduction of too many Gaussian latent variables.

Most importantly, both approaches encounter the problematic issues of assessing convergence to the stationary distribution. These results in serious practical problems such as determining the "burn-in" time and the correlation between two successive samples are used to compute variance of the estimate (Casella *et al.*, 2001).

From a Bayesian perspective, the hierarchical model further specify prior distributions for the regression coefficients of the fixed effects and for the hyperparameter in the distribution of the random effects of the GLMM (Tan *et al.*, 2006). In practice, noninformative or vague prior is often used so that Bayesian inference from the hierarchical model is similar to that from the GLMM whereas the whole posterior is available from the hierarchical model. The purpose of this section is to present a noniterative sampling approach for hierarchical models with correlated binary data to obtain an i.i.d. sample from the observed posterior distribution **after** the posterior mode has been obtained by an MCEM approach (e.g., in §5.6).

The probit-normal GLMM to be considered is given by (5.48) or (5.52). Let μ_i be defined by (5.51) and $\theta \hat{=} (\beta, \mathrm{D})$. The complete-data likelihood function for θ is given by (5.53). We consider independent prior distributions:

$$\begin{aligned} \beta &\sim N_p(\mu_0, \Sigma_0^{-1}), \quad \text{and} \\ D &\sim \text{IWishart}_q(\Lambda_0^{-1}, \nu_0). \end{aligned}$$

Then the complete-data posterior distribution is given by

$$f(\theta|Y_{\text{obs}}, Z, b) = f(\beta|Y_{\text{obs}}, Z, b) \times f(D|Y_{\text{obs}}, Z, b), \tag{5.69}$$

where

$$
\begin{aligned}
f(\beta|Y_{\rm obs}, Z, b) &= N_p\Big(\beta\Big|\tilde\beta,\ (\Sigma_0 + \Sigma_{i=1}^m X_i X_i^{\top})^{-1}\Big), \\
f(D|Y_{\rm obs}, Z, b) &= \text{IWishart}_q\Big(D\Big|\tilde D^{-1}/(\nu_0+q+1+m), \nu_0+m\Big),
\end{aligned}
$$

and $\tilde\beta$ and $\tilde D$ denote the complete-data posterior modes, defined by

$$
\begin{aligned}
\tilde\beta &= \left(\Sigma_0 + \sum_{i=1}^m X_i X_i^{\top}\right)^{-1}\left\{\Sigma_0\mu_0 + \sum_{i=1}^m X_i(Z_i - W_i^{\top} b_i)\right\}, \\
\tilde D &= \frac{1}{\nu_0+q+1+m}\left\{\Lambda_0 + \sum_{i=1}^m b_i b_i^{\top}\right\}.
\end{aligned}
$$

Note that $f(Z|Y_{\rm obs}, b, \theta)$ and $f(b|Y_{\rm obs}, Z, \theta)$ are given by (5.62) and (5.57), respectively. Therefore, based on (5.69), (5.62) and (5.57), we can implement the IBF algorithm proposed in §5.1.3 to obtain i.i.d. samples approximately from the observed posterior distribution $f(\beta, D|Y_{\rm obs})$.

5.8 Hybrid Algorithms: Combining the IBF Sampler with the Gibbs Sampler

Although the IBF methods introduced in §5.1 have been shown to be successful in a broad range of statistical models, they have limitations too. The IBF sampler via the EM-type algorithm may not be feasible, for instance, when

- The observed posterior $f(\theta|Y_{\rm obs})$ is multi-modal;
- It is impossible to find a latent vector Z to augment $Y_{\rm obs}$;
- Neither the augmented posterior $f(\theta|Y_{\rm obs}, Z)$ nor the conditional predictive density $f(Z|Y_{\rm obs}, \theta)$ has explicit expression;
- More than two blocks of r.v.'s are involved in the computation.

To partially overcome these difficulties, we can optimize the IBF sampler via choosing a Z_0 based on intermediate results from the Gibbs sampler or the DA algorithm. Since the IBF procedure holds for any Z_0, so do the noniterative sampling properties. The idea is to first produce outputs

$$\{\theta^{[k]}, Z^{[k]}\}_{k=1}^K$$

by using a single-path Gibbs sampler (see, e.g., Arnold, 1993) or the DA algorithm based on $f(\theta|Y_{\text{obs}}, Z)$ and $f(Z|Y_{\text{obs}}, \theta)$, and then let

$$Z_0 = \frac{1}{K-r+1} \sum_{k=r}^{K} Z^{[k]}. \tag{5.70}$$

Thus, Z_0 can be chosen using results after the MCMC has passed the burn-in period or certain convergence diagnostic approaches. In this section, we present two examples to illustrate the idea.

5.8.1 Nonlinear regression models

Consider a nonlinear regression model (Bates & Watts, 1988):

$$\begin{aligned} Y_i &= \theta_1(1 - e^{-\theta_2 x_i}) + \varepsilon_i, \quad i = 1, \ldots, n, \\ \varepsilon_i &\overset{\text{iid}}{\sim} N(0, \sigma^2), \end{aligned} \tag{5.71}$$

where $Y_{\text{obs}} = \{Y_i\}_1^n$ denote the observed data, x_i is the i-th value of the covariate x, $\theta = (\theta_1, \theta_2)^\top$ and σ^2 are parameters of interest. The likelihood function is

$$L(\theta, \sigma^2|Y_{\text{obs}}) = \frac{1}{(\sqrt{2\pi}\sigma)^n} \exp\left\{ -\frac{S(\theta)}{2\sigma^2} \right\},$$

where the sum of squared residuals is defined by

$$S(\theta) \hat{=} \sum_{i=1}^{n} (Y_i - \theta_1 \delta_i)^2, \quad \text{and} \quad \delta_i \hat{=} 1 - e^{-\theta_2 x_i}.$$

Consider independent prior distributions:

$$\begin{aligned} \theta &\sim N_2(a_0, A_0^{-1}) \quad \text{with} \quad A_0 \to 0, \quad \text{and} \\ \sigma^2 &\sim \text{IGamma}\left(\sigma^2 \Big| \frac{q_0}{2}, \frac{\lambda_0}{2}\right), \quad q_0 = \lambda_0 = 0. \end{aligned}$$

Then, the joint posterior density is

$$f(\theta, \sigma^2|Y_{\text{obs}}) \propto \sigma^{-n-2} \exp\left\{ -\frac{S(\theta)}{2\sigma^2} \right\}.$$

Therefore, we have

$$f(\sigma^2|Y_{\text{obs}}, \theta) = \text{IGamma}\left(\sigma^2 \Big| \frac{n}{2}, \frac{S(\theta)}{2}\right), \tag{5.72}$$

$$\begin{aligned} f(\theta|Y_{\text{obs}}, \sigma^2) &= f(\theta_1|Y_{\text{obs}}, \theta_2, \sigma^2) \times f(\theta_2|Y_{\text{obs}}, \sigma^2) \\ &= N\left(\theta_1 \Bigg| \frac{\sum_{i=1}^n \delta_i Y_i}{\delta^2}, \frac{\sigma^2}{\delta^2}\right) f(\theta_2|Y_{\text{obs}}, \sigma^2), \end{aligned} \tag{5.73}$$

where $\delta^2 \hat{=} \sum_{i=1}^n \delta_i^2$, and

$$f(\theta_2|Y_{\rm obs}, \sigma^2) \propto \frac{1}{\delta} \exp\left\{\frac{(\sum_{i=1}^n \delta_i Y_i)^2}{2\sigma^2\delta^2}\right\}. \tag{5.74}$$

Since (5.74) is a one-dimensional function of θ_2, the grid method (cf. Ex.2.13) can be used to draw samples from (5.74). With the sampling IBF (5.5), we obtain

$$f(\theta|Y_{\rm obs}) \propto \frac{f(\theta|Y_{\rm obs}, \sigma_0^2)}{f(\sigma_0^2|Y_{\rm obs}, \theta)}, \tag{5.75}$$

for some arbitrary $\sigma_0^2 \in \mathbb{R}_+$. For this problem, it is not possible to use an EM-type algorithm to choose σ_0^2 in (5.75) because the problem does not have a missing-data structure. Let $\{\theta^{[k]}, \sigma^{2[k]}\colon k = r, \dots, K\}$ denote the final $K - r + 1$ Gibbs outputs from (5.72) and (5.73), then from (5.70), we set

$$\sigma_0^2 = \frac{1}{K - r + 1} \sum_{k=r}^{K} \sigma^{2[k]}.$$

5.8.2 Binary regression models with t link

(a) Model formulation

The most commonly used link function for binary regression models is the logit link. If we replace the standard Gaussian cdf $\Phi(\cdot)$ by the logistic cdf

$$L(x) = \frac{e^x}{1 + e^x}, \qquad x \in \mathbb{R}, \tag{5.76}$$

then, the probit regression model (5.44) becomes the logistic regression model:

$$\begin{aligned} Y_i &\overset{\rm ind}{\sim} \text{Bernoulli}(p_i), \quad i = 1, \dots, n, \\ p_i &= L(x_i^\top \beta), \quad \text{or} \quad \text{logit}(p_i) = x_i^\top \beta. \end{aligned} \tag{5.77}$$

Since the cdf $L(\cdot)$ in (5.76) can well be approximated[6] by the cdf of a t-distribution with 8 or 9 degrees of freedom, we approximate the

[6]In fact, Mudholkar & George (1978) show that the logistic distribution has the same kurtosis as the t-distribution with 9 degrees of freedom. Albert & Chib (1993) show that logistic quantiles are approximately a linear function of quantiles of t-distribution with 8 degrees of freedom by plotting quantiles of the logistic distribution against quantiles of a t-distribution for various degrees of freedom.

logistic regression model (5.77) by a binary regression model with t link:

$$\begin{aligned} Y_i &\overset{\text{ind}}{\sim} \text{Bernoulli}(p_i), \quad i = 1, \ldots, n, \\ p_i &= \Pr(Y_i = 1|\beta) = T_\nu(x_i^\top \beta), \end{aligned} \tag{5.78}$$

where $T_\nu(\cdot)$ denotes the cdf of t-distribution with ν ($\nu = 8$ or 9) degrees of freedom.

(b) Full conditional distributions

We augment the observed binary data $Y_{\text{obs}} = \{Y_i\}_1^n$ with a latent vector $Z = (Z_1, \ldots, Z_n)^\top$ by defining

$$Y_i = I_{(Z_i>0)}, \quad \text{where} \quad \{Z_i\} \overset{\text{ind}}{\sim} t(x_i^\top \beta, 1, \nu).$$

Note that Z_i is a scale mixture of normal distribution (cf. Appendix A.3.5), we have

$$Z_i|\lambda_i \sim N(x_i^\top \beta,\, \lambda_i^{-1}) \quad \text{and} \quad \lambda_i \sim \text{Gamma}\Big(\frac{\nu}{2}, \frac{\nu}{2}\Big).$$

Using a flat prior for β, then the joint posterior density is

$$\begin{aligned} f(\beta, Z, \lambda|Y_{\text{obs}}) \;\propto\; & \prod_{i=1}^n \Big\{ I_{(Z_i>0)} I_{(Y_i=1)} + I_{(Z_i \le 0)} I_{(Y_i=0)} \Big\} \\ & \times N\Big(z_i \Big| x_i^\top \beta,\, \lambda_i^{-1}\Big) \times \text{Gamma}\Big(\lambda_i \Big| \frac{\nu}{2}, \frac{\nu}{2}\Big). \end{aligned}$$

We obtain the following full conditional distributions:

$$f(\beta|Y_{\text{obs}}, Z, \lambda) = N_r(\beta|(X^\top \Lambda X)^{-1} X^\top \Lambda Z,\, (X^\top \Lambda X)^{-1}), \tag{5.79}$$

$$\begin{aligned} f(Z|Y_{\text{obs}}, \beta, \lambda) &= \prod_{i=1}^m TN(Z_i|x_i^\top \beta, \lambda_i^{-1}, \mathbb{R}_+) \\ &\quad \times \prod_{i=m+1}^n TN(Z_i|x_i^\top \beta, \lambda_i^{-1}, \mathbb{R}_-), \end{aligned} \tag{5.80}$$

$$f(\lambda|Y_{\text{obs}}, \beta, Z) = \prod_{i=1}^n \text{Gamma}\Big(\lambda_i \Big| \frac{\nu+1}{2}, \frac{\nu + (Z_i - x_i^\top \beta)^2}{2}\Big), \tag{5.81}$$

where $X_{n \times r} = (x_1, \ldots, x_n)^\top$, $\Lambda = \text{diag}(\lambda_1, \ldots, \lambda_n)$, and the observed responses are ordered so that $Y_1 = \cdots = Y_m = 1$ and $Y_{m+1} = \cdots = Y_n = 0$.

(c) Implementing IBF sampler utilizing the Gibbs sampler

Using the sampling (5.5), we have

$$f(\beta|Y_{\text{obs}}) \propto \frac{f(\beta|Y_{\text{obs}}, Z_0, \lambda_0)}{f(Z_0, \lambda_0|Y_{\text{obs}}, \beta)}, \tag{5.82}$$

for arbitrary $Z_0 \in \mathcal{S}_{(Z|Y_{\text{obs}})}$, $\lambda_0 \in \mathcal{S}_{(\lambda|Y_{\text{obs}})}$, and all $\beta \in \mathcal{S}_{(\beta|Y_{\text{obs}})}$. The denominator of the right-hand side of (5.82) can be evaluated at a given point $\beta \in \mathcal{S}_{(\beta|Y_{\text{obs}})}$ by

$$f(Z_0, \lambda_0|Y_{\text{obs}}, \beta) = f(Z_0|Y_{\text{obs}}, \beta, \lambda_0) \times f(\lambda_0|Y_{\text{obs}}, \beta), \tag{5.83}$$

where

$$\begin{aligned} f(\lambda_0|Y_{\text{obs}}, \beta) &= \left\{ \int \frac{f(Z|Y_{\text{obs}}, \beta, \lambda_0)}{f(\lambda_0|Y_{\text{obs}}, \beta, Z)}\, dZ \right\}^{-1} \\ &\doteq \left\{ \frac{1}{L} \sum_{\ell=1}^{L} \frac{1}{f(\lambda_0|Y_{\text{obs}}, \beta, Z^{(\ell)})} \right\}^{-1}, \end{aligned} \tag{5.84}$$

here $\{Z^{(\ell)}\} \overset{\text{iid}}{\sim} f(Z|Y_{\text{obs}}, \beta, \lambda_0)$. Based on (5.79), (5.80) and (5.81), the Gibbs sampler can be used to obtain the desired Z_0 and λ_0.

5.9 Assessing Convergence of MCMC Methods

It is well recognized that MCMC methods can give misleading answers because after any finite number of iterations, the generated samples may not represent the stationary distribution. Therefore, monitoring convergence to the stationary distribution[7] is a key step in implementing an MCMC method. However, assessing convergence of the sequence of draws/samples generated by the DA or Gibbs sampler to the target distribution is more difficult than assessing convergence of an EM-type algorithm to the MLE. It is whether the MCMC has converged to the whole stationary distribution that has to be assessed. In practice, convergence diagnostics built on successive iterations is used as a tool to indicate the convergence to the true stationary distribution. Comprehensive reviews on convergence diagnostics are given by Cowles & Carlin (1996), Brooks & Roberts

[7]In the sense of a stopping rule to guarantee that the number of iterations is sufficient.

(1998) and Mengersen *et al.* (1999). Several books also include the subject (Gamerman, 1997; Robert, 1998; Robert & Casella, 1999; Carlin & Louis, 2000; Chen *et al.*, 2000; Little & Rubin, 2002).

In this section, we first introduce the monitoring approach based on a so-called *potential scale reduction* (PSR) statistic proposed by Gelman & Rubin (1992). Then we present two alternative methods by using the outputs from the IBF sampler.

5.9.1 Gelman and Rubin's PSR statistic

Gelman & Rubin (1992) developed a control strategy based on an explicit PSR statistic to monitor the convergence of the Gibbs sampler. Their procedure is as follows:

1) Generate $L \geq 2$ parallel chains $\{\theta_\ell^{[k]}\colon 1 \leq \ell \leq L,\ 1 \leq k \leq K\}$[8] with starting points dispersed over the parameter space;

2) For each quantity of interest $\xi = h(\theta)$, calculate the variance between the L sequence means and the average of the L within-sequence variances:

$$\begin{aligned} B &= \frac{K}{L-1}\sum_{\ell=1}^{L}(\bar{\xi}_\ell - \bar{\xi}\,)^2, \quad \text{and} \\ W &= \frac{1}{L}\sum_{\ell=1}^{L}\left\{\frac{1}{K-1}\sum_{k=1}^{K}(\xi_\ell^{[k]} - \bar{\xi}_\ell)^2\right\}, \end{aligned}$$

where $\xi_\ell^{[k]} \hat{=} h(\theta_\ell^{[k]})$, $\bar{\xi}_\ell = \frac{1}{K}\sum_{k=1}^{K}\xi_\ell^{[k]}$ and $\bar{\xi} = \frac{1}{L}\sum_{\ell=1}^{L}\bar{\xi}_\ell$;

3) Estimate $\text{Var}(\xi|Y_{\text{obs}})$, the posterior variance of ξ, by a weighted average of B and W, i.e.,

$$\widehat{\text{Var}}(\xi|Y_{\text{obs}}) = \frac{1}{K}B + \frac{K-1}{K}W,$$

which overestimates the variance of $\xi_\ell^{[k]}$ (Gelman, 1996a) while W underestimates this variance;

4) The PSR is estimated by[9]

$$\sqrt{\hat{R}} = \sqrt{\widehat{\text{Var}}(\xi|Y_{\text{obs}})/W}, \tag{5.85}$$

[8]The real length of each chain is $2K$ and just the last K draws of each chain are retained to diminish the effect of the starting distribution.

[9]Here we adopt the simplified formula of Little & Rubin (2002, p.207). For the original formula, please see Gelman & Rubin (2002).

which declines to 1 as $K \to \infty$. Once $\sqrt{\hat{R}}$ is near[10] 1 for all scalar estimands of interest, it is typically desirable to terminate the sampling process and to summarize the target distribution by a set of simulations.

5.9.2 The difference and ratio criteria

Based on the point-wise IBF (1.3) or (1.6), we can develop useful procedures for determining whether the Gibbs sampler not only has converged but also has converged to its true stationary distribution. We focus on the two-block case. The more general situations can be handled similarly. As in Ritter & Tanner (1992) and Zellner & Min (1995), we also use the Rao–Blackwellized estimators. Let

$$\{x^{[k]}, y^{[k]}\}_{k=1}^{K} \tag{5.86}$$

denote the Gibbs outputs from the full conditional pdfs $f_{(X|Y)}(x|y)$ and $f_{(Y|X)}(y|x)$. For the marginal density $f_X(x)$, we can calculate its Rao-Blackwellized estimator (cf. (1.11))

$$f_X(x) \doteq \hat{f}_{4,X}(x) = \frac{1}{K}\sum_{k=1}^{K} f_{(X|Y)}(x|y^{[k]}), \quad \forall\, x \in \mathcal{S}_X.$$

On the other hand, for a given $x \in \mathcal{S}_X$, we first generate

$$\{y^{(i)}\}_{i=1}^{n} \overset{\text{iid}}{\sim} f_{(Y|X)}(y|x).$$

Then we approximate $f_X(x)$ by (cf. (1.6))

$$f_X(x) \doteq \hat{f}_{1,X}(x) = \left\{\frac{1}{n}\sum_{i=1}^{n}\frac{1}{f_{(X|Y)}(x|y^{(i)})}\right\}^{-1}.$$

The difference and ratio criteria are defined by

$$d(x) = \hat{f}_{1,X}(x) - \hat{f}_{4,X}(x), \quad \text{and} \tag{5.87}$$

$$r(x) = \frac{\hat{f}_{1,X}(x)}{\hat{f}_{4,X}(x)}, \tag{5.88}$$

respectively, where $x \in \mathcal{S}_X$. If the Gibbs chain has converged, then $d(x)$ will be close to zero, and $r(x)$ will be close to 1. The stopping rule is based on testing whether $r(x)$ is around 1 by graphical methods.

[10]For most practical problems, values below 1.2 are acceptable. But for an important dataset, a higher level of precision may be required.

5.9.3 The Kullback–Leibler divergence criterion

Since the KL divergence defined in (1.42) provides a measure of discrepancy between two density functions, the outputs from the exact IBF sampling in §4.1 or the IBF sampler in §5.1 can be used as a benchmark to check the convergence of the DA algorithm or the Gibbs sampler based on the KL divergence criterion.

Based on $f(\theta|Y_{\text{obs}}, Z)$ and $f(Z|Y_{\text{obs}}, \theta)$, let

$$\{Z^{(i)}, \theta^{(i)}\}_{i=1}^{I} \quad \text{and} \quad \{Z^{[k]}, \theta^{[k]}\}_{k=1}^{K}$$

denote the outputs from the IBF sampler and the DA algorithm, respectively. Then, we can estimate the observed posterior density $f(\theta|Y_{\text{obs}})$ by

$$f^{\text{IBF}}(\theta|Y_{\text{obs}}) \doteq \frac{1}{I}\sum_{i=1}^{I} f(\theta|Y_{\text{obs}}, Z^{(i)}) \quad \text{and} \tag{5.89}$$

$$f^{\text{DA}}(\theta|Y_{\text{obs}}) \doteq \frac{1}{K}\sum_{k=1}^{K} f(\theta|Y_{\text{obs}}, Z^{[k]}), \tag{5.90}$$

respectively. For a fixed I, from (1.42), the KL divergence between $f^{\text{IBF}}(\theta|Y_{\text{obs}})$ and $f^{\text{DA}}(\theta|Y_{\text{obs}})$ is

$$\text{KL}_K[f^{\text{IBF}}(\theta|Y_{\text{obs}}), f^{\text{DA}}(\theta|Y_{\text{obs}})] \doteq \frac{1}{L}\sum_{\ell=1}^{L} \log \frac{f^{\text{IBF}}(\theta^{\{\ell\}}|Y_{\text{obs}})}{f^{\text{DA}}(\theta^{\{\ell\}}|Y_{\text{obs}})}, \tag{5.91}$$

which declines to 0 as $K \to \infty$, where $\{\theta^{\{\ell\}}\} \overset{\text{iid}}{\sim} f^{\text{IBF}}(\theta|Y_{\text{obs}})$.

Although from a Bayesian inference point of view, such development is in fact not of interest as the posterior can be computed using the IBF sampler. The point here is to use the IBF sampler as a validation tool in high-dimensional problems, where we may want to build confidence in a simpler model of lower dimension with both the IBF and the Gibbs sampler and then switch to the high-dimensional problem using the Gibbs sampler.

5.10 Remarks

Although the Bayesian approach offers flexibility and gives full posterior distribution, proving the existence of the posterior (Arnold & Press, 1989; Gelman & Speed, 1993) and checking the convergence of the MCMC may hinder its application despite of the great progresses made in establishing the convergence. As Gelfand (1994) pointed out that "it seems clear that cutting-edge work will always require individually tailored code with careful diagnostic work to obtain results that can be confidently presented." It would be desirable to have an explicit solution or one based on noniterative sampling approach without elaborate convergence diagnosis if possible.

In this chapter, we presented such a noniterative sampling approach for obtaining i.i.d. samples approximately from an observed posterior by combining IBF with SIR and EM as an alternative to perfect sampling. Although both perfect sampling and the IBF sampler generate i.i.d. samples and eliminate problems in monitoring convergence and mixing of the Markov chain, we have shown that the IBF sampler is a simple yet highly efficient algorithm that performs well in more complicated models such as the (generalized) linear mixed model with longitudinal data. Practically, IBF sampling is a method to quickly generate i.i.d. samples approximately from the posterior once the posterior model is identified.

The IBF sampler under the framework of EM-type algorithms has several distinct features: First, it utilizes the strengths of SIR, EM-type algorithms and Gibbs sampler, while bypasses their potential limitations. In fact, SIR generates independent samples but it does not provide an efficient ISD directly from the model specification of a practical problem. It is easy to check if the EM algorithm has converged to the posterior mode or not, but it is difficult to calculate its standard errors. For the Gibbs sampler, its advantage is easy to draw from full conditional distributions whereas the difficulty is to monitor the stochastic convergence. The IBF sampler generates i.i.d. samples, provides a built-in class of ISDs, requires the posterior mode by running an EM or needs a Z_0 by implementing a Gibbs sampler, where the diagnosis of stochastic convergence can be ignored.

Second, the EM or DA algorithm and the IBF sampler share the structure of augmented posterior/conditional predictive distributions, thus, no extra derivations are needed for the IBF sampler. In fact, even when Gibbs sampler is used, the posterior mode via EM is sometimes also required, e.g., in model selection with Bayes factor or marginal likelihood based on Gibbs outputs.

The second feature implies that the IBF sampler is applicable to problems wherever the EM-type algorithms can be applied, thus solving a wide range of practical problems.

Problems

5.1 Posterior predictive density $f(Z|Y_{\rm obs})$ can be used to predict missing values, which are needed in some important applications. Based on (5.17) and (5.18), show that

(a) For $i = n_1+1, \dots, n_1+n_2$, $x_{2i}|x_{1i}$ follows normal distribution with mean $x_{1i}\rho\sigma_2/\sigma_1 + (-\rho\sigma_2/\sigma_1,\, 1)q$ and variance $\sigma_2^2(1-\rho^2) + (-\rho\sigma_2/\sigma_1,\, 1)Q(-\rho\sigma_2/\sigma_1,\, 1)^{\top}$, where Q and q are defined by (5.19) and (5.20), respectively.

(b) For $i = n_1 + n_2 + 1, \dots, n$, $x_{1i}|x_{2i}$ is also normally distributed with mean $x_{2i}\rho\sigma_1/\sigma_2 + (1,\, -\rho\sigma_1/\sigma_2)q$ and variance $\sigma_1^2(1-\rho^2) + (1,\, -\rho\sigma_2/\sigma_1)Q(1,\, -\rho\sigma_2/\sigma_1)^{\top}$.

(*Hint*: $f(x_{2i}|x_{1i}) = f(x_{2i}|Y_{\rm obs}) = \int f(x_{2i}|Y_{\rm obs}, \mu) \cdot f(\mu|Y_{\rm obs})\, d\mu$. Note that both $f(x_{2i}|Y_{\rm obs}, \mu)$ and $f(\mu|Y_{\rm obs})$ are normal. Using (A.1) and (A.2), we know that $(x_{2i}, \mu)|Y_{\rm obs}$ have a joint normal distribution. Thus, the marginal distribution of $x_{2i}|Y_{\rm obs}$ is still normal. Its mean and variance can be calculated by $E\{E(x_{2i}|Y_{\rm obs}, \mu)|Y_{\rm obs}\}$ and $E\{\text{Var}(x_{2i}|Y_{\rm obs}, \mu)|Y_{\rm obs}\} + \text{Var}\{E(x_{2i}|Y_{\rm obs}, \mu)|Y_{\rm obs}\}$, respectively.)

5.2 **Censored data from an exponential density** (McLachlan & Krishnan, 1997). In survival or reliability analysis, a study to observe a random sample $y = (y_1, \dots, y_m)^{\top} \overset{\text{iid}}{\sim} \text{Exponential}(\theta)$ is generally terminated before all of them are completely observed. Suppose that the first r observations of y are uncensored and the remaining $m - r$ are censored (c_i denotes a censoring time) so that the observed data $Y_{\rm obs} = \{y_1, \dots, y_m; c_{r+1}, \dots, c_m\}$. Augment the $Y_{\rm obs}$ with latent failure times $Z = (z_{r+1}, \dots, z_m)^{\top}$, where $z_i > c_i$ for $i = r+1, \dots, m$.

(a) Show that the complete-data likelihood is given by

$$L(\theta|Y_{\rm obs}, Z) \propto \theta^m \exp\{-\theta(\textstyle\sum_{i=1}^r y_i + \mathbf{1}^{\top}Z)\}.$$

(b) If the Gamma(α_0, β_0) prior is put on θ, then

$$\begin{aligned} \theta|(Y_{\rm obs}, Z) &\sim \text{Gamma}(m + \alpha_0,\ y^* + \mathbf{1}^{\top}Z + \beta_0), \\ \mathbf{1}^{\top}Z - c.|(Y_{\rm obs}, \theta) &\sim \text{Gamma}(m - r, \theta), \end{aligned}$$

where $y^* \hat{=} \sum_{i=1}^r y_i$ and $c. \hat{=} \sum_{i=r+1}^m c_i$.

(c) Write down the IBF sampling procedure for this example.

5.3 Failures of nuclear pumps (Gaver & O'Muircheartaigh, 1987). Table 5.9 gives multiple failures of pumps in a nuclear plant. Assume that the failures in time interval $(0, t_i]$ for the i-th pump follow a homogeneous Poisson process with rate λ_i. Then, the number of failures $N_i \hat{=} N(t_i) \overset{\text{ind}}{\sim} \text{Poisson}(\lambda_i t_i)$. Let $Y_{\text{obs}} = \{t_i, N_i\}_{i=1}^m$ and $\lambda = (\lambda_1, \dots, \lambda_m)^\top$.

(a) If prior distributions are specified by $\lambda_i \overset{\text{iid}}{\sim} \text{Gamma}(\alpha_0, \beta)$ and $\beta \sim \text{Gamma}(a_0, b_0)$, then

$$
\begin{aligned}
f(\lambda|Y_{\text{obs}}, \beta) &= \textstyle\prod_{i=1}^m \text{Gamma}(\lambda_i|N_i + \alpha_0,\ t_i + \beta), \\
f(\beta|Y_{\text{obs}}, \lambda) &= \text{Gamma}(\beta|a_0 + m\alpha_0,\ b_0 + \textstyle\sum_{i=1}^m \lambda_i).
\end{aligned}
$$

(b) For the data in Table 5.9, implement the Gibbs sampler. Devise and implement the hybrid algorithm described in §5.8.

Table 5.9 *Numbers of failures and times for 10 pumps in a nuclear plant*

Pump i	1	2	3	4	5	6	7	8	9	10
Failures N_i	5	1	5	14	3	19	1	1	4	22
Time t_i	94.32	15.72	62.88	125.76	5.24	31.44	1.05	1.05	2.10	10.48

Source: Gaver & O'Muircheartaigh (1987).

5.4 Hierarchical models for clinical mastitis data (Schukken *et al.*, 1991). Table 7.5.1 of Robert & Casella (1999, p.334) displays counts of the number of cases of clinical mastitis[11] in 127 dairy cattle herds over a one-year period. Let X_i denote the number of cases in herd i $(i = 1, \dots, m)$. Assume that $X_i \sim \text{Poisson}(\lambda_i)$, where λ_i is the rate of infection in herd i. However, the data lack of independence because mastitis is infectious. To account for this overdispersion, Schukken *et al.* (1991) presented a complete hierarchical model by specifying $\lambda_i \sim \text{Gamma}(\alpha_0, \beta_i)$, $\beta_i \sim \text{Gamma}(a_0, b_0)$. Let $Y_{\text{obs}} = \{X_i\}_1^m$. Show that

$$
\begin{aligned}
\lambda_i|(Y_{\text{obs}}, \beta_i) &\sim \text{Gamma}(\lambda_i|X_i + \alpha_0,\ 1 + \beta_i), \\
\beta_i|(Y_{\text{obs}}, \lambda_i) &\sim \text{Gamma}(\beta|a_0 + \alpha_0,\ b_0 + \lambda_i).
\end{aligned}
$$

For this dataset, implement the Gibbs sampler. Devise and implement the hybrid algorithm described in §5.8.

[11]Mastitis is an inflammation usually caused by infection.

5.5 Biochemical oxygen demand data (Marske, 1967). The model (5.71) was derived from a study to determine the *biochemical oxygen demand* (BOD), where a sample of stream water was mixed with soluble organic matter, inorganic nutrients and dissolved oxygen, and then subdivided into BOD bottles. Each one of them was inoculated with a mixed culture of microorganisms, sealed and incubated at a fixed temperature. The bottles were opened periodically and assayed for dissolved oxygen concentration, from which the BOD was calculated in milligrams per liter. Measurments are taken at days 1, 2, 3, 4, 5 and 7. The BOD values which are averages of two analyses on each bottle are given by 8.3, 10.3, 19.0, 16.0, 15.6 and 19.8. Write a program to compute the posterior distributions of θ_1, θ_2 and σ^2 for the nonlinear regression model (5.71) using the BOD data.

5.6 Based on the method described in §5.8.2, write a computer program to fit the prostatic cancer data in Table 5.5 (cf. Ex.5.6) using the binary regression model (5.78) with t link:

$$p_i = T_8(\beta_1 + \beta_2 x_{i2} + \beta_3 x_{i3} + \beta_4 x_{i4}), \quad i = 1, \ldots, 53.$$

5.7 Design and implement the hybrid algorithm described in §5.8 for the capture-recapture model in Problem 4.9.

5.8 Hierarchical Poisson changepoint models (Maguire *et al.*, 1952). Carlin *et al.* (1992) analyzed British coal-mining disaster data (see Table 1 therein) from 1851–1962 by use a hierarchical Poisson changepoint model. At the first stage, they let

$$\begin{aligned} y_i &\sim \text{Poisson}(\theta_1 t_i), \quad i = 1, \ldots, r, \\ y_i &\sim \text{Poisson}(\theta_2 t_i), \quad i = r+1, \ldots, n, \end{aligned}$$

where θ_1 and θ_2 are unknown parameters. At the second stage, they consider independent prior distributions: k is assumed to follow a discrete uniform distribution on $\{1, \ldots, n\}$,

$$\theta_j | b_j \sim \text{Gamma}(a_{j0}, b_j), \quad j = 1, 2.$$

At the third stage, they let

$$b_j \sim \text{Gamma}(c_{j0}, d_{j0}), \quad j = 1, 2,$$

and b_1 is independent of b_2. Denoted the observed data by $Y_{\text{obs}} = \{y_i\}_1^n$. Define

$$\begin{aligned} Y_1 &\hat{=} \textstyle\sum_{i=1}^r y_i, \quad Y_2 \hat{=} \sum_{i=r+1}^n y_i, \\ T_1 &\hat{=} \textstyle\sum_{i=1}^r t_i, \quad T_2 \hat{=} \sum_{i=r+1}^n t_i. \end{aligned}$$

Prove that the three full conditionals are given by

$$f(\theta_1, \theta_2 | Y_{\text{obs}}, r, b_1, b_2) = \textstyle\prod_{j=1}^2 \text{Gamma}(\theta_j | a_{j0} + Y_j,\ b_j + T_j),$$
$$f(b_1, b_2 | Y_{\text{obs}}, r, \theta_1, \theta_2) = \textstyle\prod_{j=1}^2 \text{Gamma}(b_j | a_{j0} + c_{j0},\ \theta_j + d_{j0}),$$
$$f(k | Y_{\text{obs}}, \theta_1, \theta_2, b_1, b_2) \propto (\theta_1/\theta_2)^{Y_1} \exp\{(\theta_2 - \theta_1)T_1\}.$$

For the data (Table 1 of Carlin *et al.*, 1992), implement the IBF sampling described in §5.1.2.

5.9 Item response model (Albert, 1992). Assume that n students take an examination with J items. The answer for each item is true (T) or false (F). Let Y_{ij} equal 1 if the i-th student correctly answers the j-th item and 0 otherwise. For $i = 1, \ldots, n$ and $j = 1, \ldots, J$, let

$$Y_{ij} \stackrel{\text{ind}}{\sim} \text{Bernoulli}(p_{ij}), \quad p_{ij} = \Phi(\alpha_j b_i - \beta_j),$$

where b_i denotes the unobserved[12] "ability" for the i-th student, $\alpha_j > 0$ measures the discriminatory power (to discriminate between strong and weak students) of the j-th item and β_j represents the difficulty of the j-th item.

(a) Mimic the technique presented in §5.5 to introduce a vector of independent latent r.v.'s $Z = \{Z_{ij}\}$. Derive the three full conditionals

$$f(\theta | Y_{\text{obs}}, Z, b), \quad f(Z | Y_{\text{obs}}, \theta, b) \quad \text{and} \quad f(b | Y_{\text{obs}}, Z, \theta),$$

where $\theta = \{\alpha_j, \beta_j\}$.

(b) Design an IBF sampler by following §5.7.

(c) Tanner (1996, p.190–191) gives scores for 39 college students in a quiz of an introductory statistics course consisting of six questions. A correct answer was scored 1 and an incorrect answer was scored 0. Using the IBF sampling, apply the item response model to these data.

[12]Usually, we treat b_i as latent random variable and (α_j, β_j) as parameters.

CHAPTER 6

Constrained Parameter Problems

Constrained parameter problems refer to statistical models where some of the model parameters are constrained, e.g., by certain order. Such problems arise in a variety of applications including, for example, ordinal categorical data, sample surveys (Chiu & Sedransk, 1986), bioassay (Ramgopal *et al.*, 1993), dose finding (Gasparini & Eisele, 2000) and variance components and factor analysis models (Dempster *et al.*, 1977; Rubin & Thayer, 1982). The most common parameter restriction is an ordering of the model parameters, namely, the order restrictions (Barlow *et al.*, 1972; Robertson *et al.*, 1988; Silvapulle & Sen, 2005).

From a frequentist perspective, model fitting methods for isotonic regression such as the pool–adjacent–violators procedure provide explicit MLEs of parameters of interest for some simple cases while for more general cases the solution is obtained by nonlinear programming approach (Schmoyer, 1984; Geyer, 1991). One alternative method for fitting the isotonic regression is to use EM-type algorithms (Meng & Rubin, 1993; Liu, 2000; Tan, Tian & Fang, 2003; Tan, Tian, Fang & Ng, 2007; Tian, Ng & Tan, 2008).

This chapter describes how the EM and the DA algorithms can be used for maximum likelihood and Bayesian estimation in normal distribution subject to linear inequality constraints (§6.1 and §6.2), Poisson distribution (§6.3) and binomial distribution (§6.4) with a class of simplex constraints.

6.1 Linear Inequality Constraints

6.1.1 Motivating examples

To motivate statistical models with linear inequality constraints, we consider several examples. For example, toxicities or responses at ordered doses of a drug are often ordered. Let $d_1, \ldots, d_m$ denote the dose levels of the drug and n_i mice be treated at dose d_i ($i = 1, \ldots, m$), where the first $(m-1)$ groups are the treatment groups and the last one is the control group without the drug (i.e., $d_m = 0$).

We assume $d_1 > \cdots > d_m$. Denote by Y_{ij} the logarithm of the tumor volume for mouse j ($j = 1, \ldots, n_i$) under dose d_i. Suppose that all outcomes are independent and the outcomes in group i have the same normal distribution, that is,

$$Y_{i1}, \ldots, Y_{in_i} \stackrel{\text{iid}}{\sim} N(\mu_i, \sigma_i^2), \qquad i = 1, \ldots, m. \tag{6.1}$$

Since it is expected that higher doses yield greater response (greater tumor reduction), it is reasonable to impose a monotonic constraint on the means by

$$\mu_1 \le \cdots \le \mu_m, \tag{6.2}$$

which is called simple ordering in the setting of isotonic regression/inference.

Similarly, other ordered constraints on the means may arise in different designed experiments. For example, an experiment where several treatments are expected to reduce the response (e.g., systolic blood pressure) in the control would result in a simple tree ordering on the means of the form

$$\mu_i \le \mu_m, \qquad i = 1, \ldots, m-1. \tag{6.3}$$

Some authors study the so-called umbrella orderings (Shi, 1988; Geng & Shi, 1990), i.e., the means satisfy a unimodal trend

$$\mu_1 \le \cdots \le \mu_h \ge \mu_{h+1} \ge \cdots \ge \mu_m. \tag{6.4}$$

For a class of discrete distributions without nuisance parameters, Liu (2000) considers a general increasing convex ordering: $\mu_1 \le \mu_2 \le \cdots \le \mu_m$ and $\mu_2 - \mu_1 \le \mu_3 - \mu_2 \le \cdots \le \mu_m - \mu_{m-1}$, which is equivalent to

$$0 \le \mu_2 - \mu_1 \le \mu_3 - \mu_2 \le \cdots \le \mu_m - \mu_{m-1}. \tag{6.5}$$

He also considers the increasing concave ordering: $\mu_1 \le \mu_2 \le \cdots \le \mu_m$ and $\mu_2 - \mu_1 \ge \mu_3 - \mu_2 \ge \cdots \ge \mu_m - \mu_{m-1}$, which are equivalent to

$$\mu_2 - \mu_1 \ge \mu_3 - \mu_2 \ge \cdots \ge \mu_m - \mu_{m-1} \ge 0. \tag{6.6}$$

6.1.2 Linear transformation

From a Bayesian perspective, parameters are r.v.'s. Let $\mathbb{S}(\mu_i)$ denote the support of μ_i and $\mathbb{S}(\mu)$ the joint support of $\mu = (\mu_1, \ldots, \mu_m)^\top$. In §1.3.1 and §3.9, we defined two useful notions: *product measurable space* (PMS) and *nonproduct measurable space* (NPMS). Namely, if $\mathbb{S}(\mu) = \prod_{i=1}^m \mathbb{S}(\mu_i)$, then $\mathbb{S}(\mu)$ is called a PMS; otherwise, it is called an NPMS.

In simple ordering (6.2), $\mathbb{S}(\mu)$ is an NPMS. Making a one-to-one linear transformation on the simple ordering, we have $\mu = B_1\theta$, where θ belongs to

$$\mathbb{R} \times \mathbb{R}_+^{m-1} = \{(\theta_1, \dots, \theta_m)^\top\colon\ \theta_1 \in \mathbb{R},\ \theta_i \geq 0,\ i = 2, \dots, m\}, \quad (6.7)$$

$B_1 = \Delta_m$ and Δ_m is an $m \times m$ matrix defined by

$$\Delta_m \hat{=} \begin{pmatrix} 1 & 0 & \cdots & 0 \\ 1 & 1 & \cdots & 0 \\ \vdots & \vdots & \ddots & \vdots \\ 1 & 1 & \cdots & 1 \end{pmatrix}. \quad (6.8)$$

Obviously, $\mathbb{R} \times \mathbb{R}_+^{m-1}$ is a PMS. In other words, an NPMS is transformed into a PMS via a linear mapping. Such a linear mapping exists for all other types of constraints considered in §6.1.1. For simple tree ordering (6.3), such a transformation is $\mu = B_2\theta$, where $\theta \in \mathbb{R} \times \mathbb{R}_+^{m-1}$ and

$$B_2 = \begin{pmatrix} \mathbf{1}_{m-1} & -\mathbf{I}_{m-1} \\ 1 & \mathbf{0}_{m-1}^\top \end{pmatrix}.$$

For umbrella ordering (6.4), we obtain $\mu = B_3\theta$, where $\theta \in \mathbb{R} \times \mathbb{R}_+^{m-1}$ and

$$B_3 = \begin{pmatrix} \Delta_h & O \\ \mathbf{1}_{m-h}\mathbf{1}_h^\top & -\Delta_{m-h} \end{pmatrix}$$

with Δ_k defined in (6.8). For the increasing convex ordering (6.5), we have $\mu = B_4\theta$, where $\theta \in \mathbb{R} \times \mathbb{R}_+^{m-1}$,

$$B_4 = \begin{pmatrix} 1 & \mathbf{0}_{m-1}^\top \\ \mathbf{1}_{m-1} & \Omega_{m-1} \end{pmatrix}, \quad \text{and} \quad (6.9)$$

$$\Omega_{m-1} = \begin{pmatrix} 1 & 0 & \cdots & 0 & 0 \\ 2 & 1 & \cdots & 0 & 0 \\ \vdots & \vdots & \ddots & \vdots & \vdots \\ m-2 & m-3 & \cdots & 1 & 0 \\ m-1 & m-2 & \cdots & 2 & 1 \end{pmatrix}. \quad (6.10)$$

For the increasing concave ordering (6.6), we have $\mu = B_5\,\theta$, where $\theta \in \mathbb{R} \times \mathbb{R}_+^{m-1}$ and

$$B_5 = \begin{pmatrix} \mathbf{1}_{m-1} & -\Omega_{m-1}^{\top} \\ 1 & \mathbf{0}_{m-1}^{\top} \end{pmatrix}.$$

6.2 Constrained Normal Models

In this section, we introduce a unified framework for estimating normal means subject to order restrictions when the variances are known or unknown. This unified approach encompasses various classes of restrictions such as simple ordering, simple tree ordering, umbrella ordering, increasing convex and increasing concave ordering. The MLEs and Bayesian estimates of the parameters in the univariate normal model (6.1) with these restrictions are derived by using EM-type algorithms and the IBF sampler. We illustrate the methods with two real examples.

6.2.1 Estimation when variances are known

In model (6.1), we first assume that $\sigma^2 = (\sigma_1^2, \dots, \sigma_m^2)^{\top}$ is a known vector. The aim is to estimate the mean vector $\mu = (\mu_1, \dots, \mu_m)^{\top}$ subject to a linear constraint

$$\mu = B\,\theta \quad \text{or} \quad \mu_i = \sum_{k=1}^{q} b_{ik}\theta_k, \quad i = 1, \dots, m. \tag{6.11}$$

Based on the discussion in §6.1.2, we assume without loss of generality that $B = (b_{ik})$ is a known $m \times q$ scalar matrix and θ belongs to the following domain

$$\mathbb{R}^r \times \mathbb{R}_+^{q-r} = \{(\theta_1, \dots, \theta_q)^{\top}\colon\ \theta_k \in \mathbb{R},\ k = 1, \dots, r,$$

$$\theta_k \in \mathbb{R}_+,\ k = r+1, \dots, q\}. \tag{6.12}$$

(a) Data augmentation

Since σ^2 is known, for each i, the sample mean $\overline{Y}_i = \frac{1}{n_i}\sum_{j=1}^{n_i} Y_{ij}$ is a sufficient statistic of μ_i. Thus, we denote the observed data by

$Y_{\rm obs} = \{\overline{Y}_i\}_{i=1}^m$. Noting the linear invariant property[1] of the normal distribution, we augment the $Y_{\rm obs}$ by latent variables

$$Z(\sigma^2) = \Big\{Z_{ik}(\sigma^2)\colon\ 1 \le i \le m,\ 1 \le k \le q-1\Big\}$$

to obtain the complete-data

$$Y_{\rm com}(\sigma^2) = \Big\{Y_{\rm obs}, Z(\sigma^2)\Big\} = \Big\{Z_{ik}(\sigma^2)\colon\ 1 \le i \le m,\ 1 \le k \le q\Big\},$$

where

$$\begin{aligned} Z_{ik}(\sigma^2) &\overset{\rm ind}{\sim} N(b_{ik}\theta_k,\ \sigma_i^2/(qn_i)), \quad 1 \le i \le m, \quad 1 \le k \le q, \\ \overline{Y}_i &= \sum_{k=1}^{q} Z_{ik}(\sigma^2), \qquad\qquad 1 \le i \le m. \end{aligned} \tag{6.13}$$

By mapping $Y_{\rm com}(\sigma^2)$ to $Y_{\rm obs}$, the transformation (6.13) preserves the observed-data likelihood

$$\textstyle\prod_{i=1}^m N(\overline{Y}_i|\mu_i, \sigma_i^2/n_i).$$

To derive the conditional predictive distribution of the latent data $Z(\sigma^2)$ given $Y_{\rm obs}$ and θ, we first prove the following result.

Theorem 6.1 (Tan, Tian & Fang, 2003). Let r.v.'s $W_1, \dots, W_q$ be independent and $W_k \sim N(\beta_k, \delta_k^2)$, $k = 1, \dots, q$, then

$$\begin{aligned} &(W_1, \dots, W_{q-1})^{\top}|(\textstyle\sum_{k=1}^q W_k = w) \\ &\sim N_{q-1}\left(\beta_{-q} + \dfrac{w - \sum_{k=1}^q \beta_k}{\sum_{k=1}^q \delta_k^2} \cdot \delta_{-q}^2,\ {\rm diag}(\delta_{-q}^2) - \dfrac{\delta_{-q}^2 \delta_{-q}^{2\top}}{\sum_{k=1}^q \delta_k^2}\right), \end{aligned} \tag{6.14}$$

where $\beta_{-q} = (\beta_1, \dots, \beta_{q-1})^{\top}$ and $\delta_{-q}^2 = (\delta_1^2, \dots, \delta_{q-1}^2)^{\top}$. Especially, if $\delta_1^2 = \cdots = \delta_q^2 = \delta^2$, then

$$\begin{aligned} &(W_1, \dots, W_{q-1})^{\top}|(\textstyle\sum_{k=1}^q W_k = w) \\ &\sim N_{q-1}\left(\beta_{-q} + \dfrac{w - \sum_{k=1}^q \beta_k}{q}\mathbf{1}_{q-1},\ \delta^2\left(\mathbf{I}_{q-1} - \dfrac{\mathbf{1}_{q-1}\mathbf{1}_{q-1}^{\top}}{q}\right)\right). \quad ¶ \end{aligned} \tag{6.15}$$

[1]The linear invariant property indicates that linear combinations of independent r.v.'s from a particular family of distributions still have distribution in that family.

PROOF. Let $\beta = (\beta_1, \ldots, \beta_q)^\top$ and $\delta^2 = (\delta_1^2, \ldots, \delta_q^2)^\top$. Since $W = (W_1, \ldots, W_q)^\top \sim N_q(\beta, \text{diag}(\delta^2))$,

$$\begin{pmatrix} W \\ \sum_{k=1}^q W_k \end{pmatrix} = \begin{pmatrix} \mathbf{I}_q \\ \mathbf{1}_q^\top \end{pmatrix} W \sim N_{q+1}\left(\begin{pmatrix} \beta \\ \mathbf{1}_q^\top \beta \end{pmatrix}, \begin{pmatrix} \text{diag}(\delta^2) & \delta^2 \\ \delta^{2\top} & \mathbf{1}_q^\top \delta^2 \end{pmatrix} \right).$$

From the property of multivariate normal distribution, we have

$$(W_1, \ldots, W_q)^\top | (\textstyle\sum_{k=1}^q W_k = w)$$
$$\sim N_q\left(\beta + \frac{w - \sum_{k=1}^q \beta_k}{\mathbf{1}_q^\top \delta^2} \cdot \delta^2,\ \text{diag}(\delta^2) - \frac{\delta^2 \delta^{2\top}}{\mathbf{1}_q^\top \delta^2} \right). \tag{6.16}$$

Let

$$\Sigma = \text{diag}(\delta^2) - \frac{\delta^2 \delta^{2\top}}{\mathbf{1}_q^\top \delta^2},$$

then

$$\Sigma = D^{1/2}(\mathbf{I}_q - \Sigma_1) D^{1/2},$$

where

$$D = \text{diag}(\delta^2) \quad \text{and} \quad \Sigma_1 = D^{1/2}\mathbf{1}_q(\mathbf{1}_q^\top D \mathbf{1}_q)^{-1}\mathbf{1}_q^\top D^{1/2}.$$

Note that $\mathbf{I}_q - \Sigma_1$ is a projection matrix and the rank of a projection matrix equals its trace. So rank $(\mathbf{I}_q - \Sigma_1) = q - 1$, implying rank $(\Sigma) = q - 1 < q$. That is, the distribution in (6.16) is a degenerate q-dimensional normal distribution. From (6.16), we immediately obtain (6.14) and (6.15). ||END||

(b) MLE via the EM algorithm

The likelihood function of θ for the complete-data $Y_{\text{com}}(\sigma^2)$ is

$$L(\theta | Y_{\text{com}}(\sigma^2)) \propto \prod_{i=1}^m (\sigma_i^2)^{-q/2}$$
$$\times \exp\left\{ -\frac{1}{2} \sum_{i=1}^m \left[\frac{q n_i}{\sigma_i^2} \sum_{k=1}^q (Z_{ik}(\sigma^2) - b_{ik}\theta_k)^2 \right] \right\},$$

where $\theta \in \mathbb{R}^r \times \mathbb{R}_+^{q-r}$ defined by (6.12). Therefore, the sufficient statistics for θ_k are

$$S_k = \sum_{i=1}^m \left(\frac{n_i b_{ik}}{\sigma_i^2} \right) Z_{ik}(\sigma^2), \quad k = 1, \ldots, q.$$

The complete-data MLEs of θ_k are given by

$$\begin{aligned}
\hat{\theta}_k &= \frac{S_k}{\sum_{i=1}^m n_i b_{ik}^2/\sigma_i^2}, \qquad k = 1, \dots, r, \quad \text{and} \\
\hat{\theta}_k &= \max\left\{0,\ \frac{S_k}{\sum_{i=1}^m n_i b_{ik}^2/\sigma_i^2}\right\}, \qquad k = r+1, \dots, q.
\end{aligned}$$

Let $Z_i(\sigma^2) = (Z_{i1}(\sigma^2), \dots, Z_{i,q-1}(\sigma^2))^\top$, then from (6.13) and (6.15), the conditional predictive distribution of $Z(\sigma^2)|(Y_{\text{obs}}, \theta)$ is

$$\begin{aligned}
f(Z(\sigma^2)|Y_{\text{obs}}, \theta) &= \prod_{i=1}^m f\left(Z_i(\sigma^2)\middle|\left(\textstyle\sum_{k=1}^q Z_{ik}(\sigma^2) = \overline{Y}_i\right), \theta\right) \\
&= \prod_{i=1}^m N_{q-1}(Z_i(\sigma^2)|E_i,\ V_i), \qquad (6.17)
\end{aligned}$$

where

$$\begin{aligned}
E_i &= (b_{i1}\theta_1, \dots, b_{i,q-1}\theta_{q-1})^\top + \mathbf{1}_{q-1}\frac{\overline{Y}_i - \sum_{k=1}^q b_{ik}\theta_k}{q}, \qquad (6.18) \\
V_i &= \frac{\sigma_i^2}{qn_i}\left(\mathbf{I}_{q-1} - \frac{\mathbf{1}_{q-1}\mathbf{1}_{q-1}^\top}{q}\right). \qquad (6.19)
\end{aligned}$$

Given Y_{obs} and the current estimate $\theta^{(t)} = (\theta_1^{(t)}, \dots, \theta_q^{(t)})^\top$, the E-step is to calculate the conditional expectation of the complete-data sufficient statistic S_k,

$$\begin{aligned}
S_k^{(t)} &= E\left(S_k|Y_{\text{obs}}, \theta^{(t)}\right) \\
&= \sum_{i=1}^m \left(\frac{n_i b_{ik}}{\sigma_i^2}\right) \cdot \left(b_{ik}\theta_k^{(t)} + \frac{\overline{Y}_i - \sum_{\ell=1}^q b_{i\ell}\theta_\ell^{(t)}}{q}\right) \qquad (6.20)
\end{aligned}$$

for $k = 1, \dots, q$. The M-step is to update the estimates of θ

$$\begin{aligned}
\theta_k^{(t+1)} &= \frac{S_k^{(t)}}{\sum_{i=1}^m n_i b_{ik}^2/\sigma_i^2}, \qquad k = 1, \dots, r, \quad \text{and} \\
\theta_k^{(t+1)} &= \max\left\{0,\ \frac{S_k^{(t)}}{\sum_{i=1}^m n_i b_{ik}^2/\sigma_i^2}\right\}, \quad k = r+1, \dots, q. \qquad (6.21)
\end{aligned}$$

The standard errors of θ can be obtained by using the method of Louis (1982). Therefore, with the δ-method (see, e.g., Tanner, 1996, p.34), we can obtain the restricted MLE and standard errors of μ via the linear transformation (6.11).

Remark 6.1 The choice of the initial value $\theta^{(0)}$ is crucial. Denote the restricted MLE of μ by $\hat{\mu} = (\hat{\mu}_1, \ldots, \hat{\mu}_m)^{\top}$. Theorem 1.6 of Barlow *et al.* (1972, p.29–30) shows that

$$\min\{\overline{Y}_1, \ldots, \overline{Y}_m\} \le \hat{\mu}_i \le \max\{\overline{Y}_1, \ldots, \overline{Y}_m\}, \quad i = 1, \ldots, m.$$

Hence, $\mu^{(0)}$ can be chosen from a partial ordering of $\{\overline{Y}_i\}_{i=1}^m$ such that $\mu^{(0)} \in \mathbb{S}(\mu)$. For example, if $\mathbb{S}(\mu) = \{(\mu_1, \ldots, \mu_m)^{\top}: \mu_1 \le \cdots \le \mu_m\}$, then we take $\mu^{(0)} = (\overline{Y}_{(1)}, \ldots, \overline{Y}_{(m)})^{\top}$, where $\overline{Y}_{(1)}, \ldots, \overline{Y}_{(m)}$ denote the ordered values of $\overline{Y}_1, \ldots, \overline{Y}_m$. Hence, the initial value $\theta^{(0)} = B^{+} \mu^{(0)}$, where B^{+} denotes the Moore–Penrose inverse matrix of $B_{m \times q}$. Especially, when $q = m$, we have $B^{+} = B^{-1}$. ¶

(c) Bayesian estimation via the IBF sampler

Obviously, the statistical inferences on μ such as CIs and hypothesis testing depend on the large sample theory. Thus, for small sample size, Bayesian method is an appealing alternative.

In the Bayesian model, conjugate priors of θ exist and will be used. More specifically, the components of the θ are assumed to be independent and for $k = 1, \ldots, r$, $\theta_k \sim N(\theta_{k0}, \sigma_{k0}^2)$, and for $k = r+1, \ldots, q$, θ_k is normally distributed with mean θ_{k0} and variance σ_{k0}^2 but truncated to the interval $[0, +\infty)$, denoted by $\theta_k \sim TN(\theta_{k0}, \sigma_{k0}^2; \mathbb{R}_+)$, where θ_{k0} and σ_{k0}^2 are known scalars. With prior distribution

$$\pi(\theta) = \prod_{k=1}^{r} N(\theta_k|\theta_{k0}, \sigma_{k0}^2) \cdot \prod_{k=r+1}^{q} TN(\theta_k|\theta_{k0}, \sigma_{k0}^2;\ \mathbb{R}_+), \tag{6.22}$$

the complete-data posterior distribution of θ is

$$\begin{aligned} f(\theta|Y_{\rm obs}, Z(\sigma^2)) &= \prod_{k=1}^{r} N(\theta_k|u_k(\sigma^2), v_k^2(\sigma^2)) \\ &\quad \times \prod_{k=r+1}^{q} TN\Big(\theta_k\Big|u_k(\sigma^2), v_k^2(\sigma^2);\ \mathbb{R}_+\Big), \end{aligned} \tag{6.23}$$

where

$$\begin{aligned} u_k(\sigma^2) &= v_k^2(\sigma^2)\left(\frac{\theta_{k0}}{\sigma_{k0}^2} + \sum_{i=1}^{m} \frac{q n_i b_{ik} Z_{ik}(\sigma^2)}{\sigma_i^2}\right), \quad \text{and} \\ v_k^2(\sigma^2) &= \left(\frac{1}{\sigma_{k0}^2} + \sum_{i=1}^{m} \frac{q n_i b_{ik}^2}{\sigma_i^2}\right)^{-1}, \quad k = 1, \ldots, q. \end{aligned} \tag{6.24}$$

The conditional predictive distribution of the latent data $Z(\sigma^2)$ given $Y_{\rm obs}$ and θ is given exactly by (6.17).

To obtain i.i.d. posterior samples of μ ($\mu = B\theta$), we only need to obtain i.i.d. samples of θ from $f(\theta|Y_{\rm obs})$. It suffices to generate i.i.d. samples of $Z(\sigma^2)$ from $f(Z(\sigma^2)|Y_{\rm obs})$. From the sampling IBF (5.1), we have

$$f(Z(\sigma^2)|Y_{\rm obs}) \propto \frac{f(Z(\sigma^2)|Y_{\rm obs}, \tilde{\theta})}{f(\tilde{\theta}|Y_{\rm obs}, Z(\sigma^2))}, \tag{6.25}$$

where $\tilde{\theta}$ is the mode of the observed posterior $f(\theta|Y_{\rm obs})$. If we use diffuse priors, i.e., $\sigma_{k0}^2 \to +\infty$ for $k = 1, \ldots, q$, then the posterior mode is the same as the MLE, we have $\tilde{\theta} = \hat{\theta}$. Therefore, the IBF sampler presented in §5.1.1 can be readily applied.

6.2.2 Estimation when variances are unknown

From the assumption of (6.1), the observed data can be denoted by $Y_{\rm obs} = \{Y_{ij}\colon i = 1, \ldots, m,\ j = 1, \ldots, n_i\}$. The goal of this subsection is to estimate the mean vector $\mu = (\mu_1, \ldots, \mu_m)^{\top}$ and the variance vector $\sigma^2 = (\sigma_1^2, \ldots, \sigma_m^2)^{\top}$, where μ is estimated subject to a linear restriction (6.11), and $\theta = (\theta_1, \ldots, \theta_q)^{\top} \in \mathbb{R}^r \times \mathbb{R}_+^{q-r}$. Denote the unknown parameter vector by $\psi = (\theta, \sigma^2)$.

(a) MLE via the EM-type algorithm

The likelihood function of ψ for the observed data $Y_{\rm obs}$ is given by

$$\begin{aligned} L(\psi|Y_{\rm obs}) &= \prod_{i=1}^m \prod_{j=1}^{n_i} \frac{1}{(2\pi\sigma_i^2)^{\frac{1}{2}}} \exp\left\{ -\frac{(Y_{ij} - \mu_i)^2}{2\sigma_i^2} \right\} \\ &= \prod_{i=1}^m \prod_{j=1}^{n_i} \frac{1}{(2\pi\sigma_i^2)^{\frac{1}{2}}} \exp\left\{ -\frac{(Y_{ij} - \sum_{k=1}^q b_{ik}\theta_k)^2}{2\sigma_i^2} \right\}, \end{aligned} \tag{6.26}$$

where $\theta \in \mathbb{R}^r \times \mathbb{R}_+^{q-r}$ and $\sigma^2 \in \mathbb{R}_+^m$. Given $Y_{\rm obs}$ and $\theta \in \mathbb{R}^r \times \mathbb{R}_+^{q-r}$, the MLE of σ^2 maximizes the conditional likelihood function $L(\sigma^2|Y_{\rm obs}, \theta)$, we obtain

$$\sigma_i^2 = \frac{1}{n_i} \sum_{j=1}^{n_i} \left(Y_{ij} - \sum_{k=1}^q b_{ik}\theta_k \right)^2, \qquad i = 1, \ldots, m. \tag{6.27}$$

Similarly, given $Y_{\rm obs}$ and $\sigma^2 \in \mathbb{R}^m_+$, the MLE of θ maximizes the conditional likelihood function

$$L(\theta|Y_{\rm obs}, \sigma^2) = \prod_{i=1}^m N\left(\overline{Y}_i \,\middle|\, \sum_{k=1}^q b_{ik}\theta_k,\; \frac{\sigma_i^2}{n_i}\right), \quad \theta \in \mathbb{R}^r \times \mathbb{R}^{q-r}_+, \tag{6.28}$$

resulting in

$$\theta = \arg \max_{\theta \in \mathbb{R}^r \times \mathbb{R}^{q-r}_+} L(\theta|Y_{\rm obs}, \sigma^2). \tag{6.29}$$

Thus, we are back to the case considered in §6.2.1. In other words, after introducing the same latent data $Z(\sigma^2)$ as in §6.2.1 (cf. (6.13)), we can utilize (6.20) and (6.21) to find θ satisfying (6.29).

Remark 6.2 In the absence of missing data, the ECM algorithm is a special case of the cyclic coordinate ascent method for function optimization. In fact, the formulae (6.27) and (6.29) can be viewed as the first CM-step and the second CM-step of an ECM algorithm without missing data. In each CM-step 2, we use the EM algorithm to find the conditional MLE of θ given σ^2 by introducing latent data $Z(\sigma^2)$, which varies with σ^2. ¶

(b) Bayesian estimation via the IBF sampling

We use independent priors on θ and σ^2: $\theta \sim \pi(\theta)$ and $\sigma_i^2 \sim$ IGamma $(q_{i0}/2, \lambda_{i0}/2)$ with known q_{i0} and λ_{i0}, $i = 1, \ldots, m$. The observed-data posterior distribution $f(\psi|Y_{\rm obs})$ is proportional to the joint prior $\pi(\theta)\prod_{i=1}^m \pi(\sigma_i^2)$ times the observed likelihood $L(\psi|Y_{\rm obs})$ given by (6.26). We obtain

$$\begin{aligned} f(\sigma^2|Y_{\rm obs}, \theta) &= \prod_{i=1}^m \text{IGamma}\left(\sigma_i^2 \,\middle|\, \frac{q_{i0}+n_i}{2},\; \frac{\lambda_i(\theta)}{2}\right), \qquad (6.30)\\ f(\theta|Y_{\rm obs}, \sigma^2) &\propto \pi(\theta) L(\theta|Y_{\rm obs}, \sigma^2), \quad \theta \in \mathbb{R}^r \times \mathbb{R}^{q-r}_+, \end{aligned}$$

where

$$\lambda_i(\theta) \,\hat{=}\, \lambda_{i0} + \sum_{j=1}^{n_i}\left[Y_{ij} - \sum_{k=1}^q b_{ik}\theta_k\right]^2,$$

$\pi(\theta)$ and $L(\theta|Y_{\rm obs}, \sigma^2)$ are given by (6.22) and (6.28), respectively. Since $f(\theta|Y_{\rm obs}, \sigma^2)$ is quite intractable, we augment the observed data

Y_{obs} by the latent data $Z(\sigma^2)$ defined in (6.13). Similar to (6.23) and (6.17), we have

$$
\begin{aligned}
f(\theta|Y_{\text{obs}}, Z(\sigma^2), \sigma^2) &= \prod_{k=1}^{r} N(\theta_k|u_k(\sigma^2), v_k^2(\sigma^2)) \\
&\quad \times \prod_{k=r+1}^{q} TN\Big(\theta_k \Big| u_k(\sigma^2), v_k^2(\sigma^2); \mathbb{R}_+\Big), \quad (6.31) \\
f(Z(\sigma^2)|Y_{\text{obs}}, \theta, \sigma^2) &= \prod_{i=1}^{m} N_{q-1}(Z_i(\sigma^2)|E_i,\ V_i), \quad (6.32)
\end{aligned}
$$

where $u_k(\sigma^2)$, $v_k^2(\sigma^2)$, E_i and V_i are given by (6.24), (6.18) and (6.19), respectively.

To implement the IBF sampler, we first need to find the posterior mode $\tilde{\psi} = (\tilde{\theta}, \tilde{\sigma}^2)$. Let $\hat{\psi} = (\hat{\theta}, \hat{\sigma}^2)$ denote the MLE obtained in §6.2.2(a). If we use flat priors, i.e., $\sigma_{k0}^2 \to +\infty$ for $k = 1, \dots, q$ and $(q_{i0}, \lambda_{i0}) = (-2, 0)$ for $i = 1, \dots, m$, then the posterior mode $\tilde{\psi}$ is the same as the MLE $\hat{\psi}$. However, in practice, a flat prior on θ and noninformative priors on σ_i^2 are commonly used, that is, $(q_{i0}, \lambda_{i0}) = (0, 0)$ for $i = 1, \dots, m$. Hence, we have

$$\tilde{\theta} = \hat{\theta}, \qquad \tilde{\sigma}_i^2 = \left(\frac{n_i}{n_i + 2}\right) \hat{\sigma}_i^2, \quad i = 1, \dots, m. \tag{6.33}$$

Having obtained $(\tilde{\theta}, \tilde{\sigma}^2)$, by (6.32) we can easily compute

$$Z_0 = E(Z(\tilde{\sigma}^2)|Y_{\text{obs}}, \tilde{\theta}). \tag{6.34}$$

Now we consider sampling from

$$f(\theta, \sigma^2|Y_{\text{obs}}) = f(\theta|Y_{\text{obs}}) \cdot f(\sigma^2|Y_{\text{obs}}, \theta).$$

Since sampling from $f(\sigma^2|Y_{\text{obs}}, \theta)$ given by (6.30) is straightforward, we elaborate sampling from $f(\theta|Y_{\text{obs}})$. Note that

$$f(\theta|Y_{\text{obs}}, \tilde{\sigma}^2) \propto \frac{f(\theta|Y_{\text{obs}}, Z_0, \tilde{\sigma}^2)}{f(Z_0|Y_{\text{obs}}, \theta, \tilde{\sigma}^2)}, \tag{6.35}$$

where Z_0 is determined by (6.34), we can obtain i.i.d. samples from $f(\theta|Y_{\text{obs}}, \tilde{\sigma}^2)$ by the IBF sampler based on (6.31) and (6.32). Furthermore,

$$f(\theta|Y_{\text{obs}}) \propto \frac{f(\theta|Y_{\text{obs}}, \tilde{\sigma}^2)}{f(\tilde{\sigma}^2|Y_{\text{obs}}, \theta)}. \tag{6.36}$$

Then, by combining (6.35) with (6.30), we can obtain i.i.d. samples from $f(\theta|Y_{\text{obs}})$ via the IBF sampler.

6.2.3 Two examples

We analyze two real datasets to illustrate the proposed method. The first involves binomial data where an arcsin transformation is used to derive normal distribution with known variances. The second is to demonstrate the case of unknown variances. Since both examples involve small sample sizes, the Bayesian analysis is presented.

Example 6.1 (*Diesel fuel aerosol experiment*). An experiment was conducted by Dalbey & Lock (1982) to assess the lethality of diesel fuel aerosol smoke screens on rats. Rats were enclosed in chambers in which a specified dose of diesel fuel aerosol could be monitored and controlled. Let p_i denote the proportion of rats that died at dose d_i, $i = 1, \ldots, m$. If r_i, the number of rats tested at dose d_i, is reasonably large, then $\arcsin(\sqrt{p_i})$ can be considered normal with mean μ_i and variance $\sigma_i^2 = 1/(4r_i)$ (see, e.g., Schoenfeld, 1986, p.187). Table 6.1 lists the proportions of rats that died at the various doses and the corresponding values of $\arcsin(\sqrt{p_i})$. Schmoyer (1984) analyzed this data set and obtained MLEs of p_i subject to a sigmoid constraint.

Table 6.1 *Data from the diesel fuel aerosol experiment*

Group i	Dose d_i (h·mg/L)	r_i	p_i, proportion of dead	$\arcsin(\sqrt{p_i}) = \overline{Y}_i$	Variance $\sigma_i^2 = \frac{1}{4r_i}$
1	8	30	0.000	0.000	1/120
2	16	40	0.025	0.158	1/160
3	24	40	0.050	0.225	1/160
4	28	10	0.500	0.785	1/40
5	32	30	0.400	0.684	1/120
6	48	20	0.800	1.107	1/80
7	64	10	0.600	0.886	1/40
8	72	10	1.000	1.571	1/40

Source: Schmoyer (1984). Note: r_i is the number of rats tested at dose d_i.

We use the normal model (6.1) to fit the tranformed data. Now we have $m = 8$, all $n_i = 1$,

$$\overline{Y}_i = \arcsin(\sqrt{p_i}) \sim N(\mu_i, \sigma_i^2),$$

where $\overline{Y}_1, \ldots, \overline{Y}_m$ are independent and $\sigma_i^2 = 1/(4r_i)$ are known. The objective is to estimate the mean vector $\mu = (\mu_1, \ldots, \mu_m)^\top$ subject to (i) the monotonic ordering (6.2) and (ii) the increasing convex ordering (6.5).

Case 1: Monotonic ordering. In (6.12), set $r = 1$ and $q = m = 8$, we have $\mu = B\,\theta$, where $B = (b_{ik}) = \Delta_8$ given by (6.8) and $\theta = (\theta_1, \ldots, \theta_8)^{\top} \in \mathbb{R} \times \mathbb{R}^7_+$ given by (6.7). Let $\mu^{(0)}$ be the ordered values of $\overline{Y}_1, \ldots, \overline{Y}_8$, we take

$$\begin{aligned}\theta^{(0)} &= B^{-1}\,\mu^{(0)} \\ &= (0.000, 0.158, 0.067, 0.459, 0.101, 0.101, 0.221, 0.464)^{\top}.\end{aligned}$$

Using (6.20) and (6.21), the EM with the initial value $\theta^{(0)}$ converged to the restricted MLE $\hat{\theta}$ given in the second column of Table 6.2 after 180 iterations with precision 10^{-3}. The corresponding restricted MLE $\hat{\mu}$ are displayed in the third column of Table 6.2.

Table 6.2 *ML and Bayes estimates for the monotonic ordering*

Group i	MLE of θ_i	MLE of μ_i	Posterior mean of μ_i	Posterior std of μ_i	95% Posterior CI of μ_i
1	0.000	0.000	0.000	0.018	[-0.036, 0.037]
2	0.158	0.158	0.158	0.026	[0.106, 0.210]
3	0.067	0.225	0.225	0.033	[0.160, 0.289]
4	0.484	0.709	0.708	0.040	[0.629, 0.788]
5	0.000	0.709	0.727	0.042	[0.646, 0.811]
6	0.324	1.033	1.051	0.055	[0.943, 1.159]
7	0.000	1.033	1.085	0.061	[0.965, 1.210]
8	0.538	1.571	1.621	0.095	[1.438, 1.809]

Source: Tan, Tian & Fang (2003). Note: $\mu = B\,\theta$ and $B = \Delta_8$ given by (6.8).

In Bayesian setting, we use diffuse priors, i.e., $\sigma^2_{k0} \to +\infty$ for $k = 1, \ldots, 8$. Therefore, the posterior mode is the same as the MLE, we have $\tilde{\theta} = \hat{\theta}$. Based on (6.25) and (6.23), we conduct the IBF sampler (J = 30,000, I = 10,000, without replacement) to obtain posterior samples of θ. The posterior samples of μ can be obtained via $\mu = B\,\theta$. The corresponding Bayes estimates of μ are given in Table 6.2. From the third column and the fourth column in Table 6.2, the MLE or posterior mode of μ_i is slightly different from the posterior mean of μ_i for $i = 2, \ldots, 8$. This is true since the mode of a truncated normal distribution is different from its expectation.

Case 2: The increasing convex ordering (6.5). From (6.10), we have $\mu = B\,\theta$, where $B = (b_{ik}) = B_4$ is given by (6.10) and $\theta = (\theta_1, \ldots, \theta_8)^\top \in \mathbb{R} \times \mathbb{R}^7_+$ is given by (6.7). Let $\mu^{(0)}$ be the ordered values of $\overline{Y}_1, \ldots, \overline{Y}_8$, we have

$$B^{-1}\,\mu^{(0)} = (0, 0.158, -0.091, 0.392, -0.358, 0, 0.120, 0.243)^\top.$$

Replacing the above two negatives by 0, we let the initial value

$$\theta^{(0)} = (0, 0.158, 0, 0.392, 0, 0, 0.120, 0.243)^\top.$$

Using (6.20) and (6.21), the EM with this initial value $\theta^{(0)}$ converged to the restricted MLE $\hat{\theta}$ given in the second column of Table 6.3 after 2,000 iterations with precision 10^{-3}. The corresponding restricted MLE $\hat{\mu}$ is displayed in the third column of Table 6.3.

For Bayesian analysis, we use the same diffuse priors as in Case 1, the corresponding Bayesian estimates of μ are given in the last three columns of Table 6.3. Figure 6.1 shows a comparison among the unrestricted, the monotone ordered and the increasing convex MLEs of μ. There are apparent differences between the unrestricted and the restricted estimates.

Table 6.3 *ML and Bayes estimates for the increasing convex ordering*

Group i	MLE of θ_i	MLE of μ_i	Posterior mean of μ_i	Posterior std of μ_i	95% Posterior CI of μ_i
1	0.007	0.007	0.007	0.018	[-0.030, 0.042]
2	0.141	0.148	0.147	0.018	[0.109, 0.184]
3	0.000	0.289	0.292	0.020	[0.250, 0.333]
4	0.075	0.505	0.512	0.025	[0.460, 0.562]
5	0.000	0.721	0.740	0.033	[0.673, 0.807]
6	0.000	0.937	0.981	0.044	[0.895, 1.070]
7	0.000	1.153	1.244	0.060	[1.127, 1.362]
8	0.201	1.571	1.604	0.103	[1.507, 1.911]

Source: Tan, Tian & Fang (2003). Note: $\mu = B\,\theta$ and $B = B_4$ is given by (6.9).

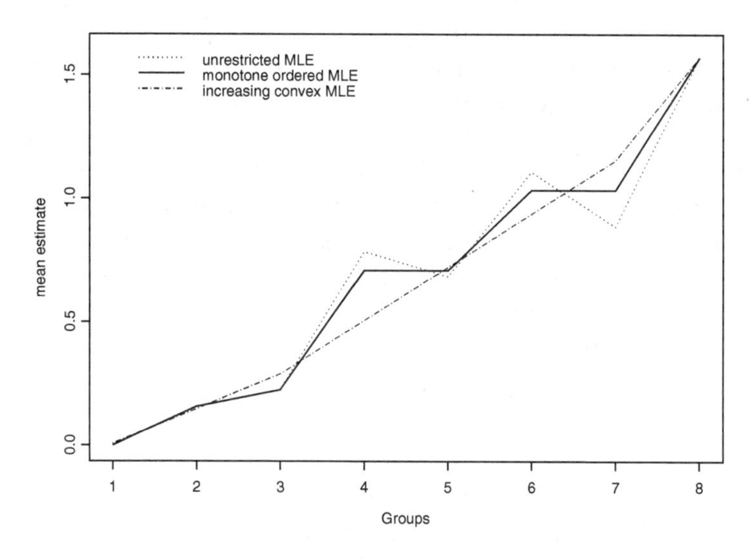

Figure 6.1 Comparison among the unrestricted MLE of μ, MLE with monotonic ordering and MLE with the increasing convex ordering. ||

Example 6.2 (*Half-life of an antibiotic drug*). The effects of an antibiotic drug are estimated by an experiment in which increasing doses are administered to $m = 5$ groups of rats and the outcomes are measurements of the half-life of the antibiotic drug, listed in Table 6.4.

Table 6.4 *Half-life of an antibiotic drug in rats*

Group i	Dose d_i (mg/kg)	n_i	Outcome (hour) Y_{ij}					Average $\overline{Y}_i$	Sample variance
1	5	5	1.17	1.12	1.07	0.98	1.04	1.076	0.005
2	10	5	1.00	1.21	1.24	1.14	1.34	1.186	0.016
3	25	4	1.55	1.63	1.49	1.53	–	1.550	0.004
4	50	5	1.21	1.63	1.37	1.50	1.81	1.504	0.054
5	200	5	1.78	1.93	1.80	2.07	1.70	1.856	0.021

Source: Hirotsu (1998). Note: n_i is the number of rats given the drug.

The usual analysis of variance is not adequate, because of the ordering of the doses. Hirotsu (1998) applies the cumulative χ^2 test to this data set and his testing result is in favor of a monotone relationship in the mean half-life, i.e., $\mu_1 \le \cdots \le \mu_5$. Let $Y_{i1}, \ldots, Y_{in_i} \overset{\text{iid}}{\sim} N(\mu_i, \sigma_i^2)$, $i = 1, \ldots, 5$. The aim is to estimate the mean vector

$\mu = (\mu_1, \ldots, \mu_5)^\top$ and the variance vector $\sigma^2 = (\sigma_1^2, \ldots, \sigma_5^2)^\top$ subject to the monotone restriction (6.2).

Let $\mu^{(0)}$ be the ordered values of $\overline{Y}_1, \ldots, \overline{Y}_5$, we set $\theta^{(0)} = B^{-1}\mu^{(0)}$ $= (1.076, 0.110, 0.318, 0.046, 0.306)^\top$, where $B = (b_{ik}) = \Delta_5$ is given by (6.8). Given $\theta^{(0)}$, we first implement the CM-step 1 to compute $\sigma^{2(0)} = (\sigma_1^2, \ldots, \sigma_5^2)^\top$ using (6.27). Given $\sigma^{2(0)}$, we then implement the CM-step 2 to find $\theta^{(1)}$ using (6.29), which consists of one E-step and one M-step. This EM-type algorithm converged after 150 iterations with precision 10^{-3}. The restricted MLE $\hat{\mu}$ and $\hat{\sigma}^2$ are given in the third column of Table 6.5 and the second column of Table 6.6, respectively.

Table 6.5 *ML and Bayes estimates of μ for the monotonic ordering*

Group i	MLE of θ_i	MLE of μ_i	Posterior mean of μ_i	Posterior std of μ_i	95% Posterior CI of μ_i
1	1.076	1.076	1.076	0.006	[1.062, 1.088]
2	0.110	1.186	1.185	0.010	[1.165, 1.207]
3	0.361	1.547	1.546	0.013	[1.520, 1.574]
4	0.000	1.547	1.562	0.018	[1.529, 1.601]
5	0.308	1.856	1.871	0.029	[1.813, 1.928]

Source: Tan, Tian & Fang (2003). Note: $\mu = B\,\theta$ and $B = \Delta_5$ is given by (6.8).

To implement the IBF sampling, we first find the posterior mode $\tilde{\theta}$ and $\tilde{\sigma}^2$. Again the flat prior on θ and the noninformative priors on σ_i^2 are used. Therefore, from (6.33), we obtain $\tilde{\theta} = \hat{\theta}$ (the second column of Table 6.5) and $\tilde{\sigma}^2$ (the third column of Table 6.6). Then we compute Z_0 by using (6.34). The first IBF sampling is implemented by drawing an i.i.d. sample of size J = 30,000 of θ from $f(\theta|Y_{\text{obs}}, Z_0, \tilde{\sigma}^2)$ and, then, obtaining an i.i.d. sample of size J_1 = 20,000 of θ from $f(\theta|Y_{\text{obs}}, \tilde{\sigma}^2)$ based on (6.35). Based on (6.36), the second IBF sampling is implemented by generating an i.i.d. sample of size I = 10,000 of θ from $f(\theta|Y_{\text{obs}})$, denoted by $\theta^{(\ell)}$, $\ell = 1, \ldots, I$. Finally, we generate $\sigma^{2(\ell)}$ from $f(\sigma^2|Y_{\text{obs}}, \theta^{(\ell)})$ for given $\theta = \theta^{(\ell)}$. Then $\sigma^{2(1)}, \ldots, \sigma^{2(I)}$ are i.i.d. samples of σ^2 from $f(\sigma^2|Y_{\text{obs}})$. The posterior samples of μ can be obtained by $\mu = B\,\theta$. The corresponding Bayesian estimates of μ and σ^2 are given in Tables 6.5 and 6.6, respectively.

Table 6.6 *ML and Bayes estimates of σ^2 for the monotonic ordering*

Group i	MLE of σ_i^2	Posterior mode of σ_i^2	Posterior mean of σ_i^2	Posterior std of σ_i^2	95% Posterior CI of σ_i^2
1	0.004	0.003	0.007	0.011	[0.001, 0.024]
2	0.013	0.009	0.021	0.025	[0.004, 0.073]
3	0.003	0.002	0.005	0.008	[0.001, 0.023]
4	0.045	0.032	0.077	0.092	[0.017, 0.291]
5	0.017	0.012	0.030	0.044	[0.006, 0.108]

Source: Tan, Tian & Fang (2003). ||

6.2.4 Discussion

Apparently, the EM algorithm in Case 2 of Ex.6.1 converges slowly requiring 2,000 iterations. To accelerate the EM, one way is to apply the parameter expanded-EM algorithm (Liu *et al.*, 1998). Another way is to reduce the number of latent variables introduced. In (6.13), we introduced a total of $m(q-1)$ normal latent variables, which are universal for arbitrarily known $m \times q$ scalar matrix $B = (b_{ik})$. For some specific B, e.g., $B = \Delta_m$ given by (6.8), we only need to introduce latent data

$$Z(\sigma^2) = \{Z_{ik}(\sigma^2)\colon\ i = 2, \ldots, m,\ k = 1, \ldots, i-1\}$$

and to obtain a complete-data $Y_{\text{com}}(\sigma^2) = \{Y_{\text{obs}}, Z(\sigma^2)\} = \{Z_{ik}(\sigma^2)\colon$ $i = 1, \ldots, m,\ k = 1, \ldots, i\}$, where

$$Z_{ik}(\sigma^2) \stackrel{\text{ind}}{\sim} N\Big(\theta_k,\ \frac{\sigma_i^2}{i\,n_i}\Big), \quad i = 1, \ldots, m,\ \ k = 1, \ldots, i, \tag{6.37}$$

and $\sum_{k=1}^{i} Z_{ik}(\sigma^2) = \overline{Y}_i$ $(i = 1, \ldots, m)$. Then there are only $m(m-1)/2$ latent variables introduced in (6.37) and the EM is expected to converge faster.

The IBF sampler cannot be directly applied to constrained parameter models because of the nonproduct parameter space. The main point of this section is to show that the IBF sampler can still be applied by getting rid of the constraints imposed on the parameters through, e.g., a linear mapping (Liu, 2000). The simplicity of the IBF sampling built on the EM algorithm makes the IBF sampler very appealing in a Bayesian framework.

6.3 Constrained Poisson Models

6.3.1 Simplex restrictions on Poisson rates

Let $\lambda = (\lambda_1, \dots, \lambda_m)^\top$ and $\lambda_i > 0$ for $i = 1, \dots, m$. Liu (2000) considered the following constrained Poisson model

$$n_i|\lambda_i \overset{\text{ind}}{\sim} \text{Poisson}(\lambda_i), \quad i = 1, \dots, m, \tag{6.38}$$

subject to

$$\lambda = B\theta \quad \text{or} \quad \lambda_i = \sum_{k=1}^{q} b_{ik}\theta_k, \quad i = 1, \dots, m, \tag{6.39}$$

where $\theta = (\theta_1, \dots, \theta_q)^\top$ with $\theta_k \geq 0$ are unknown parameters, $B = (b_{ik})$ is a known $m \times q$ scalar matrix with

$$b_{ik} \geq 0 \quad \text{and} \quad \max_{1 \leq i \leq m} b_{ik} > 0, \quad k = 1, \dots, q. \tag{6.40}$$

Since all entries in the transformation matrix B are nonnegative, the constrained λ lies in the convex cone

$$\mathbb{C} = \{\lambda \colon \lambda = B\theta, \ \theta \in \mathbb{R}^q_+\}.$$

Based on the discussions in §6.1, it is easy to see that only monotonicity restrictions[2] and the increasing convex ordering on λ are special cases of the constraint (6.39).[3] The objective is to estimate θ.

6.3.2 Data augmentation

Let $Y_{\text{obs}} = \{n_i\}_{i=1}^m$ denote the observed counts. The observed-data likelihood function is

$$L(\lambda|Y_{\text{obs}}) = \prod_{i=1}^{m} \text{Poisson}(n_i|\lambda_i) = \prod_{i=1}^{m} \frac{\lambda_i^{n_i}}{n_i!} e^{-\lambda_i}. \tag{6.41}$$

[2]Including both the increasing ordering and the decreasing ordering.

[3]However, the simple tree ordering, the umbrella ordering, the sigmoid ordering (Schmoyer, 1984), the bell-shaped ordering, and the increasing concave restriction on λ are excluded in (6.39), since some entries in these transformation matrices are negative. These facts imply that the scope of application for the proposed methods in this section is limited.

Because of the convolution property[4] of the Poisson distribution, we augment the observed data $Y_{\rm obs}$ by latent variables

$$Z = \{Z_{ik}\colon 1 \le i \le m,\ 1 \le k \le q-1\}$$

to obtain a complete-data set

$$Y_{\rm com} = \{Y_{\rm obs}, Z\} = \{Z_{ik}\colon 1 \le i \le m,\ 1 \le k \le q\},$$

where

$$\begin{aligned} Z_{ik} &\stackrel{\rm ind}{\sim} \text{Poisson}(b_{ik}\theta_k), \quad 1 \le i \le m, \quad 1 \le k \le q, &(6.42)\\ n_i &= \sum_{k=1}^{q} Z_{ik}, \qquad 1 \le i \le m. &(6.43)\end{aligned}$$

The transformation (6.43) from $Y_{\rm com}$ to $Y_{\rm obs}$ preserves the observed-data likelihood (6.41).

To derive the conditional predictive distribution of the latent variables Z given $Y_{\rm obs}$ and θ, we require the following fact (cf. Problem 6.1).

Theorem 6.2 Let $\{X_k\}_{k=1}^q$ be independent r.v.'s and for each k, $X_k \sim \text{Poisson}(\gamma_k)$, then

$$(X_1, \dots, X_q)^\top | (\textstyle\sum_{k=1}^q X_k = n) \sim \text{Multinomial}_q(n,\ p)$$

where $p = (p_1, \dots, p_q)^\top$ and $p_k = \gamma_k / \sum_{j=1}^q \gamma_j$, $k = 1, \dots, q$. ¶

6.3.3 MLE via the EM algorithm

The complete-data likelihood function is given by

$$\begin{aligned} L(\theta|Y_{\rm obs}, Z) &= \prod_{i=1}^{m}\prod_{k=1}^{q} \text{Poisson}(Z_{ik}|b_{ik}\theta_k)\\ &\propto \prod_{k=1}^{q} \theta_k^{S_k} \exp\Big\{ -\theta_k \sum_{i=1}^{m} b_{ik}\Big\}, \quad \theta \in \mathbb{R}_+^q,\end{aligned}$$

where $S_k = \sum_{i=1}^m Z_{ik}$ is a sufficient statistic of θ_k. Therefore, the complete-data MLE of θ_k is given by

$$\hat\theta_k = \frac{S_k}{\sum_{i=1}^m b_{ik}}, \quad k = 1, \dots, q.$$

[4]The convolution property indicates that sums of independent r.v.'s having this particular distribution come from the same distribution family.

Let $Z_i = (Z_{i1}, \ldots, Z_{iq})^\top$, then from (6.42), (6.43) and Theorem 6.2, the conditional predictive distribution of $Z|(Y_{\text{obs}}, \theta)$ is

$$\begin{aligned} f(Z|Y_{\text{obs}}, \theta) &= \prod_{i=1}^{m} f\Big(Z_i \Big| (\Sigma_{k=1}^{q} Z_{ik} = n_i), \theta\Big) \\ &= \prod_{i=1}^{m} \text{Multinomial}_q(Z_i|n_i,\ p_i), \end{aligned} \qquad (6.44)$$

where

$$p_i = (p_{i1}, \ldots, p_{iq})^\top, \quad p_{ik} = \frac{b_{ik}\theta_k}{\sum_{j=1}^{q} b_{ij}\theta_j}, \quad k = 1, \ldots, q. \qquad (6.45)$$

Given Y_{obs} and the current estimate $\theta^{(t)} = (\theta_1^{(t)}, \ldots, \theta_q^{(t)})^\top$, the E-step computes the conditional expectation of the sufficient statistic S_k,

$$\begin{aligned} S_k^{(t)} &= E\Big(\Sigma_{i=1}^{m} Z_{ik} \Big| Y_{\text{obs}}, \theta^{(t)}\Big) \\ &= \theta_k^{(t)} \sum_{i=1}^{m} \frac{n_i b_{ik}}{\sum_{j=1}^{q} b_{ij}\theta_j^{(t)}}, \quad k = 1, \ldots, q. \end{aligned} \qquad (6.46)$$

The M-step updates the estimates of θ

$$\theta_k^{(t+1)} = \frac{S_k^{(t)}}{\sum_{i=1}^{m} b_{ik}}, \quad k = 1, \ldots, q. \qquad (6.47)$$

6.3.4 Bayes estimation via the DA algorithm

For Bayesian estimation, with prior distribution

$$\pi(\theta) = \prod_{k=1}^{q} \text{Gamma}(\theta_k|\alpha_{k0}, \beta_{k0}), \qquad (6.48)$$

the complete-data posterior distribution of θ is

$$f(\theta|Y_{\text{obs}}, Z) = \prod_{k=1}^{q} \text{Gamma}(\theta_k|\alpha_{k0} + S_k,\ \beta_{k0} + \Sigma_{i=1}^{m} b_{ik}). \qquad (6.49)$$

The predictive distribution for the missing values is given by (6.44). This leads to the following DA algorithm:

I-step: Given the current sample of θ, impute the missing values Z by generating a sample from (6.44);

P-step: Given the current imputed complete data, generate θ from (6.49).

6.3.5 Life insurance data analysis

Broffitt (1988) considered the estimation of mortality rate in life insurance. Table 6.7 displays the age t_i from 35 to 64 years, the number N_i of people insured under a certain policy and the number

Table 6.7 *Mortality rate data in life insurance*

Index i	Age t_i	N_i, number insured	n_i, number died	n_i/N_i	Restricted MLE of p_i
1	35	1771.5	3	0.00169	0.00098
2	36	2126.5	1	0.00047	0.00098
3	37	2743.5	3	0.00109	0.00098
4	38	2766.0	2	0.00072	0.00099
5	39	2463.0	2	0.00081	0.00127
6	40	2368.0	4	0.00168	0.00156
7	41	2310.0	4	0.00173	0.00186
8	42	2306.5	7	0.00303	0.00216
9	43	2059.5	5	0.00242	0.00245
10	44	1917.0	2	0.00104	0.00275
11	45	1931.0	8	0.00414	0.00304
12	46	1746.5	13	0.00744	0.00334
13	47	1580.0	8	0.00506	0.00364
14	48	1580.0	2	0.00126	0.00393
15	49	1467.5	7	0.00477	0.00423
16	50	1516.0	4	0.00263	0.00453
17	51	1371.5	7	0.00510	0.00482
18	52	1343.0	4	0.00297	0.00512
19	53	1304.0	4	0.00306	0.00613
20	54	1232.5	11	0.00892	0.00727
21	55	1204.5	11	0.00913	0.00842
22	56	1113.5	13	0.01167	0.00956
23	57	1048.0	12	0.01145	0.01070
24	58	1155.0	12	0.01038	0.01185
25	59	1018.5	19	0.01865	0.01299
26	60	945.0	12	0.01269	0.01413
27	61	853.0	16	0.01875	0.01528
28	62	750.0	12	0.01600	0.01642
29	63	693.0	6	0.00865	0.01756
30	64	594.0	10	0.01683	0.01871

Source: Liu (2000).

n_i of insured who died ($i = 1, \ldots, m$ and $m = 30$). Anyone who started or ended a policy in the middle of a year is counted as half. Let p_i denote the true mortality rate (i.e., the probability of death) at age t_i. It is reasonable to assume that $\{p_i\}$ follows an increasing convex ordering over the observed range, that is,

$$0 \leq p_2 - p_1 \leq p_3 - p_2 \leq \cdots \leq p_m - p_{m-1} \leq 1.$$

From (6.5) and (6.9), the above increasing convex constraints can be written as

$$p = (p_1, \ldots, p_m)^\top = B_4\theta, \tag{6.50}$$

where B_4 is defined by (6.9) and $\theta = (\theta_1, \ldots, \theta_m)^\top \in \mathbb{R}_+^m$. The aim is to estimate the unknown mortality rates p subject to the constraints (6.50). The observed mortality rates ($= n_i/N_i$) against the ages are shown in Figure 6.2 as a solid line. The observed deaths n_i at each age are assumed to follow independent binomial distributions with unknown mortality rates p_i and known population sizes N_i (cf. (6.51)). Using Poisson approximation, Gelman (1996b) obtained the MLEs of p_i under the restriction (6.50) with a direct optimization routine.

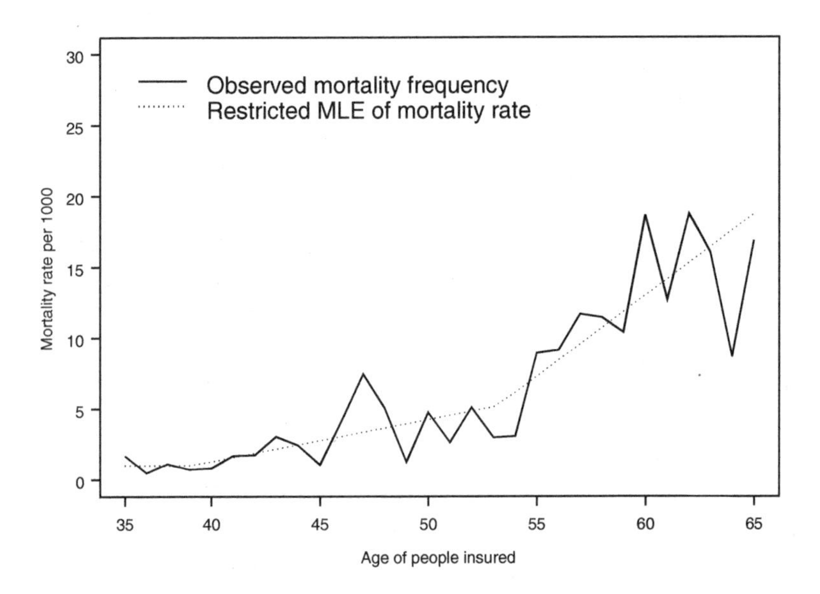

Figure 6.2 The observed mortality frequencies and the MLE of the mortality rate under the increasing convex constraints.

Furthermore, Liu (2000) assumes that

$$n_i|\lambda_i \overset{\text{ind}}{\sim} \text{Poisson}(\lambda_i), \quad i = 1, \dots, m,$$

where $\lambda_i = N_i p_i$ and $\{p_i\}$ are subject to the constraints (6.50). We have

$$\lambda = (\lambda_1, \dots, \lambda_m)^\top = \text{diag}(N_1, \dots, N_m)p = B\theta,$$

where $B_{m\times m} \hat{=} \text{diag}(N_1, \dots, N_m)B_4$ and $\theta \in \mathbb{R}^m_+$. Thus, the conditions (6.39) and (6.40) are satisfied.

Let $\theta^{(0)} = 0.0001 \cdot \mathbf{1}_m$ be the initial value of θ. Using (6.47) and (6.48), the EM algorithm converged to the restricted MLE after 3,000 iterations. The restricted MLEs $\{\hat{p}_i\}$ are given in the sixth column of Table 6.7 and are dotted in Figure 6.2.

6.4 Constrained Binomial Models

6.4.1 Statistical model

Let N_i be known positive integers, $0 \le p_i \le 1$, $i = 1, \dots, m$, and $p = (p_1, \dots, p_m)^\top$. Liu (2000) considers the following binomial model

$$n_i|(N_i, p_i) \overset{\text{ind}}{\sim} \text{Binomial}(N_i,\ p_i), \quad i = 1, \dots, m, \tag{6.51}$$

subject to simplex constraints

$$p = B\theta \quad \text{or} \quad p_i = \sum_{k=1}^{q} b_{ik}\theta_k, \quad i = 1, \dots, m, \tag{6.52}$$

and

$$\sum_{k=1}^{q} B_k^* \theta_k \le 1, \tag{6.53}$$

where $\theta = (\theta_1, \dots, \theta_q)^\top$ with $\theta_k \ge 0$ are unknown parameters, $B_{m\times q} = (b_{ik})$, $b_{ik} \ge 0$ are known scalars, and

$$B_k^* \ge \max_{1\le i\le m} b_{ik} > 0, \quad k = 1, \dots, q,$$

are known scalars. For convenience, we define

$$\theta_0 \hat{=} 1 - \sum_{k=1}^{q} B_k^*\theta_k, \quad b_{i0} \hat{=} 0, \quad \text{and} \quad B_0^* \hat{=} 1.$$

It follows from (6.53) that $0 \le \theta_0 = B_0^*\theta_0 = 1 - \sum_{k=1}^q B_k^*\theta_k$, i.e., $\sum_{k=0}^q B_k^*\theta_k = 1$. Therefore, from (6.52), we obtain

$$0 \le p_i = \sum_{k=0}^q b_{ik}\theta_k \le \sum_{k=0}^q B_k^*\theta_k = 1, \tag{6.54}$$

for all $i = 1, \dots, m$.

Liu (2000) states that monotone increasing, monotone decreasing, increasing convex, decreasing convex, increasing concave and decreasing concave constraints on p_i are special cases of (6.52) and (6.53). It is useful to set $n_i' = N_i - n_i$ and $p_i' = 1 - p_i$ for some restrictions.

6.4.2 A physical particle model

Motivated by the EM implementation of Shepp & Vardi (1982) and Lange & Carson (1984) for the Poisson emission tomography, Liu (2000) establishes a physical particle model, which suggests a DA scheme for the constrained binomial model (6.51).

Table 6.8 *Illustration for the physical particle model*

Particle •	$\underbrace{1,\dots,N_1}_{N_1}$	$\underbrace{1,\dots,N_2}_{N_2}$	$\cdots$	$\underbrace{1,\dots,j,\dots,N_i}_{N_i}$	$\cdots$	$\underbrace{1,\dots,N_m}_{N_m}$
Location ⋃	0	1	$\cdots$	k	$\cdots$	q
Probability	$B_0^*\theta_0$	$B_1^*\theta_1$	$\cdots$	$B_k^*\theta_k$	$\cdots$	$B_q^*\theta_q$
Detector ⊙	1	2	$\cdots$	i	$\cdots$	m
# detected	n_1	n_2	$\cdots$	n_i	$\cdots$	n_m

The physical particle model is described in Table 6.8. There are a total of $N = \sum_{i=1}^m N_i$ particles, where each particle is emitted at one of $1+q$ locations at random with probabilities $\{B_k^*\theta_k\}_{k=0}^q$. When emitted at location k, the particle is detected by detector i with probability b_{ik}/B_k^*. Among the N_i particles, we observed n_i particles detected by the detector i. Therefore, the observed data set is $Y_{\text{obs}} = \{N_i, n_i\}_{i=1}^m$.

(a) MLEs based on complete observations

Note that the counts emitted at the $1+q$ locations are not available. Had the counts emitted at the $1+q$ locations been available, estimation of the unknown parameters θ would be trivial.

For $1 \le i \le m$, $1 \le j \le N_i$, $k = 0, 1, \ldots, q$, we introduce binary latent variables

$$Z_{ij}(k) = \begin{cases} 1, & \text{if particle } j \text{ is emitted at location } k \\ & \text{and is detected by detector } i, \\ 0, & \text{otherwise,} \end{cases} \tag{6.55}$$

and define $Z_{ij} \hat{=} (Z_{ij}(0), Z_{ij}(1), \ldots, Z_{ij}(q))^\top$, then

$$Z_{ij}|\theta \sim \text{Multinomial}(1; B_0^*\theta_0, B_1^*\theta_1, \ldots, B_q^*\theta_q), \tag{6.56}$$

where $\sum_{k=0}^{q} Z_{ij}(k) = 1$. Therefore, the likelihood function for the complete-data $Y_{\text{com}} = \{Y_{\text{obs}}, Z\} = Y_{\text{obs}} \cup \{Z_{ij}\colon 1 \le i \le m,\ 1 \le j \le N_i\}$ is given by

$$\begin{aligned} L(\theta|Y_{\text{com}}) &\propto \prod_{i=1}^{m}\prod_{j=1}^{N_i} (B_0^*\theta_0)^{Z_{ij}(0)} \cdots (B_q^*\theta_q)^{Z_{ij}(q)} \\ &= \prod_{k=0}^{q} (B_k^*\theta_k)^{S_k}, \end{aligned}$$

so that the complete-data MLEs of θ are[5]

$$\hat{\theta}_k = \frac{S_k}{NB_k^*}, \quad k = 0, 1, \ldots, q, \tag{6.57}$$

and $S_k = \sum_{i=1}^{m}\sum_{j=1}^{N_i} Z_{ij}(k)$ is the sufficient statistic of θ_k.

(b) Consistency of the statistical model and the physical model

Next, we verify that the statistical model (6.51) with simplex constraints (6.52) and (6.53) can describe the physical particle model. In fact, by further introducing the unobservable variables

$$Y_{ij} = \begin{cases} 1, & \text{if particle } j \text{ is detected by detector } i, \\ 0, & \text{otherwise,} \end{cases}$$

we obtain

$$Y_{ij}|(Z_{ij}(k) = 1, \theta) \sim \text{Bernoulli}(b_{ik}/B_k^*). \tag{6.58}$$

[5]Since $\sum_{k=0}^{q} Z_{ij}(k) = 1$, we have $\sum_{k=0}^{q} S_k = \sum_{i=1}^{m}\sum_{j=1}^{N_i}\{\sum_{k=0}^{q} Z_{ij}(k)\} = \sum_{i=1}^{m} N_i = N$.

By using (6.58) and (6.56), we have

$$\begin{aligned}
\Pr\{Y_{ij}=1|\theta\} &= \sum_{k=0}^{q}\Pr\{Y_{ij}=1|Z_{ij}(k)=1,\theta\}\Pr\{Z_{ij}(k)=1|\theta\} \\
&= \sum_{k=0}^{q}\frac{b_{ik}}{B_k^*}(B_k^*\theta_k) \\
&= \sum_{k=0}^{q} b_{ik}\theta_k \overset{(6.54)}{=} p_i, \quad \forall\, j=1,\dots,N_i. \qquad (6.59)
\end{aligned}$$

Finally, let $n_i=\sum_{j=1}^{N_i}Y_{ij}$ $(0\le n_i\le N_i)$, then n_i denotes the number of particles detected by detector i among the N_i particles. It is clear that $n_1,\dots,n_m$ are independent and satisfy (6.51).

6.4.3 MLE via the EM algorithm

The conditional predictive distribution is given by

$$\begin{aligned}
f(Z|Y_{\rm obs},\theta) = \prod_{i=1}^{m}\prod_{j=1}^{N_i} f(Z_{ij}|Y_{\rm obs},\theta) \\
&= \prod_{i=1}^{m}\prod_{j=1}^{N_i}\sum_{y=0}^{1} f(Z_{ij},Y_{ij}=y|Y_{\rm obs},\theta) \\
&= \prod_{i=1}^{m}\prod_{j=1}^{N_i}\sum_{y=0}^{1} f(Z_{ij}|Y_{\rm obs},Y_{ij}=y,\theta)\cdot\Pr(Y_{ij}=y|Y_{\rm obs},\theta) \\
&= \prod_{i=1}^{m}\prod_{j=1}^{N_i}\sum_{y=0}^{1} f(Z_{ij}|Y_{ij}=y,\theta)\cdot\Pr(Y_{ij}=y|Y_{\rm obs},\theta), \qquad (6.60)
\end{aligned}$$

where[6]

$$\begin{aligned}
Y_{ij}|(Y_{\rm obs},\theta) &\sim \text{Hgeometric}(1,\ N_i-1,\ n_i), \qquad (6.61)\\
Z_{ij}|(Y_{ij}=1,\theta) &\sim \text{Multinomial}_{q+1}(1,\boldsymbol{\pi}_i^{(1)}), \qquad (6.62)\\
Z_{ij}|(Y_{ij}=0,\theta) &\sim \text{Multinomial}_{q+1}(1,\boldsymbol{\pi}_i^{(0)}), \qquad (6.63)\\
\boldsymbol{\pi}_i^{(1)} &= (b_{i0}\theta_0,\dots,b_{iq}\theta_q)^{\top}/p_i, \quad \text{and}\\
\boldsymbol{\pi}_i^{(0)} &= ((B_0^*-b_{i0})\theta_0,\dots,(B_q-b_{iq})\theta_q)^{\top}/(1-p_i).
\end{aligned}$$

[6]Liu (2000) does not give formulae such as (6.60) and (6.61). It seems to us that he assumes that $\{Y_{ij}\}$ are observable.

(a) Two useful theorems

To derive (6.61)–(6.63), we need the following results.

Theorem 6.3 Let $\{X_k\}_{k=1}^q$ be independent r.v.'s and for each k, $X_k \sim \text{Binomial}(n_k, p)$, then

$$X_k|(\textstyle\sum_{k'=1}^q X_{k'} = x_+) \sim \text{Hgeometric}(n_k,\ n_+ - n_k,\ x_+), \tag{6.64}$$

where $n_+ = \sum_{k=1}^q n_k$. ¶

PROOF. Let $X_+ = \Sigma_{k=1}^q X_k$ and $X_{-k} = X_+ - X_k$, then

$$\begin{aligned} X_+ &\sim \text{Binomial}(n_+,\ p), \quad \text{and} \\ X_{-k} &\sim \text{Binomial}(n_+ - n_k,\ p). \end{aligned}$$

Thus, we have

$$\begin{aligned} \Pr\{X_k = x_k | X_+ = x_+\} &= \frac{\Pr\{X_k = x_k,\ X_{-k} = x_+ - x_k\}}{\Pr\{X_+ = x_+\}} \\ &= \frac{\binom{n_k}{x_k}\binom{n_+ - n_k}{x_+ - x_k}}{\binom{n_+}{x_+}}, \end{aligned}$$

where $x_k = \max(0,\ x_+ - n_+ + n_k), \ldots, \min(n_k, x_+)$. According to the notation in Appendix A.1.2, we obtain (6.64). ||END||

Theorem 6.4

$$\Pr\{Y_{ij} = 1|Z_{ij}, \theta) = \prod_{k=0}^{q} \left(\frac{b_{ik}}{B_k^*}\right)^{Z_{ij}(k)}, \quad \text{and} \tag{6.65}$$

$$\Pr\{Y_{ij} = 0|Z_{ij}, \theta) = \prod_{k=0}^{q} \left(1 - \frac{b_{ik}}{B_k^*}\right)^{Z_{ij}(k)}. \quad ¶ \tag{6.66}$$

PROOF. From (6.58), we have

$$\begin{aligned} \Pr\{Y_{ij} = 1|Z_{ij}(k) = 1,\ \theta\} &= b_{ik}/B_k^*, \quad \text{and} \\ \Pr\{Y_{ij} = 0|Z_{ij}(k) = 1,\ \theta\} &= 1 - b_{ik}/B_k^*. \end{aligned}$$

Note that $\sum_{k=0}^q Z_{ij}(k) = 1$, we obtain (6.65) and (6.66). ||END||

(b) Derivation of (6.61)–(6.63)

First, from (6.59), we have $Y_{ij}|\theta \overset{\text{ind}}{\sim} \text{Binomial}(1,\ p_i)$, $j = 1, \ldots, N_i$. Since

$$Y_{ij}|(Y_{\text{obs}},\ \theta) \overset{d}{=} Y_{ij}|(\textstyle\sum_{j=1}^{N_i} Y_{ij} = n_i,\ \theta),$$

from (6.64), we immediately obtain (6.61).

Next, from (6.65), (6.56) and (6.59),

$$\begin{aligned}
\Pr\{Z_{ij}|Y_{ij} = 1,\ \theta\} &= \frac{\Pr\{Z_{ij}, Y_{ij} = 1|\theta\}}{\Pr\{Y_{ij} = 1|\theta\}} \\
&= \frac{\Pr\{Y_{ij} = 1|Z_{ij}, \theta\} \cdot \Pr\{Z_{ij}|\theta\}}{\Pr\{Y_{ij} = 1|\theta\}} \\
&= \frac{\{\prod_{k=0}^{q} (b_{ik}/B_k^*)^{Z_{ij}(k)}\} \cdot \Pr\{Z_{ij}|\theta\}}{p_i} \\
&= \frac{1!}{\prod_{k=0}^{q} Z_{ij}(k)!} \cdot \prod_{k=0}^{q} (b_{ik}\theta_k/p_i)^{Z_{ij}(k)} \\
&= \text{Multinomial}_{q+1}(Z_{ij}|1,\ \boldsymbol{\pi}_i^{(1)}),
\end{aligned}$$

which implies (6.62). Similarly, we can prove (6.63).

(c) The E-step and M-step

On the one hand, from (6.62) and (6.63), we obtain

$$\begin{aligned}
E(Z_{ij}(k)|Y_{ij} = 1, \theta) &= \frac{b_{ik}\theta_k}{p_i}, \quad \text{and} \\
E(Z_{ij}(k)|Y_{ij} = 0, \theta) &= \frac{(B_k^* - b_{ik})\theta_k}{1 - p_i}.
\end{aligned}$$

Rewriting them in a unified equation, we have

$$E(Z_{ij}(k)|Y_{ij}, \theta) = \frac{b_{ik}\theta_k}{p_i} \cdot Y_{ij} + \frac{(B_k^* - b_{ik})\theta_k}{1 - p_i} \cdot (1 - Y_{ij}). \tag{6.67}$$

On the other hand, from (6.61) and Appendix A.1.2, we have

$$E(Y_{ij}|Y_{\text{obs}}, \theta) = \frac{n_i}{N_i}, \quad \text{and} \quad E(1 - Y_{ij}|Y_{\text{obs}}, \theta) = 1 - \frac{n_i}{N_i}. \tag{6.68}$$

Therefore, the E-step is to compute the conditional expectation of the sufficient statistic

$$S_k = \sum_{i=1}^{m} \sum_{j=1}^{N_i} Z_{ij}(k),$$

that is,

$$\begin{aligned}
S_k^{(t)} &= \sum_{i=1}^{m}\sum_{j=1}^{N_i} E\Big(Z_{ij}(k)\Big|Y_{\rm obs},\, \theta^{(t)}\Big) \\
&= \sum_{i=1}^{m}\sum_{j=1}^{N_i} E\Big\{E\Big(Z_{ij}(k)\Big|Y_{\rm obs}, Y_{ij}, \theta^{(t)}\Big)\Big|Y_{\rm obs}, \theta^{(t)}\Big\} \\
&= \sum_{i=1}^{m}\sum_{j=1}^{N_i} E\Big\{E\Big(Z_{ij}(k)\Big|Y_{ij}, \theta^{(t)}\Big)\Big|Y_{\rm obs}, \theta^{(t)}\Big\} \\
&\overset{(6.67)}{=} \sum_{i=1}^{m}\sum_{j=1}^{N_i} E\left\{\frac{b_{ik}\theta_k^{(t)}Y_{ij}}{p_i^{(t)}} + \frac{(B_k^* - b_{ik})\theta_k^{(t)}(1-Y_{ij})}{1-p_i^{(t)}}\right|Y_{\rm obs}, \theta^{(t)}\Bigg\} \\
&\overset{(6.68)}{=} \sum_{i=1}^{m}\sum_{j=1}^{N_i} \left\{\frac{b_{ik}\theta_k^{(t)}n_i}{p_i^{(t)}N_i} + \frac{(B_k^* - b_{ik})\theta_k^{(t)}(N_i-n_i)}{(1-p_i^{(t)})N_i}\right\} \\
&= \theta_k^{(t)}\sum_{i=1}^{m}\left\{\frac{n_i b_{ik}}{p_i^{(t)}} + \frac{(N_i-n_i)(B_k^* - b_{ik})}{1-p_i^{(t)}}\right\}, \qquad (6.69)
\end{aligned}$$

for $k = 0, 1, \ldots, q$, where $p_i^{(t)} = \sum_{k=0}^{q} b_{ik}\theta_k^{(t)}$.

From (6.57), the M-step updates the estimates of θ

$$\theta_k^{(t+1)} = \frac{S_k^{(t)}}{NB_k^*}, \quad k = 0, 1, \ldots, q. \qquad (6.70)$$

6.4.4 Bayes estimation via the DA algorithm

For Bayesian estimation, with the conjugate prior distribution

$$\pi(\theta) \propto \prod_{k=0}^{q} \theta_k^{c_k - 1}, \quad \theta_k \geq 0, \quad \sum_{k=0}^{q} B_k^*\theta_k = 1, \qquad (6.71)$$

the complete-data posterior of $(B_0^*\theta_0, \ldots, B_q^*\theta_q)^\top$ is

$$(B_0^*\theta_0, \ldots, B_q^*\theta_q)^\top|(Y_{\rm obs}, Z) \sim \text{Dirichlet}(c_0 + S_0, \ldots, c_q + S_q). \quad (6.72)$$

The predictive distribution for the missing values is given by (6.60). This leads to the following DA algorithm:

I-step: Given the current sample of θ, impute the missing values Z by generating a sample from (6.60);

P-step: Given the current imputed complete data, generate θ from (6.72).

Problems

6.1 Isotonic regression under simple order (Silvapulle & Sen, 2005, p.47–49). Consider the weighted least squares

$$\min_{\mu_1 \le \cdots \le \mu_m} \sum_{i=1}^{m} w_i (y_i - \mu_i)^2,$$

where $\{w_i\}$, $\{y_i\}$ and $\{\mu_i\}$ are known positive numbers, known observations, and parameters of interest, respectively. Let $\mu^{\rm RLSE} = (\mu_1^{\rm RLSE}, \ldots, \mu_m^{\rm RLSE})^\top$ denote the restricted LSE of μ, $\mu^{\rm RLSE}$ is called the isotonic regression of $y = (y_1, \ldots, y_m)^\top$ with respect to the weights $\{w_i\}$ and the simple order. Show that $\mu^{\rm RLSE}$ has the following explicit forms:

$$\begin{aligned} \mu_i^{\rm RLSE} &= \min_{t \ge i} \max_{s \le t} \frac{w_s y_s + \cdots + w_t y_t}{w_s + \cdots + w_t}, \quad i = 1, \ldots, m, \\ &= \max_{s \le i} \max_{t \ge s} \frac{w_s y_s + \cdots + w_t y_t}{w_s + \cdots + w_t}, \quad i = 1, \ldots, m. \end{aligned}$$

This algorithm is known as the *pool adjacent violators algorithm* (PAVA).

6.2 Prove Theorem 6.2.

6.3 Based on (6.44) and (6.49), devise an IBF sampler to generate i.i.d. posterior samples of θ.

6.4 Using the DA algorithm in §6.3.4 to compute Bayesian estimates of $\{p_i\}$ for the life insurance data in Table 6.7.

6.5 Mimic Ex.6.1, using normal approximation to obtain the MLEs of p_i under the restriction (6.50) for the life insurance data in Table 6.7.

6.6 Prove (6.63).

6.7 By using the EM algorithm ((6.69) and (6.70)) and the DA algorithm ((6.71) and (6.72)) to compute the restricted MLEs and Bayesian estimates of p_i for the life insurance data in Table 6.7.

CHAPTER 7

Checking Compatibility & Uniqueness

7.1 Introduction

Checking compatibility for two given conditional distributions and identifying the corresponding unique compatible marginal distributions are important problems in mathematical statistics, especially in Bayesian statistical inferences.

Definition 7.1 Two conditional distributions $f_{(X|Y)}$ and $f_{(Y|X)}$ are said to be **compatible** if there exists **at least** one joint distribution for (X, Y) with them being its conditional distributions. ¶

A considerable literature has been spawned on the discussions of checking the compatibility of conditional densities in the past 30 years (e.g., Besag, 1974; Arnold & Strauss, 1988; Casella & George, 1992; Gelman & Speed, 1993, 1999; Hobert & Casella, 1996, 1998; Robert & Casella, 1999). Amongst the Gibbs sampler may perhaps be one of the most widely discussed MCMC sampling algorithms in the Bayesian computation literature for generating joint distribution via individual conditional distributions. This chapter mainly concerns the following three issues:

- First, how do we check the compatibility of two given conditional distributions?
- Moreover, if $f_{(X|Y)}$ and $f_{(Y|X)}$ are compatible, is the associated joint density $f_{(X,Y)}$ unique?
- Finally, when $f_{(X,Y)}$ is unique, how do we find it?

For a two-dimensional random vector (X, Y) taking values in the sample space $(\mathcal{X}, \mathcal{Y})$, a fundamental issue in probability and statistics is to use some combinations of marginal and/or conditional densities to determine the joint density function of (X, Y). Given the marginal density f_X and the conditional density $f_{(Y|X)}$ (or symmetrically, given both f_Y and $f_{(X|Y)}$), we can uniquely characterize the joint density as follows:

$$f_{(X,Y)}(x,y) = f_X(x) f_{(Y|X)}(y|x), \quad (x,y) \in (\mathcal{X}, \mathcal{Y}), \tag{7.1}$$
$$= f_Y(y) f_{(X|Y)}(x|y), \quad (x,y) \in (\mathcal{X}, \mathcal{Y}). \tag{7.2}$$

Second, it is well known that marginal densities f_X and f_Y are not sufficient to determine the joint density $f_{(X,Y)}$ uniquely. For example, let f_X and f_Y be two positive densities defined in the real line $\mathbb{R}$ and F_X and F_Y be the corresponding cdfs, then, for any given $\alpha \in [-1, 1]$,

$$f^{\alpha}_{(X,Y)}(x,y) = \Big\{1 + \alpha[2F_X(x) - 1][2F_Y(y) - 1]\Big\} \times f_X(x) f_Y(y), \quad (x,y) \in \mathbb{R}^2, \tag{7.3}$$

is a joint pdf of (X, Y) with marginal pdfs f_X and f_Y (Gumbel, 1960, p.704). Moreover, marginal normality is not enough to characterize a bivariate normal distribution. The simplest example (Arnold *et al.*, 1999, p.54) perhaps is

$$f_{(X,Y)}(x,y) = \begin{cases} \frac{1}{\pi} e^{-(x^2+y^2)/2}, & \text{if } xy > 0, \\ 0, & \text{otherwise}, \end{cases} \tag{7.4}$$

which has standard normal marginals. Obviously, (7.4) is not a bivariate normal density.

Third, it is well known that (see, e.g., Theorem 7.4 in §7.2) two full conditional distributions can over-determine (i.e., contain more than necessary information to characterize) the joint distribution.

Fourth, two conditional means, say $E(X|Y = y)$ and $E(Y|X = x)$, are not enough to characterize the joint density. As a result, some statisticians turned to determining whether $E(X|Y = y)$ and $f_{Y|X}$ are sufficient to characterize the joint density (e.g., Papageorgiou, 1983; Wesolowski, 1995a, 1995b; Arnold *et al.*, 1999, 2001).

In this chapter, we consider compatibility in the following three situations:

(a) given $f_{(X|Y)}$ and $f_{(Y|X)}$;

(b) given $E(X|Y = y)$ and $f_{(Y|X)}$; and

(c) given f_Y and $f_{(Y|X)}$.

Moreover, we further distinguish the *product measurable space* (PMS) from the *nonproduct measurable space* (NPMS), and the **continuous** case from the **discrete** case. Can we characterize the marginal density f_X (hence, the joint density $f_{(X,Y)}$) for the above cases with different combinations? To our knowledge, such materials and related examples have not been introduced in the current textbooks of probability and statistics. One aim of this chapter is to bridge this gap.

In §7.2, we consider the case of two continuous conditional distributions (i.e., Case (a)) under PMS. In §7.3, we focus on finite discrete conditional distributions (i.e., Cases (a) and (b)) under PMS. The NPMS case is presented in §7.4. Finally, we discuss Case (c) under PMS in §7.5.

7.2 Two Continuous Conditionals: PMS

7.2.1 Several basic notions

Let two random variables/vectors (X, Y) be absolutely continuous with respect to some measure μ on the joint support

$$\mathcal{S}_{(X,Y)} = \Big\{(x, y)\colon\ f_{(X,Y)}(x, y) > 0,\ (x, y) \in (\mathcal{X}, \mathcal{Y})\Big\}.$$

The absolute continuous assumption allows discussion of a continuous variable (i.e., its pdf is Lebesgue measurable) with a discrete variable (i.e., its pmf gives rise to a counting measure).

Definition 7.2 If $\mathcal{S}_{(X,Y)} = \mathcal{S}_X \times \mathcal{S}_Y$, then the measure μ is said to be **product measurable** and μ can be written as $\mu_1 \times \mu_2$; otherwise, it is said to be **nonproduct measurable**, where

$$\begin{aligned} \mathcal{S}_X &= \Big\{x\colon\ f_X(x) > 0,\ x \in \mathcal{X}\Big\} \quad \text{and} \\ \mathcal{S}_Y &= \Big\{y\colon\ f_Y(y) > 0,\ y \in \mathcal{Y}\Big\} \end{aligned}$$

denote the supports of X and Y, respectively. ¶

For example, from (7.3) we have

$$\mathcal{S}_{(X,Y)} = \mathbb{R}^2 = \mathcal{S}_X \times \mathcal{S}_Y;$$

while from (7.4) we obtain

$$\mathcal{S}_{(X,Y)} = \{(x, y)\colon\ xy > 0\} \neq \mathbb{R}^2 = \mathcal{S}_X \times \mathcal{S}_Y.$$

Next, we define 2 two-dimensional domains:[1]

$$\mathcal{S}_{(X|Y)} = \Big\{(x,y)\colon f_{(X|Y)}(x|y) > 0,\ x \in \mathcal{X},\ y \in \mathcal{Y}\Big\}, \quad \text{and}$$
$$\mathcal{S}_{(Y|X)} = \Big\{(x,y)\colon f_{(Y|X)}(y|x) > 0,\ x \in \mathcal{X},\ y \in \mathcal{Y}\Big\}.$$

7.2.2 A review on existing methods

In PMS, Arnold & Press (1989) obtained the following necessary and sufficient conditions for the compatibility of two conditional distributions.

Theorem 7.1 (Arnold & Press, 1989). A joint pdf $f_{(X,Y)}$ with conditional densities $f_{(X|Y)}$ and $f_{(Y|X)}$ exist iff

(i) $\mathcal{S}_{(X|Y)} = \mathcal{S}_{(Y|X)} = \mathcal{S}_{(X,Y)}$; and

(ii) there exist two functions $u(x)$ and $v(y)$ such that $\int_{\mathcal{S}_X} u(x)dx < +\infty$ and

$$\frac{f_{(X|Y)}(x|y)}{f_{(Y|X)}(y|x)} = \frac{u(x)}{v(y)}, \quad \forall\, x \in \mathcal{S}_X \quad \text{and} \quad y \in \mathcal{S}_Y. \qquad ¶$$

It can be readily shown that $f_X(x) \propto u(x)$ and $f_Y(y) \propto v(y)$. In addition, the condition $\int_{\mathcal{S}_X} u(x)dx < \infty$ is equivalent (via Tonelli's theorem) to the condition $\int_{\mathcal{S}_Y} v(y)dy < \infty$ and only one of them is required to be checked in practice. However, this theorem does not show how to identify the functions $u(x)$ and $v(y)$, especially for the cases of multiple solutions.

To prove the uniqueness of f_X, consider a Markov chain with state space $\mathcal{S}_X$ and transition kernel

$$K(x,x') = \int_{\mathcal{S}_Y} f_{(X|Y)}(x|y) f_{(Y|X)}(y|x')\, dy. \tag{7.5}$$

Given the existence of f_X, Arnold & Press (1989) provided the following necessary and sufficient conditions for the uniqueness of f_X.

Theorem 7.2 (Arnold & Press, 1989). Let $f_{(X|Y)}$ and $f_{(Y|X)}$ be compatible, then the marginal density f_X can be uniquely determined iff the Markov chain with state space $\mathcal{S}_X$ and transition kernel $K(x,x')$ defined in (7.5) is indecomposable. ¶

[1]It is quite important to distinguish $\mathcal{S}_{(X|Y)}$ from the conditional support $\mathcal{S}_{(X|Y)}(y)$ defined in (7.25).

It is noteworthy that it is difficult to check the above condition for uniqueness in practice. Second, Theorem 7.2 itself cannot provide the expression of $f_X(x)$. Theorem 7.3 provides a positivity condition which is a sufficient condition for f_X (hence for $f_{(X,Y)}$) being unique (Hammersley & Clifford, 1970; Besag, 1974) and the unique solution f_X is given explicitly (Ng, 1997a; Tian & Tan, 2003).

Theorem 7.3 (Ng, 1997a). Suppose that $f_{(X|Y)}$ and $f_{(Y|X)}$ are compatible. If $f_{(X|Y)}(x|y) > 0$ and $f_{(Y|X)}(y|x) > 0$ for all $x \in \mathcal{X}$ and $y \in \mathcal{Y}$, then the marginal density f_X is uniquely determined by the point-wise IBF:

$$f_X(x) = \left\{ \int_{\mathcal{S}(Y)} \frac{f_{Y|X}(y|x)}{f_{X|Y}(x|y)} \, dy \right\}^{-1}, \quad \text{for any given } x \in \mathcal{S}_X. \qquad \P \ (7.6)$$

PROOF. Under the assumptions, we have $\mathcal{X} = \mathcal{S}_X$ and $\mathcal{Y} = \mathcal{S}_Y$. By combining (7.1) with (7.2), we have

$$f_Y(y) = \frac{f_{(Y|X)}(y|x)}{f_{(X|Y)}(x|y)} f_X(x), \quad x \in \mathcal{S}_X, \; y \in \mathcal{S}_Y. \qquad (7.7)$$

Integrating this identity with respect to y, we immediately obtain (7.6). ||END||

In practice, uniqueness can be readily determined via Theorem 7.3 than via Theorem 7.2 (see §7.3 for more details). However, the positivity condition in Theorem 7.3 is still too stringent to be practically satisfied (e.g., see Ex.7.4 in §7.3.3). By relaxing the positivity assumption, the following theorem gives another sufficient condition for uniqueness (Patil, 1965; Gelman & Speed, 1993; Ng, 1997a; Arnold *et al.*, 1999).

Theorem 7.4 (Ng, 1997a). Suppose that $f_{X|Y}$ and $f_{Y|X}$ are compatible. If there exists some $y_0 \in \mathcal{Y}$ such that $f_{Y|X}(y_0|x) > 0$ for all $x \in \mathcal{X}$, then the marginal density $f_X(x)$ is uniquely determined by the sampling IBF:

$$f_X(x) \propto \frac{f_{X|Y}(x|y_0)}{f_{Y|X}(y_0|x)}. \qquad \P \ (7.8)$$

The above theorem suggests that two fully specified conditional densities can overly determine (i.e., contain more than necessary information to characterize) the joint distribution. Although the sampling IBF (7.8) is easy to apply in practice, Theorem 7.4 cannot be applied to situations (see, Ex.7.5 and Ex.7.6 in §7.3.3) in which there is no $y_0 \in \mathcal{Y}$ such that $f_{Y|X}(y_0|x) > 0$ for all $x \in \mathcal{X}$.

7.2.3 Two examples

Example 7.1 (*Measurement error models*). Let an r.v. Y of interest be unobservable. We are only able to observe

$$X = Y + \varepsilon_1,$$

where ε_1 is a Gaussian error. By exchanging the role of Y for X, the question is whether it is possible to have $X = Y + \varepsilon_1$ and

$$Y = X + \varepsilon_2$$

simultaneously (Arnold & Press, 1989). Let $h_i(\cdot)$ denote the pdf of ε_i for $i = 1, 2$. The proposed model, if exists, will have conditional distributions in location family

$$f_{(X|Y)}(x|y) = h_1(x - y) \quad \text{and} \quad f_{(Y|X)}(y|x) = h_2(y - x).$$

Using (7.8) and setting $y_0 = 0$, we have

$$f_X(x) \propto \frac{h_1(x)}{h_2(-x)}, \quad -\infty < x < +\infty. \tag{7.9}$$

If both $h_1(\cdot)$ and $h_2(\cdot)$ are standard normal densities, then

$$X|(Y = y) \sim N(y, 1) \quad \text{and} \quad Y|(X = x) \sim N(x, 1).$$

From (7.9), we have $f_X(x) \propto 1$ for $x \in \mathbb{R}$, which is not a density. Therefore, the two conditionals are incompatible.

Similarly, if the distribution of $X|(Y = y)$ is a Student's t-distribution with 5 degrees of freedom with location y, then

$$h_1(z) = \frac{1}{\sqrt{5}B(1/2, 5/2)} \left(1 + \frac{z^2}{5}\right)^{-3}.$$

From (7.9), we obtain

$$f_X(x) \propto (1 + x^2/5)^{-3} e^{x^2/2}, \quad x \in \mathbb{R}.$$

It is easy to verify that

$$\int_{-\infty}^{\infty} (1 + x^2/5)^{-3} e^{x^2/2}\, dx = +\infty,$$

indicating that $f_X(x)$ is not a density. Hence the two conditionals are also incompatible. ||

Example 7.2 (*Restricted exponential distributions*). Casella and George (1992) considered two conditional distributions that are exponential distributions restricted to the interval $[0, b)$, that is,

$$\begin{aligned} f_{(X|Y)}(x|y) &\propto y\exp(-yx), & 0 \le x < b < +\infty, \quad (7.10) \\ f_{(Y|X)}(y|x) &\propto \frac{x\exp(-xy)}{\int_0^b x\exp(-xy)\,dy}, & 0 \le y < b < +\infty. \quad (7.11) \end{aligned}$$

Applying (7.8) and setting $y_0 = 1$, the marginal distribution of X is given by

$$f_X(x) \propto \frac{1-\exp(-bx)}{x} \mathrel{\hat{=}} h(x), \quad 0 \le x < b < +\infty. \tag{7.12}$$

Note that $h(x)$ is a strict decreasing function in $[0, b)$, we have

$$h(x) \le h(0) = b, \quad \text{and} \quad \int_0^b h(x)dx \le b^2 < +\infty.$$

Hence, $f_X(x)$ exists, i.e., (7.10) and (7.11) are compatible.

If let $b = +\infty$, then from (7.12),

$$f_X(x) \propto 1/x, \quad 0 \le x < +\infty.$$

Obviously, $f_X(x)$ is not a density. In other words, the two conditionals are incompatible when $b = +\infty$. ||

7.3 Finite Discrete Conditionals: PMS

In this section, we focus on finite discrete conditional distributions. For $i = 1, \ldots, m$ and $j = 1, \ldots, n$, we define the joint distribution matrix $P_{m\times n}$, and conditional probability matrices $A_{m\times n}$ and $B_{n\times m}$ as follows:

$$\begin{aligned} P &= (p_{ij}) = (\Pr\{X = x_i, Y = y_j\}), \quad (7.13) \\ A &= (a_{ij}) = (\Pr\{X = x_i | Y = y_j\}), \quad \text{and} \\ B &= (b_{ij}) = (\Pr\{Y = y_j | X = x_i\}), \quad (7.14) \end{aligned}$$

where $\sum_{i=1}^m \sum_{j=1}^n p_{ij} = 1$, and all column totals for A and all row totals for B are identical to 1.

Definition 7.3 Two conditional distribution matrices A and B are said to be **compatible** if there exists **at least** one joint distribution matrix P such that

$$p_{ij} = a_{ij}p_{\cdot j} = b_{ij}p_{i\cdot}, \quad \forall\, i,\ j, \tag{7.15}$$

where $p_{\cdot j} = \sum_{i=1}^{m} p_{ij}$ and $p_{i\cdot} = \sum_{j=1}^{n} p_{ij}$. ¶

In addition, we let

$$\begin{aligned} \xi &= (\xi_1, \ldots, \xi_m)^{\top} \in \mathbb{T}_m \quad \text{with} \quad \xi_i = \Pr\{X = x_i\}, \\ \eta &= (\eta_1, \ldots, \eta_n)^{\top} \in \mathbb{T}_n \quad \text{with} \quad \eta_j = \Pr\{Y = y_j\}. \end{aligned} \tag{7.16}$$

7.3.1 The formulation of the problems

The aim is to find possible solutions to the system of linear equations in (7.15) subject to the complex constraints $P \in \mathbb{T}_{mn}$. In fact, we only need to find a compatible marginal distribution of X, say, ξ. Once we obtain ξ, we have $P = \text{diag}(\xi)B$. Equivalently, we only need to find $\xi \in [0,1]^m$ that satisfies

$$\begin{aligned} 1 &= \xi_1 + \cdots + \xi_m, \quad \text{and} \\ 0 &= \xi_i b_{ij} - a_{ij} \sum_{k=1}^{m} \xi_k b_{kj}, \quad \forall\, i,\ j. \end{aligned} \tag{7.17}$$

This system can be rewritten in the following matrix form

$$e_1 = D\xi, \qquad \xi \in [0,1]^m, \tag{7.18}$$

where $e_1 = (1, 0, \ldots, 0)^{\top}$ is the unit vector of N-dimensional with $N = 1 + mn$, and D is an $N \times m$ matrix with its first row being $\mathbf{1}_m^{\top}$ and the $(i-1)n + j + 1$-th row ($i = 1, \ldots, m$ and $j = 1, \ldots, n$) is given by

$$(\mathbf{0}_{i-1}^{\top}, b_{ij}, \mathbf{0}_{m-i}^{\top}) - a_{ij}(b_{1j}, \ldots, b_{ij}, \ldots, b_{mj}).$$

7.3.2 The connection with quadratic optimization under box constraints

For any given e_1 and D, we can use the ℓ_2-norm (i.e., the Euclidean distance) to measure the discrepancy between e_1 and $D\xi$ and denote it by

$$\ell_2(e_1, D\xi) = ||e_1 - D\xi||^2.$$

Here, we consider the following quadratic optimization problem with unit cube constraints:

$$\hat{\xi} = \arg \min_{\xi \in [0,1]^m} \ell_2(e_1, D\xi). \tag{7.19}$$

In practice, the built-in S-plus function "`nlregb`" (nonlinear least squares subject to box constraints) can be used to calculate $\hat{\xi}$. For convenience, an S-plus function named "`lseb`" is given in §7.3.6.

We consider the following ways to produce initial values of ξ for our function `lseb`. We may generate random numbers $V_i^{(0)}$ ($i = 1, \dots, m$) from the chi-square distribution with n_i degrees of freedom and let

$$\xi^{(0)} = (V_1^{(0)}, \dots, V_m^{(0)})^{\top} \Big/ \sum_{i=1}^{m} V_i^{(0)}.$$

Alternatively, we notice that when $\text{rank}(D) = N \le m$ and without constraints, the solution to (7.19) is not unique and all solutions assume the form:

$$\hat{\xi}_\tau^{\text{LSE}} = D^+ e_1 + [\mathbf{I}_m - D^+ D]\tau,$$

where τ is an arbitrary vector in $\mathbb{R}^m$ and $D^+ = D^{\top}(DD^{\top})^{-1}$ denotes the Moore–Penrose generalized inverse of matrix D. When $\text{rank}(D) = N \le m$ and with constraints, the solution to (7.19) is also not unique. In general, different initial values will result in different solutions. In this case, we suggest

$$\xi_\tau^{(0)} = \min\Big\{ \max\{\mathbf{0}_m,\ \hat{\xi}_\tau^{\text{LSE}}\},\ \mathbf{1}_m \Big\}. \tag{7.20}$$

Theorem 7.5 For the constrained optimization problem (7.19), we have the following results:

(i) When the solution $\hat{\xi}$ calculated from (7.19) is unique and the resulting ℓ_2-norm $< 10^{-10}$ (say), then A and B are compatible and the unique X-marginal is specified by $\hat{\xi}$;

(ii) When $\hat{\xi}$ is unique but the corresponding ℓ_2-norm $\ge 10^{-10}$, then A and B are incompatible;

(iii) When (7.19) has multiple solutions (denoted by $\{\hat{\xi}_\tau, \tau \in \mathbb{R}^m\}$) and all ℓ_2-norms $< 10^{-10}$, then A and B are compatible and the multiple X-marginals are specified by $\{\hat{\xi}_\tau, \tau \in \mathbb{R}^m\}$. ¶

PROOF. We first note that the system of linear equations (7.18) has solution(s) iff $\ell_2(e_1, D\xi) = 0$. On the other hand, the constrained optimization problem (7.19) may have a unique solution or multiple solutions. Therefore, if $\hat{\xi}$ is unique and the resulting ℓ_2-norm is almost equal to zero, then the system of linear equations (7.18) has a unique solution. In other words, A and B are compatible and the unique X-marginal is given by $\hat{\xi}$. If $\hat{\xi}$ is unique and the corresponding ℓ_2-norm is greater than some pre-specified small constant, then solution to (7.18) does not exist. In this case, A and B are incompatible. If the constrained optimization algorithm converges to different solutions for different initial values, then (7.18) has multiple solutions. That is, A and B are compatible and have multiple compatible joint distributions. ||END||

7.3.3 Numerical examples

Four examples are used to illustrate the proposed methods. In Ex.7.3, we first apply Theorems 7.1 and 7.3 to check the compatibility and uniqueness problems, and then apply Theorem 7.5(i) for confirmation. In Ex.7.4, we apply Theorems 7.1 and 7.4 to check the compatibility and uniqueness problems, and then apply Theorem 7.5(i) for verification. Finally, we notice that Theorems 7.3 and 7.4 do not apply to Ex.7.5 and Ex.7.6, thus Theorem 7.5(ii) and 7.5(iii) are used to check the compatibility therein.

Example 7.3 (*Uniqueness*). Consider two conditional distribution matrices

$$A = \begin{pmatrix} 1/7 & 1/4 & 3/7 & 1/7 \\ 2/7 & 1/2 & 1/7 & 2/7 \\ 4/7 & 1/4 & 3/7 & 4/7 \end{pmatrix} \quad \text{and}$$

$$B = \begin{pmatrix} 1/6 & 1/6 & 1/2 & 1/6 \\ 2/7 & 2/7 & 1/7 & 2/7 \\ 1/3 & 1/12 & 1/4 & 1/3 \end{pmatrix},$$

where $\mathcal{X} = \mathcal{S}_X = \{x_1, x_2, x_3\}$ and $\mathcal{Y} = \mathcal{S}_Y = \{y_1, \ldots, y_4\}$. By using (7.6), the X-marginal is given by

X	x_1	x_2	x_3
$\xi_i = \Pr\{X = x_i\}$	0.24	0.28	0.48

Similarly, the Y-marginal is given by

Y	y_1	y_2	y_3	y_4
$\eta_j = \Pr\{Y = y_j\}$	0.28	0.16	0.28	0.28

It is easy to verify that the two conditions in Theorem 7.1 are satisfied. Therefore, A and B are compatible. Since all $a_{ij} > 0$ and $b_{ij} > 0$, the uniqueness of $f_X(x)$ is guaranteed by Theorem 7.3. The unique joint distribution of (X, Y) is given by

$$P = \begin{pmatrix} 0.04 & 0.04 & 0.12 & 0.04 \\ 0.08 & 0.08 & 0.04 & 0.08 \\ 0.16 & 0.04 & 0.12 & 0.16 \end{pmatrix}.$$

Alternatively, the system of linear equations (7.17) becomes

$$\begin{aligned} 1 &= \xi_1 + \xi_2 + \xi_3, \\ 0 &= \xi_i b_{ij} - a_{ij}(\xi_1 b_{1j} + \xi_2 b_{2j} + \xi_3 b_{3j}), \end{aligned}$$

where $i = 1, 2, 3$ and $j = 1, 2, 3, 4$. Using $\mathbf{1}_3/3$ as the initial value, from (7.19), we obtain

$$\hat{\xi} = (0.24, 0.28, 0.48)^\top,$$

and the ℓ_2-norm is 9.50928×10^{-34}. Using $(2/3, 0.5/3, 0.5/3)^\top$ as the initial value, we obtain the same $\hat{\xi}$ while the ℓ_2-norm is 2.63251×10^{-32}. Therefore, according to Theorem 7.5(i), A and B are compatible and the unique compatible X-marginal is specified by $\hat{\xi}$. ‖

Example 7.4 (*Uniqueness*). Consider two conditional distribution matrices

$$A = \begin{pmatrix} 1/6 & 0 & 3/14 \\ 0 & 1/4 & 4/14 \\ 5/6 & 3/4 & 7/14 \end{pmatrix} \quad \text{and} \quad B = \begin{pmatrix} 1/4 & 0 & 3/4 \\ 0 & 1/3 & 2/3 \\ 5/18 & 6/18 & 7/18 \end{pmatrix},$$

where $\mathcal{X} = \{x_1, x_2, x_3\}$ and $\mathcal{Y} = \{y_1, y_2, y_3\}$. By using (7.8) with $y_0 = y_3$, the X-marginal is given by

X	x_1	x_2	x_3
$\xi_i = \Pr\{X = x_i\}$	2/14	3/14	9/14

Similarly, letting $x_0 = x_3$ in (7.8) yields the following Y-marginal

Y	y_1	y_2	y_3
$\eta_j = \Pr\{Y = y_j\}$	3/14	4/14	7/14

The joint distribution of (X, Y) is given by

$$P = \begin{pmatrix} 1/28 & 0 & 3/28 \\ 0 & 2/28 & 4/28 \\ 5/28 & 6/28 & 7/28 \end{pmatrix}.$$

Since $\mathcal{S}_{(X|Y)} = \mathcal{S}_{(Y|X)} = \mathcal{S}_{(X,Y)} = \{(x_i, y_j)\colon i, j = 1, 2, 3, \ (i, j) \neq (1, 2), (2, 1)\}$, the first condition in Theorem 7.1 is satisfied. It is easy to verify that the second condition is satisfied as well. Therefore, A and B are compatible, and the uniqueness of $f_X(x)$ is ensured by Theorem 7.4.

Alternatively, using $\mathbf{1}_3/3$ as the initial value, from (7.19), we obtain

$$\hat{\xi} = (0.142857, 0.214286, 0.642857)^{\top} = (2/14, 3/14, 9/14)^{\top}$$

and the ℓ_2-norm is 7.65557×10^{-33}. Using $(2/3, 0.5/3, 0.5/3)^{\top}$ as the initial value, we obtain the same $\hat{\xi}$ while the ℓ_2-norm is 5.07964×10^{-32}. Therefore, according to Theorem 7.5(i), A and B are compatible and the unique compatible X-marginal is specified by $\hat{\xi}$. $\|$

Example 7.5 (*Incompatibility*). Consider two conditional distribution matrices

$$A = \begin{pmatrix} 1/6 & 0 & 3/14 \\ 0 & 1/4 & 4/14 \\ 5/6 & 3/4 & 7/14 \end{pmatrix} \quad \text{and} \quad B = \begin{pmatrix} 3/4 & 0 & 1/4 \\ 0 & 1/3 & 2/3 \\ 5/18 & 6/18 & 7/18 \end{pmatrix}.$$

For different τ, using (7.20) as initial values, we obtain the same $\hat{\xi} = (0.088927,\ 0.228110,\ 0.673934)^{\top}$ from (7.19) and the same ℓ_2-norm 0.00902916. Therefore, according to Theorem 7.5(ii), A and B are not compatible. $\|$

Example 7.6 (*Multiple solutions*). Consider two conditional distribution matrices

$$A = \begin{pmatrix} \frac{a}{a+b} & 1 & 0 & 0 \\ \frac{b}{a+b} & 0 & 0 & 0 \\ 0 & 0 & \frac{e}{e+f} & \frac{g}{g+h} \\ 0 & 0 & \frac{f}{e+f} & \frac{h}{g+h} \end{pmatrix} \quad \text{and}$$

$$B = \begin{pmatrix} \frac{a}{a+c} & \frac{c}{a+c} & 0 & 0 \\ 1 & 0 & 0 & 0 \\ 0 & 0 & \frac{e}{e+g} & \frac{g}{e+g} \\ 0 & 0 & \frac{f}{f+h} & \frac{h}{f+h} \end{pmatrix}. \tag{7.21}$$

Let $p > 0$ and $q > 0$ such that $p+q = 1$. If $a+b+c = e+f+g+h = 1$ with all numbers being positive, then there exist infinitely many joint distributions defined by

$$P = \begin{pmatrix} pa & pc & 0 & 0 \\ pb & 0 & 0 & 0 \\ 0 & 0 & qe & qg \\ 0 & 0 & qf & qh \end{pmatrix}$$

with A and B being its conditional matrices.

Let $a = 0.1$, $b = 0.6$, $c = 0.3$, $e = 0.2$, $f = 0.3$, $g = 0.4$ and $h = 0.1$. Using $\mathbf{1}_4/4$ as initial values, from (7.19), we obtain

$$\hat{\xi} = (0.134848, 0.202273, 0.397727, 0.265152)^\top.$$

The ℓ_2-norm is 7.82409×10^{-34} and the corresponding joint distribution is

$$P = \begin{pmatrix} 0.0337121 & 0.101136 & 0 & 0 \\ 0.2022727 & 0 & 0 & 0 \\ 0 & 0 & 0.132576 & 0.2651515 \\ 0 & 0 & 0.198864 & 0.0662879 \end{pmatrix}.$$

Using $(0.1, 0.2, 0.4, 0.3)^\top$ as the initial value, from (7.19), we obtain

$$\hat{\xi} = (0.0867424, 0.1301136, 0.4698864, 0.3132576)^\top,$$

the ℓ_2-norm is 3.18952×10^{-34}, and the corresponding joint distribution is

$$P = \begin{pmatrix} 0.0216856 & 0.0650568 & 0 & 0 \\ 0.1301136 & 0 & 0 & 0 \\ 0 & 0 & 0.156629 & 0.3132576 \\ 0 & 0 & 0.234943 & 0.0783144 \end{pmatrix}.$$

According to Theorem 7.5(iii), A and B are compatible with multiple solutions. ||

7.3.4 Extension to more than two dimensions

Theorem 7.5 can be readily extended to higher-dimensional settings. In this subsection, we will illustrate the corresponding results for the three-dimensional case. For $i = 1, \ldots, m$, $j = 1, \ldots, n$ and $k = 1, \ldots, l$, we let

$$p_{ijk} = \Pr\{X = x_i, Y = y_j, Z = z_k\},$$

$$\begin{aligned}
a_{ijk} &= \Pr\{X = x_i | Y = y_j, Z = z_k\}, \\
b_{ijk} &= \Pr\{Y = y_j | Z = z_k, X = x_i\}, \\
c_{ijk} &= \Pr\{Z = z_k | X = x_i, Y = y_j\}, \\
\xi &= (\xi_1, \ldots, \xi_m)^\top \in \mathbb{T}_m \quad \text{with} \quad \xi_i = \Pr\{X = x_i\}, \\
\Delta_{l \times m} &= (\delta_{ki}) = (\delta_1, \ldots, \delta_m) \quad \text{with} \quad \delta_{ki} = \Pr\{Z = z_k | X = x_i\},
\end{aligned}$$

where $\delta_i \in \mathbb{T}_l$ for $i = 1, \ldots, m$.

Definition 7.4 Three conditional distribution arrays (a_{ijk}), (b_{ijk}) and (c_{ijk}) are said to be **compatible** if there exists **at least** one joint distribution (p_{ijk}) such that

$$\begin{aligned}
p_{ijk} &= a_{ijk} \Pr\{Y = y_j, Z = z_k\} \\
&= b_{ijk} \Pr\{Z = z_k, X = x_i\} \\
&= c_{ijk} \Pr\{X = x_i, Y = y_j\}, \quad \forall\ i,\ j,\ k.
\end{aligned}$$

¶

Note that $p_{ijk} = b_{ijk} \times \delta_{ki} \times \xi_i$, we only need to find the X-marginal $\xi \in [0,1]^m$ and the conditional matrix $\Delta \in [0,1]^{lm}$ such that

$$\begin{aligned}
1 &= \mathbf{1}_m^\top \xi, \\
1 &= \mathbf{1}_l^\top \delta_i, \quad \forall i, \\
0 &= b_{ijk}\delta_{ki}\xi_i - a_{ijk} \textstyle\sum_{i'=1}^m b_{i'jk}\delta_{ki'}\xi_{i'}, \quad \forall\ i,\ j,\ k, \\
0 &= b_{ijk}\delta_{ki} - c_{ijk} \textstyle\sum_{k'=1}^l b_{ijk'}\delta_{k'i}, \quad \forall\ i,\ j,\ k.
\end{aligned}$$

This system of linear equations can be rewritten as

$$e = G\zeta, \qquad \xi \in [0,1]^m, \quad \Delta \in [0,1]^{lm}, \tag{7.22}$$

where $\zeta^\top = (\xi^\top, \delta_1^\top, \ldots, \delta_m^\top)$. Similar to (7.19) and Theorem 7.5, we consider the following quadratic optimization problem with unit cube constraints

$$(\hat{\xi}, \hat{\Delta}) = \arg \min_{\xi \in [0,1]^m,\ \Delta \in [0,1]^{lm}} ||e - G\zeta||^2. \tag{7.23}$$

Theorem 7.6 For the constrained optimization problem (7.23), we have the following results:

(i) If the solution $(\hat{\xi}, \hat{\Delta})$ calculated from (7.23) is unique and the resulting ℓ_2-norm $< 10^{-10}$, then (a_{ijk}), (b_{ijk}) and (c_{ijk}) are compatible, the unique X-marginal is specified by $\hat{\xi}$ and the unique $Z|X$-conditional is determined by $\hat{\Delta}$;

(ii) If $(\hat{\xi}, \hat{\Delta})$ is unique but the corresponding ℓ_2-norm $\geq 10^{-10}$, then (a_{ijk}), (b_{ijk}) and (c_{ijk}) are incompatible;

(iii) For different initial values, if (7.23) converges to different solutions:

$$\left\{(\hat{\xi}_\tau, \hat{\Delta}_\tau),\ \tau \in \mathbb{R}^{(1+l)m}\right\}$$

and all ℓ_2-norms $< 10^{-10}$, then (a_{ijk}), (b_{ijk}) and (c_{ijk}) are compatible, the multiple X-marginal are specified by

$$\left\{\hat{\xi}_\tau, \tau \in \mathbb{R}^{(1+l)m}\right\},$$

and the multiple $Z|X$-conditional are determined by

$$\left\{\hat{\Delta}_\tau, \tau \in \mathbb{R}^{(1+l)m}\right\}.$$

¶

7.3.5 The compatibility of regression function and conditional distribution

Let $\mathcal{X} = \{x_1, \ldots, x_m\}$ and $\mathcal{Y} = \{y_1, \ldots, y_n\}$ and P, B, ξ be defined in (7.13), (7.14) and (7.16), respectively. If the regression function is defined by

$$\phi = (\phi_1, \ldots, \phi_n)^\top = E(X|Y) \quad \text{with} \quad \phi_j = E(X|Y = y_j),$$

and the conditional distribution matrix B is said to be **compatible**, then there exists at least one X-marginal specified by $\xi \in \mathbb{T}_m$ such that

$$\begin{aligned}
\phi_j &= \sum_{i=1}^m x_i \Pr\{X = x_i | Y = y_j\} \\
&= \sum_{i=1}^m x_i b_{ij} \xi_i \Big/ \sum_{i=1}^m b_{ij} \xi_i, \quad j = 1, \ldots, n,
\end{aligned}$$

where $\min\{x_1, \ldots, x_m\} \leq \phi_j \leq \max\{x_1, \ldots, x_m\}$. Hence, we only need to find $\xi \in [0, 1]^m$ such that

$$\begin{aligned}
1 &= \xi_1 + \cdots + \xi_m, \text{ and} \\
0 &= \sum_{i=1}^m (\phi_j - x_i) b_{ij} \xi_i, \quad j = 1, \ldots, n. \qquad (7.24)
\end{aligned}$$

Note that system (7.24) can be expressed as the same matrix form as (7.18), where $e_1 \hat{=} (1, \mathbf{0}_n^\top)^\top$ and

$$D = \begin{pmatrix} 1 & 1 & \cdots & 1 \\ (\phi_1 - x_1)b_{11} & (\phi_1 - x_2)b_{21} & \cdots & (\phi_1 - x_m)b_{m1} \\ \vdots & \vdots & \ddots & \vdots \\ (\phi_n - x_1)b_{1n} & (\phi_n - x_2)b_{2n} & \cdots & (\phi_n - x_m)b_{mn} \end{pmatrix},$$

respectively. Similarly, we can show that system (7.24) is equivalent to the constrained quadratic optimization problem in (7.19).

Theorem 7.7 For the system (7.24), we have the following results:

(i) If the solution $\hat{\xi}$ calculated from (7.19) is unique and the resulting ℓ_2-norm $< 10^{-10}$, then ϕ and B are compatible and the unique X-marginal is specified by $\hat{\xi}$;

(ii) If $\hat{\xi}$ is unique but the corresponding ℓ_2-norm $\geq 10^{-10}$, then ϕ and B are incompatible;

(iii) If (7.19) has multiple solutions (denoted by $\{\hat{\xi}_\tau, \tau \in \mathbb{R}^m\}$) and all ℓ_2-norms $< 10^{-10}$, then ϕ and B are compatible and the multiple X-marginals are specified by $\{\hat{\xi}_\tau, \tau \in \mathbb{R}^m\}$. ¶

Example 7.7 (*Uniqueness and incompatibility*). Let $\mathcal{X} = \{x_1, x_2, x_3\} = \{1, 2, 3\}$. Consider the regression function values:

$$\phi = E(X|Y) = (\phi_1, \phi_2, \phi_3)^\top = (5/3, 2, 2)^\top$$

and the following conditional distribution matrix

$$B = \begin{pmatrix} 20/47 & 15/47 & 12/47 \\ 20/53 & 15/53 & 18/53 \\ 0 & 15/27 & 12/27 \end{pmatrix}.$$

From (7.19), using $\mathbf{1}_3/3$ as the initial value yields

$$\hat{\xi} = (0.2611, 0.5889, 0.1500)^\top = (47/180, 106/180, 27/180)^\top$$

and the ℓ_2-norm is 3.29334×10^{-32}. Using $(2/12, 4/12, 6/12)^\top$ as the initial value produces the same $\hat{\xi}$ while the ℓ_2-norm is 4.06163×10^{-32}. According to Theorem 7.7(i), ϕ and B are compatible and the unique compatible X-marginal is specified by $\hat{\xi}$. The unique joint probability matrix is given by

$$P = \begin{pmatrix} 0.1111 & 0.08333 & 0.06667 \\ 0.2222 & 0.16667 & 0.20000 \\ 0.0000 & 0.08333 & 0.06667 \end{pmatrix} = \begin{pmatrix} 1/9 & 1/12 & 1/15 \\ 2/9 & 2/12 & 3/15 \\ 0 & 1/12 & 1/15 \end{pmatrix}.$$

If we replace ϕ by $(5.5/3, 2.2, 2.5)^\top$ with other settings remaining the same, it can be shown that $\phi = (5.5/3, 2.2, 2.5)^\top$ and B are incompatible by Theorem 7.7(ii). From (7.19), using $\mathbf{1}_3/3$ as the initial value yields

$$\hat{\xi} = (0.119825, 0.569671, 0.309541)^\top$$

and the ℓ_2-norm is 0.00896194. If we use different initial values, the same $\hat{\xi}$ and ℓ_2-norm are obtained. In addition, the sum of components of $\hat{\xi}$ is $0.991037 < 1$. ||

Example 7.8 (*Multiple solutions*). Let $\mathcal{X} = \{x_1, x_2, x_3, x_4\} = \{1, 2, 3, 4\}$. Consider the following regression function values

$$\begin{aligned} \phi &= E(X|Y) = (\phi_1, \phi_2, \phi_3, \phi_4)^\top \\ &= \left(\frac{a+2b}{a+b}, 1, \frac{3e+4f}{e+f}, \frac{3g+4h}{g+h}\right)^\top. \end{aligned}$$

Let the conditional distribution matrix B be given in (7.21) with $a = 0.2$, $b = 0.3$, $c = 0.5$, $e = 0.1$, $f = 0.4$, $g = 0.3$ and $h = 0.2$. From (7.19) and using $0.25\mathbf{1}_4$ as the initial value, we obtain

$$\hat{\xi} = (0.6708,\ 0.2875,\ 0.0167,\ 0.025)^\top,$$

the ℓ_2-norm is 4.96896×10^{-32}, and the corresponding joint distribution is

$$P = \begin{pmatrix} 0.191667 & 0.479167 & 0 & 0 \\ 0.287500 & 0 & 0 & 0 \\ 0 & 0 & 0.00416667 & 0.01250000 \\ 0 & 0 & 0.01666667 & 0.00833333 \end{pmatrix}.$$

Using $(0.1, 0.2, 0.4, 0.3)^\top$ as the initial value, we get

$$\hat{\xi} = (0.6611,\ 0.2833,\ 0.0222,\ 0.0334)^\top,$$

the ℓ_2-norm is 3.4249×10^{-34}, and the corresponding joint distribution is

$$P = \begin{pmatrix} 0.188889 & 0.472222 & 0 & 0 \\ 0.283333 & 0 & 0 & 0 \\ 0 & 0 & 0.00555556 & 0.0166667 \\ 0 & 0 & 0.02222222 & 0.0111111 \end{pmatrix}.$$

According to Theorem 7.7(iii), ϕ and B are compatible with multiple solutions. ||

7.3.6 Appendix: S-plus function (lseb)

To find the least squares estimate with box constraints, we provide the following S-plus code (lseb).

```
function(y, X, a, b, th0) {
   # Function name: lseb(y, X, a, b, th0)
   # Aim:     To find \thLSE = arg min ||y - X \th ||^2
   #          subject to a <= \th <= b
   # Input:  y: m x 1;  X: m x q; a, b, th0: q x 1
   # Output: \thLSE and ||y - X \thLSE ||^2
   # ------------------------------------------------------
   # NLS<- nlregb(nres = m, start = th_0, residuals =
   #    fun.r, jacobian = fun.j, lower = 0, upper = Inf)
   #    is the S-plus function of nonlinear least
   #    squares subject to box constraints, where
   #    NLS[[1]] = \thLSE: minimizing ||y - X \th||^2
   #    NLS[[2]] = funmin = ||y - X \thLSE ||^2
   # ------------------------------------------------------
   fun.r <- function(th, y, X) { c(X %*% th - y) }
   fun.j <- function(th, y, X) { X }
   m <- length(y)
   NLS <- nlregb(nres = m, start = th0, res = fun.r,
       jac = fun.j, lower = a, upper = b, y = y, X = X)
   thLSE <- NLS[[1]]
   precise <- NLS[[2]]
   options(digits = 6)
   return(thLSE, precise)
}
```

7.3.7 Discussion

In this section, based on ℓ_2-norm criterion, we presented a unified method to check the compatibility and uniqueness for two finite discrete conditional distributions. Extension to three-dimensional cases is also introduced. Furthermore, the method can be applied to checking the compatibility and uniqueness of one finite discrete regression function and one finite discrete conditional distribution. One advantage of using the ℓ_2-norm criterion is that the built-in S-plus function can be utilized to solve the quadratic optimization problem with box constraints.

Although other criteria (e.g., ℓ_1-norm or KL divergence) are useful alternatives to the ℓ_2-norm, the corresponding optimization algorithms may be more complex. Moreover, if X and/or Y are infinite discrete random variables (e.g., Poisson, geometric variates), the proposed iterative algorithm would be more difficult to implement.

7.4 Two Conditional Distributions: NPMS

Denoted the conditional supports of $X|(Y = y)$ and $Y|(X = x)$ by

$$\mathcal{S}_{(X|Y)}(y) = \{x\colon f_{(X|Y)}(x|y) > 0,\, x \in \mathcal{S}_X\},\ \forall\, y \in \mathcal{S}_Y, \quad (7.25)$$
$$\mathcal{S}_{(Y|X)}(x) = \{y\colon f_{(Y|X)}(y|x) > 0,\, y \in \mathcal{S}_Y\},\ \forall\, x \in \mathcal{S}_X, \quad (7.26)$$

respectively. For the NPMS case, i.e., $\mathcal{S}_{(Y|X)}(x) \neq \mathcal{S}_Y$, in §3.9, we introduce a so-called **transition** method to derive the marginal density of X based on two known conditional densities. The key to the transition method is its ability to find a point y^* (y^* may not belong to $\mathcal{S}_Y$) satisfying (3.22).

However, when such a point y^* is not available, Song *et al.* (2006) extended Theorem 7.1 to the following necessary and sufficient conditions for the compatibility of two conditional distributions in the NPMS $\mathcal{S}_{(X,Y)} \subseteq \mathcal{S}_X \times \mathcal{S}_Y$.

Theorem 7.8 (Song *et al.*, 2006). The given conditionals $f_{(X|Y)}$ and $f_{(Y|X)}$ are compatible iff

(i) $\mathcal{S}_{(X|Y)} = \mathcal{S}_{(Y|X)} = \mathcal{S}_{(X,Y)}$; and

(ii) There exist functions $u(x)$ and $v(y)$ such that

$$\frac{f_{(X|Y)}(x|y)}{f_{(Y|X)}(y|x)} = \frac{u(x)}{v(y)}, \quad \forall\, (x, y) \in \mathcal{S}_{(X,Y)}, \quad (7.27)$$

where $u(x)$ and $v(y)$ are positive and integrable in $\mathcal{S}_X$ and $\mathcal{S}_Y$, respectively, and $\int_{\mathcal{S}_X} u(x)dx < \infty$. ¶

They further proved that if (7.27) holds, then $u(x)/\int_{\mathcal{S}_X} u(t)dt$ is one marginal density of X. Ex.7.9 and Ex.7.10 show how to check the compatibility of the given conditionals.

Example 7.9 (*Uniform distribution on an arc-shaped domain*). We consider the following two conditional densities:

$$f_{(X|Y)}(x|y) = \frac{I_{(1-[1-y^2]^{1/2}<x<y)}}{y - 1 + \sqrt{1-y^2}}, \quad 0 < y < 1, \quad \text{and}$$
$$f_{(Y|X)}(y|x) = \frac{I_{(x<y<[1-(x-1)^2]^{1/2})}}{\sqrt{1-(x-1)^2} - x}, \quad 0 < x < 1.$$

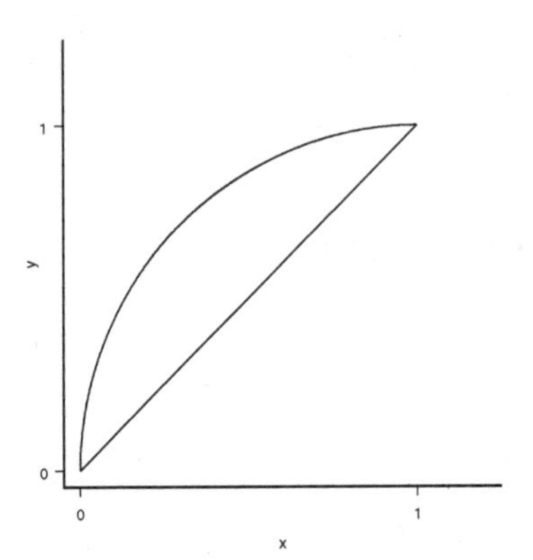

Figure 7.1 The joint support $\mathcal{S}_{(X,Y)} = \{(x,y)\colon (x-1)^2+y^2 < 1,\ y > x\}$.

From Figure 7.1, it is clear that

$$\begin{aligned}
\mathcal{S}_{(X|Y)} &= \mathcal{S}_{(Y|X)} = \mathcal{S}_{(X,Y)} \\
&= \Big\{(x,y)\colon (x-1)^2 + y^2 < 1,\ y > x\Big\}, \\
\mathcal{S}_X &= \mathcal{S}_Y = (0,1), \\
\mathcal{S}_{(X|Y)}(y) &= \Big\{x\colon 1 - \sqrt{1-y^2} < x < y\Big\}, \quad \text{and} \\
\mathcal{S}_{(Y|X)}(x) &= \Big\{y\colon x < y < \sqrt{1-(x-1)^2}\Big\}.
\end{aligned}$$

Since there is no transition point y^* satisfying (3.22), the transition method of Tian & Tan (2003) does not apply. Now, by using (7.27), we have

$$\frac{f_{(X|Y)}(x|y)}{f_{(Y|X)}(y|x)} = \frac{\sqrt{1-(x-1)^2} - x}{y - 1 + \sqrt{1-y^2}} = \frac{u(x)}{v(y)}.$$

Therefore,

$$f_X(x) = (\pi/4 - 1/2)^{-1}(\sqrt{1-(x-1)^2} - x), \quad 0 < x < 1,$$

and $f_{(X,Y)}(x,y) = (\pi/4 - 1/2)^{-1}$. ‖

Example 7.10 (*Improper models*). Let the putative conditional densities be given by

$$\begin{aligned}
f_{(X|Y)}(x|y) &= y \cdot I_{(0<x<y^{-1})}, \quad y > 0, \quad \text{and} \\
f_{(Y|X)}(y|x) &= x \cdot I_{(0<y<x^{-1})}, \quad x > 0.
\end{aligned}$$

Note that

$$\mathcal{S}_{(X|Y)} = \mathcal{S}_{(Y|X)} = \mathcal{S}_{(X,Y)} = \{(x,y)\colon x > 0,\ y > 0,\ xy < 1\}$$

and $\mathcal{S}_X = \mathcal{S}_Y = (0, \infty)$. From (7.27), we have

$$\frac{y}{x} = \frac{u(x)}{v(y)}.$$

As the function $u(x) = x^{-1}$ is not integrable, the two conditionals are not compatible. ||

The following example shows that two compatible conditionals are not able to uniquely determine the joint distribution.

Example 7.11 (*Mixture uniform distributions*). Consider two conditional densities:

$$\begin{aligned} f_{(X|Y)}(x|y) &= 0.5 \cdot I_{[0,2]|[0,1]}(x|y) + I_{(2,3]|(1,3]}(x|y) \quad \text{and} \\ f_{(Y|X)}(y|x) &= I_{[0,1]|[0,2]}(y|x) + 0.5 \cdot I_{(1,3]|(2,3]}(y|x), \end{aligned}$$

where

$$I_{\mathbb{X}|\mathbb{Y}}(x|y) = \begin{cases} 1, & \text{if } x \in \mathbb{X} \text{ given } y \in \mathbb{Y}, \\ 0, & \text{otherwise.} \end{cases}$$

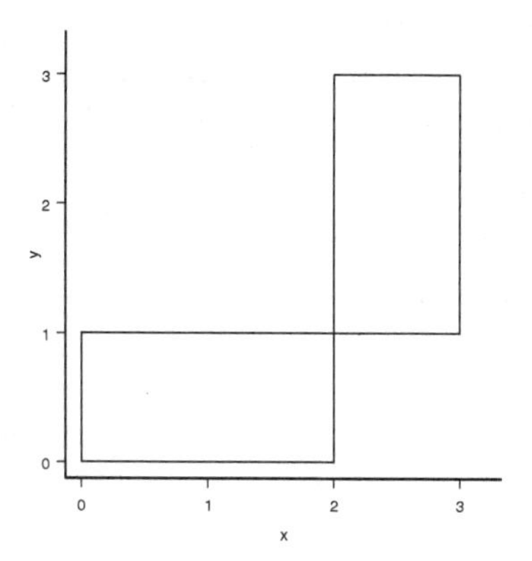

Figure 7.2 The joint support $\mathcal{S}_{(X,Y)} = \{[0,2] \times [0,1]\} \cup \{(2,3] \times (1,3]\}$.

From Figure 7.2, it is easy to see that

$$\mathcal{S}_{(X|Y)} = \mathcal{S}_{(Y|X)} = \mathcal{S}_{(X,Y)} = \{[0,2] \times [0,1]\} \cup \{(2,3] \times (1,3]\}$$

and $\mathcal{S}_X = \mathcal{S}_Y = [0,3]$. By using (7.27), we have

$$\frac{f_{(X|Y)}(x|y)}{f_{(Y|X)}(y|x)} = 0.5 \cdot I_{[0,2]\times[0,1]}(x,y) + I_{(2,3]\times(1,3]}(x,y),$$

where

$$I_{\mathbb{X}\times\mathbb{Y}}(x,y) = \begin{cases} 1, & \text{if } x \in \mathbb{X} \text{ and } y \in \mathbb{Y}, \\ 0, & \text{otherwise.} \end{cases}$$

We choose

$$\begin{aligned} u(x) &= c \cdot I_{(0\le x\le 2)} + d \cdot I_{(2<x\le 3)}, \quad \text{and} \\ v(y) &= 2c \cdot I_{(0\le y\le 1)} + 0.5d \cdot I_{(1<y\le 3)}, \end{aligned}$$

where $c > 0$ and $d > 0$. The compatibility of the two conditionals is guaranteed as $\int_{\mathcal{S}_X} u(x)dx < \infty$. The joint pdf can be shown to be

$$f_{(X,Y)}(x,y) = c \cdot I_{[0,2]\times[0,1]}(x,y) + 0.5d \cdot I_{(2,3]\times(1,3]}(x,y),$$

which is a mixture uniform distribution for any given c and d satisfying $2c + d = 1$. ||

7.5 One Marginal and Another Conditional

Suppose that we are given one marginal density f_Y and another conditional density $f_{(Y|X)}$, we ask whether there exists one or more joint pdfs, how to identify them, and under what conditions they are unique. It is obvious that the joint pdf $f_{(X,Y)}$ is unique if f_X is unique. This section will answer this question partially. We only consider the PMS case, i.e., $\mathcal{S}_{(X,Y)} = \mathcal{S}_X \times \mathcal{S}_Y$.

7.5.1 A sufficient condition for uniqueness

Let X and Y be two r.v.'s which may be continuous, discrete or mixed.

Definition 7.5 The marginal density f_Y and the conditional density $f_{(Y|X)}$ are said to be **compatible** if there exists **at least** one marginal density f_X such that

$$f_Y(y) = \int_{\mathcal{S}_X} f_{(Y|X)}(y|x) f_X(x)\, dx, \quad \forall\, y \in \mathcal{S}_Y. \qquad \P \ (7.28)$$

We summarize the implications of (7.28) as follows:

- In signal analysis, Eq.(7.28) is a general mathematical model for describing the distortion of an input signal f_X through an input–output system with linear distortion characterized by an impulse response function $f_{(Y|X)}$, resulting in a distorted signal f_Y;

- In image analysis, f_X represents the true undistorted image and f_Y represents the recorded blurred image with the blurring mechanism characterized by $f_{(Y|X)}$;
- Mathematicians know Eq.(7.28) as Fredholm's integral equation of the first kind (Vardi & Lee, 1993), if f_Y is a nonnegative real-valued function and $f_{(Y|X)}$ is a nonnegative bounded real-valued function. For example,

$$f_X(x) = e^{-x} \cdot I_{(x>0)} \tag{7.29}$$

  is a solution to the integral equation

$$\frac{\Phi(y-1)}{\phi(y-1)} = \int_0^\infty \exp[x(y-0.5x)]\, f_X(x)\, dx, \quad y \in \mathbb{R},$$

  where Φ and ϕ denote the cdf and the pdf of $N(0,1)$;
- Statisticians recognize Eq.(7.28) as the formula for a mixture of densities. Thus f_Y and $f_{(Y|X)}$ are compatible iff f_Y can be expressed as a mixture of the given conditional densities $\{f_{(Y|X)}(y|x)\colon x \in \mathcal{S}_X\}$.

Seshadri & Patil (1964) obtained the following sufficient condition for $f_X(x)$ to be unique.

Theorem 7.9 (Seshadri & Patil, 1964). Let f_Y and $f_{(Y|X)}$ be compatible, a sufficient condition for f_X (and hence for $f_{(X,Y)}$) to be unique is that the conditional density $f_{(Y|X)}$ is of the following exponential form:

$$f_{(Y|X)}(y|x) = \exp[xa(y) + b(y) + c(x)], \tag{7.30}$$

where $a(\cdot)$, $b(\cdot)$ and $c(\cdot)$ are three real-valued functions. ¶

Example 7.12 (*Uniqueness*). Let

$$\begin{aligned} f_Y(y) &= (1+y)^{-2} \cdot I_{(y>0)} \quad \text{and} \\ f_{(Y|X)}(y|x) &= xe^{-xy} \cdot I_{(y>0)}. \end{aligned}$$

It can be shown that (7.29) is a solution to (7.28) so that f_Y and $f_{(Y|X)}$ are compatible. Since

$$f_{(Y|X)}(y|x) = \exp[x(-y) + 0 + \log(x)] \cdot I_{(y>0)}$$

has the form of (7.30), the uniqueness of f_X is ensured by Theorem 7.9. Hence, the unique joint density is

$$f_{(X,Y)}(x,y) = xe^{-x(y+1)} \cdot I_{(x>0,\ y>0)}. \qquad \|$$

Example 7.13 (*Multiple solutions*). Let

$$\begin{aligned} f_Y(y) &= e^{-y} \cdot I_{(y \geq 0)} \quad \text{and} \\ f_{(Y|X)}(y|x) &= \Big\{ e^{-y}(1+\alpha-2\alpha e^{-x}) \\ &\quad -2\alpha e^{-2y}(1-2e^{-x}) \Big\} \cdot I_{(x\geq 0,\ y \geq 0)}, \end{aligned}$$

where $-1 \leq \alpha \leq 1$. When $\alpha = 0$, we have $f_{(Y|X)}(y|x) = e^{-y}$, which implies that Y and X are independent. When $-1 \leq \alpha < 0$ or $0 < \alpha \leq 1$, $f_{(Y|X)}$ does not take the form of (7.30). From (7.28), we obtain

$$\int_0^\infty [e^{-y}(1+\alpha-2\alpha e^{-x}) - 2\alpha e^{-2y}(1-2e^{-x})] f_X(x)\, dx = e^{-y}.$$

Upon simplification, we have $\int_0^\infty e^{-y} f_X(x)\, dx = 0.5$. Hence, for any given $\lambda \in (1, \infty)$,

$$f_X^\lambda(x) = \frac{(\lambda-1)^n}{\Gamma(n)} y^{n-1} e^{-(\lambda-1)y}, \quad y \geq 0,$$

is a desired solution, where $n = \log(0.5)/\log([\lambda-1]/\lambda)$. Therefore, f_Y and $f_{(Y|X)}$ are compatible. ||

Example 7.14 (*Incompatibility*). Let

$$\begin{aligned} f_Y(y) &= \text{Poisson}(y|\mu) \qquad \text{and} \\ f_{(Y|X)}(y|x) &= \text{Poisson}(y|\lambda(x)). \end{aligned}$$

Note that

$$f_{(Y|X)}(y|x) = \exp\Big\{ y \log \lambda(x) - \log y! - \lambda(x) \Big\},$$

therefore $f_{(Y|X)}$ does not have the form of (7.30) unless $\lambda(x) = e^x$. However, f_Y and $f_{(Y|X)}$ are incompatible. In fact, the moment generating functions of Y and $Y|X$ are given by

$$M_Y(t) = e^{s\mu} \quad \text{and} \quad M_{Y|X}(t) = e^{s\lambda(x)},$$

where $s \hat{=} e^t - 1 > -1$. From (7.28), it is easy to obtain $M_Y(t) = \sum_{x=0}^\infty M_{Y|X}(t) f_X(x)$. That is,

$$e^{s\mu} = \sum_{x=0}^\infty e^{s\lambda(x)} f_X(x),$$

implying that if Y and X are not independent (in which case $\lambda(x)$ depends on x), no solution exists for f_X. ||

Especially if $f_{(Y|X)}(y|x)$ is a function of $y - x$ alone ($f_{(Y|X)}$ is then said to be space invariant or position invariant), Eq.(7.28) is a convolution formula. To demonstrate this point, we consider the following example.

Example 7.15 (*Convolution*). Let $Y \sim N(0, 2)$ and $Y|(X = x) \sim N(x, 1)$. We can verify that

$$f_Y(y) = \frac{1}{2\sqrt{\pi}} e^{-y^2/4} \quad \text{and} \quad f_{(Y|X)}(y|x) = \frac{1}{\sqrt{2\pi}} e^{-(y-x)^2/2}$$

are compatible. The corresponding marginal distribution of X is $N(0, 1)$ and its uniqueness is ensured by Theorem 7.9. Hence

$$f_{(X,Y)}(x, y) = \frac{1}{2\pi} e^{-(2x^2-2xy+y^2)/2},$$

namely, (X, Y) follows a bivariate normal distribution with means 0 and 0, variances 1 and 2 and correlation coefficient $\rho = 1/\sqrt{2}$. ‖

7.5.2 The continuous case

Suppose that we are given f_Y and $f_{(Y|X)}$, how can we identify the corresponding marginal density f_X? In fact, (7.28) is exactly a mathematical inversion of a linear system with positive parameters, subject to positivity constraints on the solution.

Vardi & Lee (1993) make the connection of such linear inverse problem with positivity restrictions with statistical estimation problems from incomplete data via the famous KL divergence (cf. §1.6.2). Let $g(y)$ and $h(y)$ be two densities with the same support $\mathcal{S}_Y$, the KL divergence, $\text{KL}\{g(y), h(y)\}$, between $g(y)$ and $h(y)$ is defined in (1.42). From (1.43), we obtain

$$\text{KL}\{g(y), h(y)\} \geq 0 \quad \text{and} \quad \text{KL}\{g(y), h(y)\} = 0 \ \text{ iff } \ g(y) = h(y).$$

Instead of directly finding f_X satisfying the integral Eq.(7.28), one can find

$$\hat{f}_X(x) = \arg \min_{f_X(x) \geq 0} \text{KL}\left\{ f_Y(y), \int_{\mathcal{S}_X} f_{(Y|X)}(y|x) f_X(x)\, dx \right\}.$$

To compute $\hat{f}_X(x)$, Vardi & Lee (1993) used the EM algorithm to derive the following iterative scheme: $\forall\, x \in \mathcal{S}_X$,

$$f_X^{(t)}(x) = f_X^{(t-1)}(x) \int_{\mathcal{S}_Y} \frac{f_{(Y|X)}(y|x) \cdot f_Y(y)}{\int_{\mathcal{S}_X} f_{(Y|X)}(y|x') f_X^{(t-1)}(x')\, dx'}\, dy, \qquad (7.31)$$

where $f_X^{(0)}(x)$ is an arbitrary strictly positive density of X, and $t = 1, 2, \ldots$. If Eq.(7.28) has a nonnegative solution, then the algorithm (7.31) converges to it. Moreover, even when Eq.(7.28) does not have a nonnegative solution (i.e., f_Y and $f_{(Y|X)}$ are incompatible), the algorithm (7.31) still converges to $\hat{f}_X(x)$, which minimizes the KL divergence between f_Y and $\int_{\mathcal{S}_X} f_{(Y|X)}(y|x) f_X(x)\,dx$ over all nonnegative f_X.

Vardi & Lee (1993) presented two complicated methods to derive Eq.(7.31). We show in fact an alternative and rather straightforward derivation exists. For all $x \in \mathcal{S}_X$ and $y \in \mathcal{S}_Y$, from (7.7) and (7.28), we have

$$\begin{aligned} f_{(X|Y)}(x|y) &= \frac{f_{(Y|X)}(y|x) f_X(x)}{f_Y(y)} \\ &= \frac{f_{(Y|X)}(y|x) f_X(x)}{\int_{\mathcal{S}_X} f_{(Y|X)}(y|x') f_X(x')\,dx'} \quad \text{and} \qquad (7.32) \\ f_X(x) &= \int_{\mathcal{S}_Y} f_{(X|Y)}(x|y) f_Y(y)\,dy. \qquad (7.33) \end{aligned}$$

Given the $(t-1)$-th iteration, $f_X^{(t-1)}(x)$, of $f_X(x)$, from (7.32) and (7.33), we obtain

$$f_{(X|Y)}^{(t-1)}(x|y) = \frac{f_{(Y|X)}(y|x) f_X^{(t-1)}(x)}{\int_{\mathcal{S}_X} f_{(Y|X)}(y|x') f_X^{(t-1)}(x')\,dx'}$$

and

$$f_X^{(t)}(x) = \int_{\mathcal{S}_Y} f_{(X|Y)}^{(t-1)}(x|y) f_Y(y)\,dy,$$

which implies (7.31).

7.5.3 The finite discrete case

We assume that X and Y are discrete random variables taking values on $\mathcal{X} = \{x_1, \ldots, x_m\}$ and on $\mathcal{Y} = \{y_1, \ldots, y_n\}$, respectively and define $\xi_i = \Pr\{X = x_i\}$, $\eta_j = \Pr\{Y = y_j\}$ and

$$b_{ij} = \Pr\{Y = y_j | X = x_i\}$$

for $i = 1, \ldots, m$ and $j = 1, \ldots, n$.

Definition 7.6 The marginal probability vector $\eta = (\eta_1, \ldots, \eta_n)^\top$ and the conditional probability matrix $B_{m \times n} = (b_{ij})$ are said to be

compatible if there exists **at least** one marginal probability vector $\xi = (\xi_1, \ldots, \xi_m)^{\top}$ such that

$$\eta_j = \sum_{i=1}^{m} b_{ij}\xi_i, \quad j = 1, \ldots, n. \qquad \P \quad (7.34)$$

Therefore, the discrete version of (7.31) can be used to iteratively solve the marginal probability vector, $\xi^{(\infty)}$, of X:

$$\xi_i^{(t)} = \xi_i^{(t-1)} \sum_{j=1}^{n} \left(\frac{b_{ij}}{\sum_{i'=1}^{m} b_{i'j}\, \xi_{i'}^{(t-1)}} \right) \eta_j, \tag{7.35}$$

where $i = 1, \ldots, m$, $t \geq 1$, $\xi^{(0)} = (\xi_1^{(0)}, \ldots, \xi_m^{(0)})^{\top} \in \mathbb{T}_m$ is an initial vector. In matrix notations, Eq.(7.35) becomes

$$\xi^{(t)} = \xi^{(t-1)} \star (B\mathbf{a}), \quad \mathbf{a}_{n\times 1} \hat{=} \eta/(B^{\top}\xi^{(t-1)}), \quad t \geq 1, \tag{7.36}$$

where $\star$ and $/$ denote component-wise vector operator of multiplication and division, respectively. The corresponding joint probability distribution is given by

$$P = (p_{ij}) = (\Pr\{X = x_i, Y = y_j\}) = \text{diag}(\xi^{(\infty)})B.$$

Example 7.16 (*Incompatibility*). Let $\eta = (0.65, 0.35)^{\top}$ and

$$B = \begin{pmatrix} 1/6 & 5/6 \\ 3/8 & 5/8 \end{pmatrix}. \tag{7.37}$$

Applying the algorithm (7.36) with $\xi^{(0)} = (0.5, 0.5)^{\top}$ as the starting value, we obtain the X-marginal $\xi^{(\infty)} = \xi^{(36)} = (0, 1)^{\top}$ at the 36-th iteration and the corresponding joint probability distribution is

$$P = \begin{pmatrix} 0 & 0 \\ 0.375 & 0.625 \end{pmatrix}.$$

Since the resulting Y-marginal $\eta^* = (0.375, 0.625)^{\top}$ does not coincide with η, then the given η and B are incompatible. ‖

Example 7.17 (*Uniqueness*). Consider $\eta = (31/96, 65/96)^{\top}$ and B is still given by (7.37). Applying the algorithm (7.36) with $\xi^{(0)} = (0.5, 0.5)^{\top}$ as the starting value, we obtain the X-marginal $\xi^{(\infty)} =$

$\xi^{(272)} = (0.25, 0.75)^{\top}$ at the 272-nd iteration and the corresponding joint probability distribution is

$$P = \begin{pmatrix} 1/24 & 5/24 \\ 9/32 & 15/32 \end{pmatrix} = \begin{pmatrix} 0.041667 & 0.20833 \\ 0.281250 & 0.46875 \end{pmatrix}.$$

Since its Y-marginal $\eta^* = (0.32292, 0.67708)^{\top}$ coincides with η, it follows that η and B are compatible. In addition, different initial values yield the same final results but with varying numbers of iterations. For example, when $\xi^{(0)} = (0.1, 0.9)^{\top}$, $(0.2, 0.8)^{\top}$ and $(0.3, 0.7)^{\top}$, the numbers of iterations required for reaching convergence are 292, 248 and 251, respectively. ||

Example 7.18 (*Multiple solutions*). Let $\eta = (1/3, 2/3)^{\top}$ and

$$B = \begin{pmatrix} 1/4 & 3/4 \\ 3/5 & 2/5 \\ 1/8 & 7/8 \end{pmatrix}.$$

Applying the algorithm (7.36) with $\xi^{(0)} = \mathbf{1}_3/3$ as the starting value, we obtain the X-marginal

$$\xi^{(\infty)} = \xi^{(43)} = (0.32801, 0.35228, 0.31971)^{\top}$$

at the 43-rd iteration and the corresponding joint probability distribution is

$$P = \begin{pmatrix} 0.082002 & 0.24601 \\ 0.211367 & 0.14091 \\ 0.039964 & 0.27975 \end{pmatrix}.$$

Table 7.1 *The X-marginal $\xi^{(\infty)}$, the joint probability distribution matrix P and the resulting Y-marginal η^* using different starting values $\xi^{(0)}$*

$\xi^{(0)}$	$(0.1, 0.2, 0.7)^{\top}$	$(0.2, 0.3, 0.5)^{\top}$	$(0.4, 0.4, 0.2)^{\top}$
T	49	41	54
$\xi^{(\infty)}$	$(0.095, 0.414, 0.491)^{\top}$	$(0.189, 0.389, 0.422)^{\top}$	$(0.435, 0.324, 0.241)^{\top}$
P	$\begin{pmatrix} 0.0237 & 0.0711 \\ 0.2482 & 0.1655 \\ 0.0614 & 0.4301 \end{pmatrix}$	$\begin{pmatrix} 0.0473 & 0.1420 \\ 0.2333 & 0.1555 \\ 0.0527 & 0.3691 \end{pmatrix}$	$\begin{pmatrix} 0.1087 & 0.3261 \\ 0.1945 & 0.1297 \\ 0.0301 & 0.2109 \end{pmatrix}$
η^*	$(0.33333, 0.66667)^{\top}$	$(0.33333, 0.66667)^{\top}$	$(0.33333, 0.66667)^{\top}$

Note: T denotes the number of iterations for reaching convergence.

Since the resulting Y-marginal $\eta^* = (0.33333, 0.66667)^\top$ coincides with η, then the given η and B are compatible. However, in this example, different initial values will yield different X-marginal $\xi^{(\infty)}$ and different joint probability distribution P (see Table 7.1). Therefore, the compatibility may not be unique. ||

7.5.4 The connection with quadratic optimization under box constraints

Ex.7.18 showed that there may exist infinitely many joint distributions (or there may exist infinitely many X-marginal distributions) with the given η and B as its Y-marginal and $Y|X$-conditional distributions. Let $\{\xi^k\colon k \in \mathbb{K}\}$ denote the family of marginal distributions of X. It is then reasonable to ask whether the shortest X-marginal under ℓ_2-norm exists, i.e., if there is some $k_0 \in \mathbb{K}$ such that

$$||\xi^{k_0}|| = \min_{k \in \mathbb{K}} ||\xi^k||,$$

and if there is, how to identify it. The answer may become clear if we replace the KL entropy criterion by the standard Euclidean distance. In this section, we only consider the finite discrete case.

The system of linear equations in (7.34) can be rewritten as

$$\eta = B^\top \xi, \qquad \xi \in \mathbb{T}_m. \tag{7.38}$$

It is easy to see that if solution to Eq.(7.38) exists (i.e., the given η and B are compatible), then the solution is given by

$$\hat{\xi} = \arg \min_{\xi \in \mathbb{T}_m} ||\eta - B^\top \xi||^2. \tag{7.39}$$

Note that $\mathbb{T}_m$ is a subset of the unit cube $[0,1]^m$, if we can identify

$$\tilde{\xi} = \arg \min_{\xi \in [0,1]^m} ||\eta - B^\top \xi||^2, \tag{7.40}$$

and $\tilde{\xi} \in \mathbb{T}_m$, then $\tilde{\xi} = \hat{\xi}$. The S-plus function `lseb` in §7.3.6 can be used to calculate $\tilde{\xi}$.

Similar to the discussions in §7.3.2, when $\text{rank}\,(B^\top) = n \le m$ and there are no constraints, then the solution (7.40) is not unique and all solutions have the form

$$\tilde{\xi}_\tau^{\text{LSE}} = (B^\top)^+ \eta + [\mathbf{I}_m - (B^\top)^+ B^\top]\tau,$$

where $\tau \in \mathbb{R}^q$ is an arbitrary vector and $C^+ = C^\top(CC^\top)^{-1}$. Clearly,

$$\tilde{\xi}^{\text{LSE}} = (B^\top)^+\eta$$

is the unique solution with the shortest ℓ_2-norm among all $\tilde{\xi}_\tau^{\text{LSE}}$.

When $\text{rank}\,(B^\top) = n \le m$ but there exist constraints, then the solution (7.40) is also not unique. In general, different initial values will result in different solutions. We suggest taking

$$\xi_\tau^{(0)} = \min\{\max\{\mathbf{0},\ \tilde{\xi}_\tau^{\text{LSE}}\},\ \mathbf{1}\} \tag{7.41}$$

to run the `lseb` p times (say, $p = 100$ or 500 times) and then choose the solution with the shortest ℓ_2-norm. The following example demonstrates the idea.

Example 7.18 (*Continuation*). Note that $\text{rank}\,(B^\top) = 2$, then ξ is not unique. We apply the `lseb` to find ξ, which minimizes $||\eta - B^\top\xi||^2$ subject to $\xi \in [0,1]^3$. We used 100 different initial values (indexed by $1, 2, \ldots, 100$) of the same form as (7.41), where the first $\tau = \mathbf{0}_3$ and the other 99 τ's are i.i.d. random numbers from $[0,1]^3$.

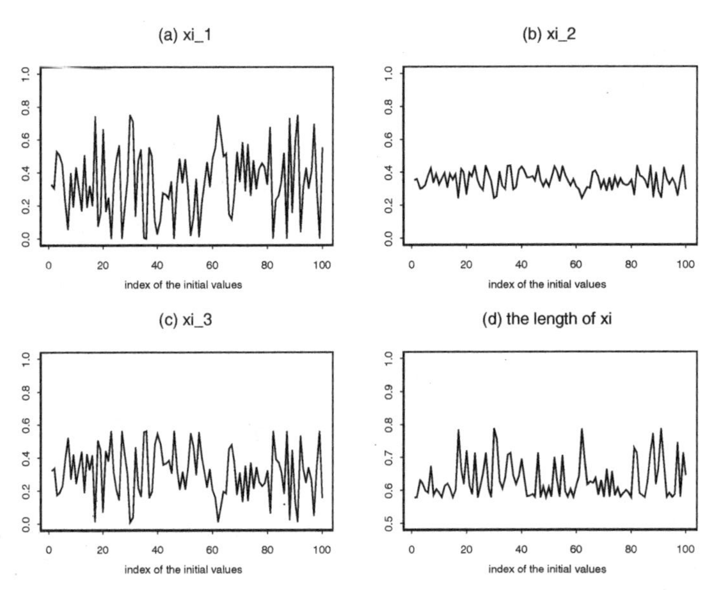

Figure 7.3 The algorithm `lseb` is used to find ξ, which minimizes $||\eta - C^\top\xi||^2$ subject to $\xi \in [0,1]^3$. Given 100 different initial values (indexed by $1, 2, \ldots, 100$), the algorithm stops with precise $||\eta - C^\top\xi||^2 \le 10^{-30}$. Plots (a), (b), (c) and (d) show the 100 different $\xi = (\xi_1, \xi_2, \xi_3)^\top$ and its length $||\xi||$ against the indexes of the initial values.

The stopping rule for the algorithm is $||\eta - B^\top\xi||^2 \le 10^{-30}$. Figure 7.3 shows the 100 different $\xi = (\xi_1, \xi_2, \xi_3)^\top$ against the indices of the initial values. The vector

$$\xi = (0.32817869, 0.352234, 0.31958763)^\top$$

has the shortest length 0.577846, which corresponds to the initial value $\xi^{(0)} = \min\{\max\{\mathbf{0},\ (B^\top)^+\eta\},\ \mathbf{1}\}$. ||

Problems

7.1 Uniqueness (Arnold *et al.*, 2002, p.238). Consider the following conditional distribution matrices

$$A = \begin{pmatrix} 1/4 & 1/2 \\ 3/4 & 1/2 \end{pmatrix} \quad \text{and} \quad B = \begin{pmatrix} 1/3 & 2/3 \\ 3/5 & 2/5 \end{pmatrix},$$

where $\mathcal{X} = \mathcal{S}_X = \{x_1, x_2\}$ and $\mathcal{Y} = \mathcal{S}_Y = \{y_1, y_2\}$. Show that

(a) The X-marginal and Y-marginal are given by

X	x_1	x_2
$\xi_i = \Pr\{X = x_i\}$	3/8	5/8

and

Y	y_1	y_2
$\eta_j = \Pr\{Y = y_j\}$	1/2	1/2

(b) The unique joint distribution of (X, Y) is

$$P = \begin{pmatrix} 1/8 & 1/4 \\ 3/8 & 1/4 \end{pmatrix}.$$

7.2 Uniqueness (Arnold *et al.*, 2004, p.142). Consider the following conditional distribution matrices

$$A = \begin{pmatrix} \frac{3}{22} & 0 & 0 & \frac{2}{11} & \frac{1}{4} \\ \frac{7}{22} & 0 & \frac{6}{31} & \frac{4}{11} & 0 \\ \frac{6}{11} & \frac{9}{22} & \frac{11}{31} & \frac{5}{11} & 0 \\ 0 & \frac{13}{22} & \frac{14}{31} & 0 & \frac{3}{4} \end{pmatrix}, B = \begin{pmatrix} \frac{1}{4} & 0 & 0 & \frac{1}{3} & \frac{5}{12} \\ \frac{1}{3} & 0 & \frac{2}{17} & \frac{8}{21} & 0 \\ \frac{2}{7} & \frac{3}{14} & \frac{11}{42} & \frac{5}{21} & 0 \\ 0 & \frac{13}{42} & \frac{1}{3} & 0 & \frac{5}{14} \end{pmatrix}.$$

Prove that the unique compatible X-marginal is

$$\hat{\xi} = (12/117, 21/117, 42/117, 42/117)^\top$$

and the joint distribution of (X, Y) is given by

$$\begin{pmatrix} 0.02564 & 0 & 0 & 0.03418 & 0.04273 \\ 0.05982 & 0 & 0.05128 & 0.06837 & 0 \\ 0.10256 & 0.07692 & 0.09401 & 0.08547 & 0 \\ 0 & 0.11111 & 0.11965 & 0 & 0.12820 \end{pmatrix}.$$

7.3 **Incompatibility** (Arnold *et al.*, 2002, p.234). Show that the following two conditional distribution

$$A = \begin{pmatrix} 0 & 0 & \frac{1}{10} & 0 & 0 \\ 0 & \frac{1}{3} & \frac{3}{10} & \frac{4}{7} & 0 \\ 1 & \frac{1}{3} & \frac{2}{10} & \frac{2}{7} & 1 \\ 0 & \frac{1}{3} & \frac{3}{10} & \frac{1}{7} & 0 \\ 0 & 0 & \frac{1}{10} & 0 & 0 \end{pmatrix} \text{ and } B = \begin{pmatrix} 0 & 0 & 1 & 0 & 0 \\ 0 & \frac{1}{5} & \frac{1}{5} & \frac{3}{5} & 0 \\ \frac{1}{9} & \frac{2}{9} & \frac{3}{9} & \frac{2}{9} & \frac{1}{9} \\ 0 & \frac{2}{5} & \frac{1}{5} & \frac{2}{5} & 0 \\ 0 & 0 & 1 & 0 & 0 \end{pmatrix}$$

are not compatible.

7.4 **Multiple solutions** (Arnold *et al.*, 2004, p.142). Show that the following two conditional distribution matrices

$$\begin{pmatrix} \frac{1}{4} & \frac{1}{3} & 0 & 0 & 0 & 0 \\ \frac{3}{4} & \frac{2}{3} & 0 & 0 & 0 & 0 \\ 0 & 0 & \frac{5}{12} & \frac{3}{7} & 0 & 0 \\ 0 & 0 & \frac{7}{12} & \frac{4}{7} & 0 & 0 \\ 0 & 0 & 0 & 0 & \frac{9}{20} & \frac{5}{11} \\ 0 & 0 & 0 & 0 & \frac{11}{20} & \frac{6}{11} \end{pmatrix} \text{ and } \begin{pmatrix} \frac{1}{3} & \frac{2}{3} & 0 & 0 & 0 & 0 \\ \frac{3}{7} & \frac{4}{7} & 0 & 0 & 0 & 0 \\ 0 & 0 & \frac{5}{11} & \frac{6}{11} & 0 & 0 \\ 0 & 0 & \frac{7}{15} & \frac{8}{15} & 0 & 0 \\ 0 & 0 & 0 & 0 & \frac{9}{19} & \frac{10}{19} \\ 0 & 0 & 0 & 0 & \frac{11}{23} & \frac{12}{23} \end{pmatrix}$$

are compatible with multiple solutions.

APPENDIX A

Basic Statistical Distributions and Stochastic Processes

In this appendix, we list some useful distributions including abbreviation, support, density, mean, variance, covariance, properties, relationship with other distributions, the random variable generation method and some existing S-plus functions. An exhaustive review of statistical distributions is provided by Johnson & Kotz (1969–1972) and Johnson *et al.* (1992, 1994, 1995). In addition, we provide a summary of the Poisson process and the nonhomogeneous Poisson process (Ross, 1983). All computer codes referred to in the following are in S-plus/R.

A.1 Discrete Distributions

A.1.1 Finite Discrete: $X \sim \text{FDiscrete}_d(\{x_i\}, \{p_i\})$, $p_i \geq 0$, $i = 1, \ldots, d$, $\sum_{i=1}^{d} p_i = 1$,

$$\Pr(X = x_i) = p_i, \quad i = 1, \ldots, d.$$

$E(X) = \sum x_i p_i$ and $\text{Var}(X) = \sum x_i^2 p_i - (\sum x_i p_i)^2$. The **uniform discrete** distribution is a special case of the finite discrete distribution with $p_i = 1/d$ for all i. The S-plus function, `sample`(x, N, prob $= p$, replace = F) produces samples from this distribution, i.e., a vector of length N randomly chosen from $\{x_1, \ldots, x_d\}$ with corresponding probabilities $\{p_1, \ldots, p_d\}$ without replacement. For example, `sample`(0:1, 100, c(0.3, 0.7), T) will produce 100 i.i.d. Bernoulli(0.3) samples.

A.1.2 Hypergeometric: $X \sim \text{Hgeometric}(m, n, k)$,

$$\text{Hgeometric}(x|m, n, k) = \binom{m}{x}\binom{n}{k-x} \bigg/ \binom{m+n}{k},$$

where $x = \max(0, k-n), \ldots, \min(m, k)$. $E(X) = km/N'$ and $\text{Var}(X) = kmn(N'-k)/[N'^2(N'-1)]$, where $N' = m+n$. The hypergeometric can be described by an urn model with m red and n black balls. Any sequences of k drawings resulting in x red and $k-x$ black balls have the same probability. It is similar to the binomial distribution but sampled from a finite population without replacement. The S-plus function, `rhyper`(N, m, n, k), can be used to generate N i.i.d. samples of X.

A.1.3 Poisson: $X \sim \text{Poisson}(\lambda)$, $\lambda > 0$,

$$\text{Poisson}(x|\lambda) = \lambda^x e^{-\lambda}/x!, \quad x \in \mathbb{N}.$$

$E(X) = \lambda$ and $\text{Var}(X) = \lambda$. If $\{X_i\}_{i=1}^d \overset{\text{ind}}{\sim} \text{Poisson}(\lambda_i)$, then

$$\begin{aligned} \textstyle\sum_{i=1}^d X_i &\sim \text{Poisson}(\textstyle\sum_{i=1}^d \lambda_i), \quad \text{and} \\ (X_1, \ldots, X_d)|(\textstyle\sum_{i=1}^d X_i = n) &\sim \text{Multinomial}_d(n, p), \end{aligned}$$

where $p = (\lambda_1, \ldots, \lambda_d)^\top / \sum_{i=1}^d \lambda_i$. The Poisson and gamma distributions have the following relationship:

$$\sum_{x=k}^{\infty} \text{Poisson}(x|\lambda) = \int_0^{\lambda} \text{Gamma}(y|k, 1)\, dy.$$

The Poisson generator in S-plus is `rpois`(N, λ).

A.1.4 Binomial: $X \sim \text{Binomial}(n, p)$, integer $n > 0$, $p \in [0, 1]$,

$$\text{Binomial}(x|n, p) = \binom{n}{x} p^x (1-p)^{n-x}, \quad x = 0, 1, \ldots, n.$$

$E(X) = np$ and $\text{Var}(X) = np(1-p)$. When $n = 1$, the binomial is also called the **Bernoulli** distribution. If

$$\{X_i\}_{i=1}^d \overset{\text{ind}}{\sim} \text{Binomial}(n_i, p),$$

then

$$\sum_{i=1}^d X_i \sim \text{Binomial}\left(\sum_{i=1}^d n_i, p\right).$$

The binomial and beta distributions have the following relationship:

$$\sum_{x=0}^{k} \text{Binomial}(x|n, p) = \int_0^{1-p} \text{Beta}(x|n-k, k+1)\, dx, \quad 0 \le k \le n.$$

The binomial generator in S-plus is `rbinom`$(N,\ n,\ p)$.

A.1.5 Multinomial: $X \sim \text{Multinomial}(n; p_1, \ldots, p_d)$ or $X \sim \text{Multinomial}_d(n, p)$, integer $n > 0$, $p = (p_1, \ldots, p_d)^\top \in \mathbb{T}_d$,

$$\text{Multinomial}_d(x|n, p) = \binom{n}{x_1, \ldots, x_d} \prod_{i=1}^{d} p_i^{x_i},$$

where $x_i \geq 0$, $\sum_{i=1}^{d} x_i = n$. $E(X_i) = np_i$, $\text{Var}(X_i) = np_i(1 - p_i)$ and $\text{Cov}(X_i, X_j) = -np_ip_j$. The binomial distribution is a special case of the multinomial with $d = 2$. The conditional sampling method (cf. §2.2.5) can be used to simulate a multivariate draw of X as follows:

- Draw $X_i \sim \text{Binomial}(n - \sum_{j=1}^{i-1} X_j, p_i / \sum_{j=i}^{d} p_j)$, $1 \leq i \leq d-1$;
- Set $X_d = n - \sum_{j=1}^{d-1} X_j$.

The corresponding S-plus code is given by

```
function(n, p) {
   # Function name: rmultinomial(n, p)
   # Generate one random vector (x_1, ..., x_d) from
   # Multinomial(n; p_1, ..., p_d) with d >= 3
   d <- length(p)
   N <- n
   S <- 1
   x <- rep(0, d)
   for(i in 1:(d - 1)) {
       if(n == 0) {  x[i] <- 0  }
       else { x[i] <- rbinom(1, n, p[i]/S) }
       n <- n - x[i]
       S <- S - p[i]   }
   x[d] <- N - sum(x)
   return(x)      }
```

A.2 Continuous Distributions

A.2.1 Uniform: $X \sim U(a, b)$, $a < b$,

$$U(x|a, b) = 1/(b - a), \quad x \in (a, b).$$

$E(X) = (a + b)/2$ and $\text{Var}(X) = (b - a)^2/12$. A noninformative distribution is obtained by letting $a \to -\infty$ and $b \to \infty$. If $Y \sim$

$U(0,1)$, then $X = a + (b-a)Y \sim U(a,b)$. The random number generator in S-plus is `runif`(N, a, b).

A.2.2 Beta: $X \sim \text{Beta}(a,b)$, $a, b > 0$,

$$\text{Beta}(x|a,b) = x^{a-1}(1-x)^{b-1}/B(a,b), \quad x \in (0,1),$$

where $B(a,b) = \Gamma(a)\Gamma(b)/\Gamma(a+b)$ denotes the beta function.

$$\begin{aligned} E(X) &= a/(a+b), \\ E(X^2) &= a(a+1)/[(a+b)(a+b+1)], \quad \text{and} \\ \text{Var}(X) &= ab/[(a+b)^2(a+b+1)]. \end{aligned}$$

When $a = b = 1$, $\text{Beta}(1,1) = U(0,1)$. The k-th order statistics from a sample of N i.i.d. $U(0,1)$ follows $\text{Beta}(k, N-k+1)$. The beta and gamma distributions have the following relationship:

$$X \stackrel{d}{=} \frac{Y}{Y+Z},$$

where $Y \sim \text{Gamma}(a,1)$, $Z \sim \text{Gamma}(b,1)$, and Y and Z are independent. The beta distribution is the conjugate prior for the binomial likelihood. A noninformative distribution is obtained as $a, b \to 0$. The beta generator is `rbeta`(N, a, b).

A.2.3 Dirichlet: $X \sim \text{Dirichlet}(a_1, \ldots, a_d)$ or $X \sim \text{Dirichlet}_d(a)$, $a = (a_1, \ldots, a_d)^\top$, $a_i > 0$, $i = 1, \ldots, d$,

$$\text{Dirichlet}_d(x|a) = \frac{1}{B_d(a)} \prod_{i=1}^{d} x_i^{a_i - 1}, \quad x = (x_1, \ldots, x_d)^\top \in \mathbb{T}_d,$$

where $B_d(a) = B(a_1, \ldots, a_d) = \prod_{i=1}^d \Gamma(a_i)/\Gamma(\sum_{i=1}^d a_i)$ denotes the multivariate beta function. Let $a. = \sum_{i=1}^d a_i$, then

$$\begin{aligned} E(X_i) &= a_i/a., \\ \text{Var}(X_i) &= a_i(a. - a_i)/[a.^2(a. + 1)], \quad \text{and} \\ \text{Cov}(X_i, X_j) &= -a_i a_j/[a.^2(a. + 1)], \quad i \neq j. \end{aligned}$$

When $d = 2$, we have $\text{Dirichlet}(a_1, a_2) = \text{Beta}(a_1, a_2)$. The Dirichlet and gamma distributions have the following relationship:

$$X_i \stackrel{d}{=} \frac{Y_i}{\sum_{j=1}^d Y_j}, \quad \text{where } \{Y_i\}_{i=1}^d \stackrel{\text{ind}}{\sim} \text{Gamma}(a_i, 1).$$

The Dirichlet is the conjugate prior for the multinomial likelihood. A noninformative distribution is obtained as $a_i \to 0$ for all i. Let

$$\{W_i\}_{i=1}^{d-1} \stackrel{\text{ind}}{\sim} \text{Beta}(a_1 + \cdots + a_i,\ a_{i+1}),$$

then, the following SR (Fang *et al.*, 1990, p.146)

- $X_i \stackrel{d}{=} (1 - W_{i-1}) \prod_{j=i}^{d-1} W_j, \quad i = 1, \ldots, d-1, \quad W_0 \hat{=} 0;$
- $X_d \stackrel{d}{=} 1 - W_{d-1}$

can be used to simulate a multivariate draw of $X = (X_1, \ldots, X_d)^\top \sim$ Dirichlet$(a_1, \ldots, a_d)$. The corresponding S-plus code is given by

```
function(a) {
    # Function name: rDirichlet(a)
    # Generate one random vector (x_1, ..., x_d) from
    # Dirichlet(a_1, ..., a_d) with d >= 3
    d <- length(a)
    w <- rep(0, d - 1)
    for(i in 1:(d - 1)) {
        w[i] <- rbeta(1, sum(a[1:i]), a[i + 1])  }
    x <- rep(0, d)
    x[1] <- prod(w)
    for(i in 2:(d - 1)) {
        x[i] <- (1 - w[i - 1]) * prod(w[i:(d - 1)]) }
    x[d] <- 1 - sum(x[1:(d - 1)])
    return(x)   }
```

A.2.4 Logistic: $X \sim \text{Logistic}(\mu, \sigma^2)$, $-\infty < \mu < \infty$, $\sigma^2 > 0$,

$$\text{Logistic}(x|\mu, \sigma^2) = \frac{\exp(-\frac{x-\mu}{\sigma})}{\sigma[1 + \exp(-\frac{x-\mu}{\sigma})]^2}, \quad x \in \mathbb{R}.$$

$E(X) = \mu$ and $\text{Var}(X) = \pi^2\sigma^2/3$. The logistic is another symmetric and unimodal distribution, more similar to the normal in appearance than the Laplace, but with even heavier tails. Both the cdf and its inverse function have closed-form expressions:

$$\begin{aligned} F(x|\mu, \sigma^2) &= \left[1 + e^{-\frac{x-\mu}{\sigma}}\right]^{-1}, \quad x \in \mathbb{R}, \\ F^{-1}(x|\mu, \sigma^2) &= \mu + \sigma \log \frac{x}{1-x}, \quad x \in (0, 1). \end{aligned}$$

The logistic generator in S-plus is **rlogis**(N, μ, σ).

A.2.5 Laplace or (**Double Exponential**): $X \sim \text{Laplace}(\mu, \sigma^2)$, $-\infty < \mu < \infty$, $\sigma^2 > 0$,

$$\text{Laplace}(x|\mu, \sigma^2) = \frac{1}{2\sigma} \exp(-|x - \mu|/\sigma), \quad x \in \mathbb{R}.$$

$E(X) = \mu$ and $\text{Var}(X) = 2\sigma^2$. Like the Gaussian distribution, the Laplace is symmetric and unimodal, but has a heavier tail. $|X - \mu| \sim \text{Exponential}(1/\sigma)$. Let $\{Y_i\}_{i=1}^4 \overset{\text{iid}}{\sim} N(0, 1)$, then $Y_1Y_4 - Y_2Y_3 \sim \text{Laplace}(0, 2^2)$ (Nyquist *et al.*, 1954). The inversion method (cf. §2.2.1) can be used to draw N i.i.d. samples from the standard Laplace$(0, 1)$ distribution. The S-plus code is given by

```
function(N){
    # Function name: rLaplace(N)
    # Generate N i.i.d. samples from the
    # standard Laplace(0, 1) distribution
    u <- runif(N)
    x <- rep(0, N)
    for(i in 1:N) {
       if(u[i] < 0.5) { x[i] <- log(2 * u[i]) }
       else { x[i] <-  - log(2 * (1 - u[i]))  }     }
    return(x) }
```

A.2.6 Exponential: $X \sim \text{Exponential}(\beta)$, rate $\beta > 0$,

$$\text{Exponential}(x|\beta) = \beta e^{-\beta x}, \quad x \in \mathbb{R}_+.$$

$E(X) = 1/\beta$ and $\text{Var}(X) = 1/\beta^2$. If $\{X_i\}_{i=1}^n \overset{\text{iid}}{\sim} \text{Exponential}(\beta)$, then $\sum_{i=1}^n X_i \sim \text{Gamma}(n, \beta)$. The exponential distribution generator in S-plus is **rexp**(N, β).

A.2.7 Gamma: $X \sim \text{Gamma}(\alpha, \beta)$, shape $\alpha > 0$, rate $\beta > 0$,

$$\text{Gamma}(x|\alpha, \beta) = \frac{\beta^\alpha}{\Gamma(\alpha)} x^{\alpha-1} e^{-\beta x}, \quad x \in \mathbb{R}_+,$$

where $\Gamma(\alpha) = \int_0^\infty y^{\alpha-1} e^{-y}\, dy$ denotes the gamma function. We have $\Gamma(\alpha + 1) = \alpha\Gamma(\alpha)$, $\Gamma(1) = 1$ and $\Gamma(1/2) = \sqrt{\pi}$. $E(X) = \alpha/\beta$ and $\text{Var}(X) = \alpha/\beta^2$. The case of $\alpha = 1$ is the exponential distribution Exponential(β). The case of $\alpha = \nu/2$ and $\beta = 1/2$ is the chi-square distribution Gamma$(\nu/2, 1/2) = \chi^2(\nu)$. If $X \sim$ Gamma(α, β) and $c > 0$, then

$$Y = cX \sim \text{Gamma}(\alpha, \beta/c).$$

If $\{X_i\}_{i=1}^n \overset{\text{ind}}{\sim}$ Gamma(α_i, β), then $\sum_{i=1}^n X_i \sim$ Gamma$(\sum_{i=1}^n \alpha_i, \beta)$. The gamma is the conjugate prior for the Poisson mean and for the inverse of the normal variance. A noninformative distribution is obtained as $\alpha, \beta \to 0$. The gamma generator in S-plus is `rgamma`(N, α, β).

A.2.8 Inverse Gamma: $X \sim$ IGamma(α, β), shape $\alpha > 0$, scale $\beta > 0$,

$$\text{IGamma}(x|\alpha, \beta) = \frac{\beta^\alpha}{\Gamma(\alpha)} x^{-(\alpha+1)} e^{-\beta/x}, \quad x \in \mathbb{R}_+.$$

$E(X) = \beta/(\alpha-1)$ (if $\alpha > 1$) and Var$(X) = \beta^2/[(\alpha-1)^2(\alpha-2)]$ (if $\alpha > 2$). Obviously, we have IGamma$(x|\alpha, \beta) =$ Gamma$(x^{-1}|\alpha, \beta)/x^2$. In addition, if $X^{-1} \sim$ Gamma(α, β), then $X \sim$ IGamma(α, β). The inverse gamma is the conjugate prior for the normal variance σ^2. A noninformative distribution is obtained as $\alpha, \beta \to 0$.

A.2.9 Chi-square: $X \sim \chi^2(\nu) \equiv$ Gamma$(\frac{\nu}{2}, \frac{1}{2})$, degree of freedom $\nu > 0$,

$$\chi^2(x|\nu) = \frac{2^{-\nu/2}}{\Gamma(\nu/2)} x^{\nu/2-1} e^{-x/2}, \quad x \in \mathbb{R}_+.$$

$E(X) = \nu$ and Var$(X) = 2\nu$. If $Y \sim N(0, 1)$, then $X = Y^2 \sim \chi^2(1)$. If $\{X_i\}_{i=1}^n \overset{\text{ind}}{\sim} \chi^2(\nu_i)$, then $\sum_{i=1}^n X_i \sim \chi^2(\sum_{i=1}^n \nu_i)$. The chi-square generator is `rchisq`(N, ν).

A.2.10 F or (**Fisher's F**): $X \sim F(\nu_1, \nu_2)$, ν_1, ν_2 positive integers,

$$F(x|\nu_1, \nu_2) = \frac{(\nu_1/\nu_2)^{\nu_1/2}}{B(\frac{\nu_1}{2}, \frac{\nu_2}{2})} x^{\frac{\nu_1}{2}-1} \left(1 + \frac{\nu_1 x}{\nu_2}\right)^{-\frac{\nu_1+\nu_2}{2}}, \quad x \in \mathbb{R}_+.$$

$E(X) = \frac{\nu_2}{\nu_2-2}$ (if $\nu_2 > 2$), Var$(X) = \frac{2\nu_2^2(\nu_1+\nu_2-2)}{\nu_1(\nu_2-4)(\nu_2-2)^2}$ (if $\nu_2 > 4$). An alternative definition of $F(\nu_1, \nu_2)$ is $X \overset{d}{=} [\chi^2(\nu_1)/\nu_1]/[\chi^2(\nu_2)/\nu_2]$. The F generator is `rf`(N, ν_1, ν_2).

A.2.11 Inverse chi-square: $X \sim \text{I}\chi^2(\nu) \equiv$ IGamma$(\frac{\nu}{2}, \frac{1}{2})$, $\nu > 0$,

$$\text{I}\chi^2(x|\nu) = \frac{2^{-\nu/2}}{\Gamma(\nu/2)} x^{-(\nu/2+1)} e^{-1/(2x)}, \quad x \in \mathbb{R}_+.$$

$E(X) = \frac{1}{\nu-2}$ (if $\nu > 2$) and $\text{Var}(X) = \frac{2}{(\nu-2)^2(\nu-4)}$ (if $\nu > 4$).

A.2.12 Normal or (**Gaussian**): $X \sim N(\mu, \sigma^2)$, $-\infty < \mu < \infty$, $\sigma^2 > 0$,

$$N(x|\mu, \sigma^2) = \frac{1}{\sqrt{2\pi}\sigma} \exp\left[-\frac{(x-\mu)^2}{2\sigma^2} \right], \quad x \in \mathbb{R}.$$

$E(X) = \mu$ and $\text{Var}(X) = \sigma^2$. If $\{X_i\} \overset{\text{ind}}{\sim} N(\mu_i, \sigma_i^2)$, then $\sum a_i X_i \sim N(\sum a_i \mu_i, \sum a_i^2 \sigma_i^2)$. If $X_1|X_2 \sim N(X_2, \sigma_1^2)$ and $X_2 \sim N(\mu_2, \sigma_2^2)$, then $X_1 \sim N(\mu_2, \sigma_1^2 + \sigma_2^2)$. A noninformative or flat distribution is obtained as $\sigma^2 \to \infty$. The normal generator is `rnorm(`N, μ, σ`)`.

A.2.13 Inverse Gaussian (or **Wald**): $X \sim \text{IGaussian}(\mu, \lambda)$, $\mu > 0$, $\lambda > 0$,

$$\text{IGaussian}(x|\mu, \lambda) = \sqrt{\frac{\lambda}{2\pi x^3}} \exp\left[-\frac{\lambda(x-\mu)^2}{2\mu^2 x} \right], \quad x \in \mathbb{R}_+.$$

$E(X) = \mu$ and $\text{Var}(X) = \mu^3/\lambda$. If $X \sim \text{IGaussian}(\mu, \lambda)$ and $c > 0$, then $cX \sim \text{IGaussian}(c\mu, c\lambda)$. If $\{X_i\}_{i=1}^n \overset{\text{ind}}{\sim} \text{IGaussian}(\mu_i, c\mu_i^2)$, then $\Sigma_{i=1}^n X_i \sim \text{IGaussian}(\Sigma_{i=1}^n \mu_i, c(\Sigma_{i=1}^n \mu_i)^2)$. Let $X \sim \text{IGaussian}(\mu, \lambda)$, then $\lambda(X-\mu)^2/(\mu^2 X) \sim \chi^2(1)$. This result first obtained by Shuster (1968) can be used to simulate N i.i.d. draws from the inverse Gaussian distribution. The corresponding S-plus code is given by

```
function(N, mu, lambda){
    # Function name: rigaussian(N, mu, lambda)
    # Generate N i.i.d. samples of x from
    # IGaussianDE(mu, lambda) with density
    # c exp[-lambda(x-mu)^2/(2 mu^2 x)], mu, lambda > 0
    # where c = [lambda/(2 \pi x^3)]^{1/2}
    y <- (rnorm(N, 0, 1))^2
    a <- (mu^2/(2 * lambda)) * y
    b <- 4 * mu * lambda * y + mu^2 * y^2
    x1 <- mu + a - (mu/(2 * lambda)) * sqrt(b)
    u <- runif(N)
    x <- rep(0, N)
    for(i in 1:N) {
       if(u[i] < mu/(mu + x1[i])) { x[i] <- x1[i] }
       else { x[i] <- mu^2/x1[i] }        }
    return(x) }
```

A.2.14 Lognormal: $X \sim LN(\mu, \sigma^2)$, $-\infty < \mu < \infty$, $\sigma^2 > 0$,

$$LN(x|\mu, \sigma^2) = \frac{1}{\sqrt{2\pi}\sigma x} \exp\left[-\frac{(\log x - \mu)^2}{2\sigma^2} \right], \quad x \in \mathbb{R}_+.$$

$E(X) = \exp(\mu + 0.5\sigma^2)$ and $\mathrm{Var}(X) = [E(X)]^2[\exp(\sigma^2) - 1]$. If $\log(X) \sim N(\mu, \sigma^2)$, then $X \sim LN(\mu, \sigma^2)$. The lognormal generator is `rlnorm`(N, μ, σ).

A.2.15 Multivariate Normal or (**Gaussian**): $X \sim N_d(\mu, \Sigma)$ or $N(\mu, \Sigma)$, $\mu \in \mathbb{R}^d$, $\Sigma_{d\times d} > 0$,

$$N_d(x|\mu, \Sigma) = \frac{1}{(\sqrt{2\pi}\,)^d |\Sigma|^{\frac{1}{2}}} \exp\Big\{ -\frac{1}{2}(x-\mu)^\top \Sigma^{-1}(x-\mu) \Big\},$$

where $x \in \mathbb{R}^d$. $E(X) = \mu$ and $\mathrm{Var}(X) = \Sigma$. Assume that

$$X|Y \sim N_d(AY,\, \Sigma_{x|y}) \quad \text{and} \quad Y \sim N_q(\mu_y,\, \Sigma_y), \tag{A.1}$$

then the joint pdf of (X, Y) is also multinormal because $E(X|Y) = AY$ is a linear function of Y. Using the following identities:

$$E(X) = E(E(X|Y)), \quad \mathrm{Var}(X) = E(\mathrm{Var}(X|Y)) + \mathrm{Var}(E(X|Y)),$$

we have $E(X) = A\mu_y$, $\mathrm{Var}(X) = \Sigma_{x|y} + A\Sigma_y A^\top$, and

$$\begin{aligned} \mathrm{Cov}(X, Y) &= E(XY^\top) - E(X)E(Y^\top) \\ &= E(E(XY^\top|Y)) - A\mu_y E(Y^\top) \\ &= A[E(YY^\top) - E(Y)E(Y^\top)] \\ &= A\Sigma_y, \end{aligned}$$

which results in

$$\begin{pmatrix} X \\ Y \end{pmatrix} \sim N_{d+q}\left(\begin{pmatrix} A\mu_y \\ \mu_y \end{pmatrix}, \begin{pmatrix} \Sigma_{x|y} + A\Sigma_y A^\top & A\Sigma_y \\ \Sigma_y A^\top & \Sigma_y \end{pmatrix} \right). \tag{A.2}$$

The multinormal generator is `rmvnorm`(N, mean $= \mu$, cov $= \Sigma$).

A.2.16 Wishart: $X \sim \mathrm{Wishart}_d(A, \nu)$, scale matrix $A_{d\times d} > 0$, degree of freedom $\nu > 0$,

$$\mathrm{Wishart}_d(X|A, \nu) = \frac{|X|^{\frac{\nu-d-1}{2}} e^{-0.5\,\mathrm{tr}\,(A^{-1}X)}}{2^{\frac{\nu d}{2}} \pi^{\frac{d(d-1)}{4}} \prod_{i=1}^d \Gamma(\frac{\nu+1-i}{2}) \cdot |A|^{\frac{\nu}{2}}},$$

where $X_{d\times d} > 0$. $E(X) = \nu A$. When $d = 1$ and $A = 1$, the Wishart reduces to the chi-square distribution: $\text{Wishart}_1(1,\nu) = \chi^2(\nu)$. The Wishart is the conjugate prior for the inverse covariance matrix Σ^{-1} of a multinormal distribution. A noninformative distribution is proportional to $|X|^{-(d+1)/2}$ obtained as $\nu \to 0$ and $|A^{-1}| \to 0$. When ν is an integer and $\nu \geq d$, the multinormal generator can be used to simulate a draw from the Wishart based on the following idea:

- Draw $Y_1, \ldots, Y_\nu \overset{\text{iid}}{\sim} N_d(\mathbf{0}, A)$;
- Set $X = \sum_{i=1}^{\nu} Y_i Y_i^\top$, then $X \sim \text{Wishart}_d(A, \nu)$.

The corresponding S-plus code is given by

```
function(d, A, v){
    # Function name: rwishart(d, A, v)
    # Generate one random matrix X from the
    # Wishart distribution Wishart_d(A, v)
    # Input:  dimension d>=2, degree of freedom v>=d,
    #         positive define matrix A of d by d
    # Output: positive define random matrix X of d by d
    D <- diag(eigen(A)$values)
    G <- eigen(A)$vectors     # A= G D G'
    Asqrt <- G %*% sqrt(D) %*% t(G)
                              # Asqrt= G D^{1/2} G'
    Z <- matrix(rnorm(d * v), ncol = v)
    X <- Asqrt %*% Z %*% t(Z) %*% t(Asqrt)
                              # X = A^{1/2} ZZ' A^{1/2}
    return(X)     }
```

Non-integral ν requires the general algorithm originally proposed by Odell & Feiveson (1966).

A.2.17 Inverse Wishart: $X \sim \text{IWishart}_d(A^{-1}, \nu)$, scale matrix $A_{d\times d} > 0$, degree of freedom $\nu > 0$,

$$\text{IWishart}_d(X|A^{-1},\nu) = \frac{|X|^{-\frac{\nu+d+1}{2}} e^{-0.5\,\text{tr}\,(AX^{-1})}}{2^{\frac{\nu d}{2}} \pi^{\frac{d(d-1)}{4}} \prod_{i=1}^{d} \Gamma(\frac{\nu+1-i}{2}) \cdot |A^{-1}|^{\frac{\nu}{2}}},$$

where $X_{d\times d} > 0$. $E(X) = (\nu - d - 1)^{-1} A$. When $d = 1$ and $A^{-1} = 1$, the inverse Wishart reduces to the inverse chi-square distribution: $\text{IWishart}_1(1,\nu) = \text{I}\chi^2(\nu)$. If $X^{-1} \sim \text{Wishart}_d(A^{-1},\nu)$, then $X \sim \text{IWishart}_d(A^{-1},\nu)$. This can be verified by using the following fact:

$$\text{If } X_{d\times d} = X^\top, \quad \text{then } J(X^{-1} \to X) = |X|^{-(d+1)},$$

where $J(Y \to X) \hat{=} |\partial Y/\partial X|$ denote the Jacobian determinant. The inverse Wishart is the conjugate prior for the covariance matrix Σ in a multinormal distribution. A noninformative distribution is proportional to $|X|^{-(d+1)/2}$ obtained as $\nu \to 0$ and $|A| \to 0$.

A.3 Mixture Distributions

A.3.1 Gamma Poisson: $X \sim \text{GPoisson}(\alpha, \beta)$, shape $\alpha > 0$, rate $\beta > 0$,

$$\text{GPoisson}(x|\alpha, \beta) = \binom{x+\alpha-1}{x}\left(\frac{\beta}{\beta+1}\right)^{\alpha}\left(\frac{1}{\beta+1}\right)^{x},$$

where $x = 0, 1, 2, \ldots$. $E(X) = \alpha/\beta$ and $\text{Var}(X) = \alpha(\beta+1)/\beta^2$. The gamma Poisson is a robust alternative to the Poisson distribution. If

$$\lambda \sim \text{Gamma}(\alpha, \beta) \quad \text{and} \quad X|\lambda \sim \text{Poisson}(\lambda),$$

then $X \sim \text{GPoisson}(\alpha, \beta)$. This mixture gives an algorithm for simulating from the gamma Poisson distribution.

A.3.2 Negative Binomial: $X \sim \text{NBinomial}(r, p)$, integer $r > 0$, $0 < p < 1$,

$$\text{NBinomial}(x|r, p) = \binom{x+r-1}{x} p^r (1-p)^x, \quad x = 0, 1, 2, \ldots.$$

$E(X) = r(1-p)/p$ and $\text{Var}(X) = r(1-p)/p^2$. The negative binomial is a special case of the gamma Poisson with $\alpha = r$ being positive integer and $\beta = p/(1-p)$. The X is the number of Bernoulli failures before r successes are achieved, where the probability of success is p. The **geometric distribution** is the special case of the negative binomial with $r = 1$. The built-in negative binomial generator is `rnbinom`(N, r, p).

A.3.3 Beta Binomial: $X \sim \text{BBinomial}(n, a, b)$, integer $n > 0$, $a, b > 0$,

$$\text{BBinomial}(x|n, a, b) = \binom{n}{x} \frac{B(x+a, n-x+b)}{B(a, b)}, \quad x = 0, 1, \ldots, n.$$

$E(X) = na/(a+b)$ and $\text{Var}(X) = nab(a+b+n)/[(a+b)^2(a+b+1)]$. The beta binomial is a robust alternative to the binomial distribution. If

$$p \sim \text{Beta}(a, b) \quad \text{and} \quad X|p \sim \text{Binomial}(n, p),$$

then $X \sim \text{BBinomial}(n, a, b)$. This result yields a sampling method to generate the beta binomial distribution.

A.3.4 Dirichlet Multinomial: $X \sim \text{DMultinomial}_d(n, a)$, n positive integer, $a = (a_1, \ldots, a_d)^\top$, $a_i > 0$ for all i,

$$\text{DMultinomial}_d(x|n, a) = \binom{n}{x_1, \ldots, x_d} \frac{B_d(x + a)}{B_d(a)},$$

where $x = (x_1, \ldots, x_d)^\top$, $x_i \geq 0$, $\sum_{i=1}^d x_i = n$.

$$\begin{aligned} E(X_i) &= na_i/a., \qquad a. \hat{=} \textstyle\sum_{i=1}^d a_i, \\ \text{Var}(X_i) &= n(a. + n)a_i(a. - a_i)/[a.^2(a. + 1)], \\ \text{Cov}(X_i, X_j) &= -n(a. + n)a_i a_j/[a.^2(a. + 1)], \quad i \neq j. \end{aligned}$$

When $d = 2$, the Dirichlet multinomial reduces to the beta binomial. The Dirichlet multinomial is a robust alternative to the multinomial distribution. If

$$p \sim \text{Dirichlet}_d(a) \quad \text{and} \quad X|p \sim \text{Multinomial}_d(n, p),$$

then $X \sim \text{DMultinomial}_d(n, a)$, which can be used to generate the distribution.

A.3.5 t or (**Student's t**): $X \sim t(\mu, \sigma^2, \nu)$, $-\infty < \mu < \infty$, $\sigma^2 > 0$, $\nu > 0$,

$$t(x|\mu, \sigma^2, \nu) = \frac{\Gamma(\frac{\nu+1}{2})}{\Gamma(\frac{\nu}{2})\sqrt{\nu\pi}\sigma} \left[1 + \frac{(x - \mu)^2}{\nu\sigma^2}\right]^{-\frac{\nu+1}{2}}, \quad x \in \mathbb{R}.$$

$E(X) = \mu$ (if $\nu > 1$) and $\text{Var}(X) = \frac{\nu}{\nu-2}\sigma^2$ (if $\nu > 2$). The case of $\nu = 1$ is called the **Cauchy distribution**. The t is a common heavy-tail alternative to the normal distribution in a robust analysis. If

$$\tau \sim \text{Gamma}(\nu/2, \nu/2) \quad \text{and} \quad X|\tau \sim N(\mu, \tau^{-1}\sigma^2),$$

then $X \sim t(\mu, \sigma^2, \nu)$. This mixture gives an algorithm to generate the t-distribution. In addition, let $Z \sim N(0, 1)$, we have the following SR:

$$\left.\frac{X - \mu}{\sqrt{\tau^{-1}\sigma^2}}\right| \tau \stackrel{d}{=} Z, \quad \text{or} \quad X \stackrel{d}{=} \mu + \frac{\sigma Z}{\sqrt{\nu\tau/\nu}} \stackrel{d}{=} \mu + \frac{N(0, \sigma^2)}{\sqrt{\chi^2(\nu)/\nu}}.$$

This SR results in an alternative method to generate the t-variate. When $\mu = 0$ and $\sigma^2 = 1$, it is called the standard t-distribution, denoted by $t(\nu)$. The $t(\nu)$ generator is $\texttt{rt}(N,\, \nu)$.

A.3.6 Multivariate t: $X \sim t_d(\mu, \Sigma, \nu)$, location parameter $\mu \in \mathbb{R}^d$, dispersion matrix $\Sigma_{d\times d} > 0$, degree of freedom $\nu > 0$,

$$t_d(x|\mu, \Sigma, \nu) = \frac{\Gamma(\frac{\nu+d}{2})}{\Gamma(\frac{\nu}{2})(\sqrt{\nu\pi})^d |\Sigma|^{\frac{1}{2}}} \left[1 + \frac{(x-\mu)^{\top}\Sigma^{-1}(x-\mu)}{\nu}\right]^{-\frac{\nu+d}{2}},$$

where $x \in \mathbb{R}^d$. $E(X) = \mu$ (if $\nu > 1$) and $\text{Var}(X) = \frac{\nu}{\nu-2}\Sigma$ (if $\nu > 2$). The multivariate t provides a heavy-tail alternative to the multinormal while accounting for correlation among the components of X. If

$$\tau \sim \text{Gamma}(\nu/2, \nu/2) \quad \text{and} \quad X|\tau \sim N_d(\mu, \tau^{-1}\Sigma),$$

then $X \sim t_d(\mu, \Sigma, \nu)$. This mixture gives a sampling method to generate the multivariate t distribution. Equivalently, we have the following SR:

$$X \stackrel{d}{=} \mu + \frac{N_d(\mathbf{0}, \Sigma)}{\sqrt{\chi^2(\nu)/\nu}},$$

which itself can be served as the definition of the multivariate t-variate.

A.4 Stochastic Processes

A.4.1 Homogeneous Poisson: $\{X_i, i \geq 1\} \sim \text{HPP}(\lambda)$, where $\lambda > 0$ denotes the rate. A counting process $\{N(t), t \geq 0\}$ with successive event times $0 < X_1 < X_2 < \cdots$ is said to be a Poisson process with rate λ, if

(a) $N(0) = 0$;

(b) The process has stationary and independent increments;

(c) $\Pr\{N(h) \geq 2\} = o(h)$;

(d) $\Pr\{N(h) = 1\} = \lambda h + o(h)$.

Property: Let $\{X_i, i \geq 1\} \sim \text{HPP}(\lambda)$, then

1. For all $s, t \geq 0$, $N(t+s) - N(s) = N(t) \sim \text{Poisson}(\lambda t)$;

2. $\{X_i - X_{i-1}\} \stackrel{\text{iid}}{\sim}$ Exponential(λ), $X_0 \hat{=} 0$;

3. The joint pdf of $X_1, \ldots, X_n$ is $\lambda^n e^{-\lambda x_n}$;

4. Given that $N(t) = n$, X_i $(i = 1, \ldots, n)$ has the same distribution as the i-th order statistic of n i.i.d. samples from $U(0, t)$.

The second property can be used to generate all the event times occurring in $(0, t]$ of a Poisson process with rate λ.

A.4.2 Nonhomogeneous Poisson: $\{X_i, i \geq 1\} \sim$ NHPP$(\lambda(t), t \geq 0)$ or $\{X_i, i \geq 1\} \sim$ NHPP$(m(t), t \geq 0)$, where $\lambda(t)$ and $m(t) \hat{=} \int_0^t \lambda(s)ds$ denote the **intensity** function and the **mean** function, respectively. A counting process $\{N(t), t \geq 0\}$ is said to be a nonhomogeneous Poisson process with intensity $\lambda(t)$, if

(a) $N(0) = 0$;

(b) The process has independent increments;

(c) $\Pr\{N(t+h) - N(t) \geq 2\} = o(h)$;

(d) $\Pr\{N(t+h) - N(t) = 1\} = \lambda(t)h + o(h)$.

Property: Let $\{X_i, i \geq 1\} \sim$ NHPP$(m(t), t \geq 0)$, then

1. $N(t+s) - N(s) \sim$ Poisson$(m(t+s) - m(t))$;

2. The joint pdf of $X_1, \ldots, X_n$ is $[\prod_{i=1}^n \lambda(x_i)]e^{-m(T)}$, where $T = x_n$ if it is failure truncated and $T = t$ if it is time truncated;

3. Conditional on $X_n = x_n$, $X_1 < \cdots < X_{n-1}$ are distributed as $n-1$ order statistics from the following cdf

$$G(x) = 0 \cdot I_{(x \leq 0)} + \frac{m(x)}{m(x_n)} \cdot I_{(0 < x \leq x_n)} + 1 \cdot I_{(x > x_n)}.$$

4. Conditional on $N(t) = n$, $X_1 < \cdots < X_n$ are distributed as n order statistics from the following cdf

$$G(x) = 0 \cdot I_{(x \leq 0)} + \frac{m(x)}{m(t)} \cdot I_{(0 < x \leq t)} + 1 \cdot I_{(x > t)}.$$

List of Figures

List of Tables

List of Acronyms

Mathematics and Statistics

a.s.	almost surely
cdf	cumulative distribution function
CE	cross-entropy
cf.	confer
CI	confidence/credible interval
CP	changepoint problem
CPU	central processing unit
CV	coefficient of variation
DA	data augmentation
ECM	expectation/conditional maximization
e.g.	for example
EM	expectation-maximization
Eq.	equation
Ex.	example
GDD	grouped Dirichlet distribution
GLM	generalized linear model
GLMM	generalized linear mixed model
HPP	homogeneous Poisson process
HS	hidden sensitivity
IBF	inverse Bayes formulae
i.e.	that is
iff	if and only if
i.i.d.	independent and identical distribution
ISD	importance sampling density
I-step	imputation step
KL	Kullback–Leibler
LSE	least squares estimate
MAR	missing at random
MCAR	missing completely at random
MCEM	Monte Carlo EM
MCMC	Markov chain Monte Carlo

MDP	missing data problem
MLE	maximum likelihood estimate
MM	minorization-maximization
MSE	mean squared error
NDD	nested Dirichlet distribution
NHPP	nonhomogeneous Poisson process
NPMS	nonproduct measurable space
NR	Newton–Raphson
NRR	nonrandomized response
PAVA	pool adjacent violators algorithm
pdf	probability density function
pmf	probability mass function
PMS	product measurable space
PSR	potential scale reduction
P-step	posterior step
QLB	quadratic lower bound
QM	quantile-maximization
RD	randomizing device
RR	randomized response
RLSE	restricted least squares estimate
r.v.	random variable
r.v.'s	random variables
SE	Shannon entropy, or standard error
SIR	sampling/importance resampling
SR	stochastic representation
std	standard deviation
VDR	vertical density representation
ZIP	zero-inflated Poisson

Medicine

AIDS	acquired immunodeficiency syndrome
BOD	biochemical oxygen demand
HIV	human immunodeficiency virus
HUS	hemolytic uremic syndrome
REE	resting energy expenditure
SCD	sickle cell disease

List of Symbols

Mathematics

$\propto$	proportional to
$\|$	end of an example
$\|$END$\|$	end of the proof of a theorem/lemma
¶	end of a theorem/lemma/definition/remark
$\gg$	much greater than
$\hat{=}$	equal by definition
$\equiv$	always equal to
$\doteq$, $\approx$	approximately equal to
$\neq$	not equal to
$\forall$	for all
a^+	$\max(a, 0)$
$\lceil a \rceil$	smallest integer larger than a
$\bar{x}$	mean of the vector $x_{d\times 1}$
$x.$	sum of all components in x
$x^\top$	transpose of x
$x^{\otimes 2}$	$xx^\top$
$\|x\|_p$	ℓ_p-norm of x, $(\lvert x_1\rvert^p + \cdots + \lvert x_d\rvert^p)^{1/p}$
$\|x\|$	$\|x\|_2$
$\mathrm{diag}(x)$	diagonal matrix with main diagonal elements $x_1, \ldots, x_d$
$\mathbf{0}_d$	d-dimensional vector of zeros
$\mathbf{1}_d$	d-dimensional vector of ones
$\mathbf{I}_d$	$d \times d$ identity matrix
$\lvert A\rvert$	determinant of the matrix A
$\mathrm{tr}\,(A)$	trace of A
$A^\top$	transpose of A
A^{-1}	inverse of A
A^+	Moore–Penrose generalized inverse of A, $A^\top(AA^\top)^{-1}$

∇f	gradient of f
$\nabla^2 f$	Hessian of f
$\nabla^{ij} f(x, y)$	$\partial^{i+j} f(x, y)/\partial x^i \partial y^j$
$\Gamma(\alpha)$	gamma function ($\alpha > 0$)
$B(\alpha_1, \ldots, \alpha_d)$	multivariate beta function
$B(\alpha_1, \alpha_2)$	beta function
$I_{(x \in \mathcal{X})}$	indicator function
$\binom{n}{k}$	binomial coefficient
$\binom{n}{n_1, \ldots, n_m}$	multinomial coefficient
$\mathbb{N}$	set of natural numbers $\{0, 1, 2, \ldots\}$
$\mathbb{R}^d$	d-dimensional Euclidean space
$\mathbb{R}$	real line $(-\infty, +\infty)$
$\mathbb{R}_+^d$	d-dimensional positive orthant
$\mathbb{R}_-^d$	d-dimensional nonpositive orthant
$\mathbb{R}_+$	positive real line $(0, +\infty)$
$\mathbb{R}_-$	nonpositive real line $(-\infty, 0]$
$\mathbb{B}_d(r)$	d-dimensional ball with radius r, $\{x\colon x \in \mathbb{R}^d,\ x^\top x \le r^2\}$
$\mathbb{B}_d$	d-dimensional unit ball, $\mathbb{B}_d(1)$
$\mathbb{S}_d(r)$	d-dimensional sphere surface with radius r, $\{x\colon x \in \mathbb{R}^d,\ x^\top x = r^2\}$
$\mathbb{S}_d$	d-dimensional unit sphere surface, $\mathbb{S}_d(1)$
$\mathbb{V}_d(c)$	d-dimensional simplex, $\{x\colon x \in \mathbb{R}_+^d,\ x^\top \mathbf{1} \le c\}$
$\mathbb{V}_n$	$\mathbb{V}_n(1)$
$\mathbb{T}_d(c)$	d-dimensional hyperplane, $\{x\colon x \in \mathbb{R}_+^d,\ x^\top \mathbf{1} = c\}$
$\mathbb{T}_d$	$\mathbb{T}_d(1)$

Probability

$\sim$	distributed as
$\overset{\text{iid}}{\sim}$	independently and identically distributed
$\overset{\text{ind}}{\sim}$	independently distributed
$\overset{d}{=}$	having the same distribution on both sides
X, Y	random variables/vectors
$\mathcal{X}, \mathcal{Y}$	sample space
x, y	realizations

$f_X, f_X(x)$	density of X
$f_{(X,Y)}, f_{(X,Y)}(x, y)$	joint density of (X, Y)
$\mathcal{S}_X, \mathcal{S}_{(X,Y)}$	supports of X and (X, Y)
$\mathcal{S}_{(X\|Y)}(y)$	support of $X\|(Y = y)$
$\text{SE}(X)$	Shannon entropy of random vector X
$\text{KL}(g, h)$	KL divergence/distance between g and h
$\phi(x)$	pdf of standard normal distribution
$\Phi(x)$	cdf of standard normal distribution
$\Psi(x)$	$\phi(x)/\{1 - \Phi(x)\}$
Pr	probability measure
$E(X)$	expectation of r.v. X
$\text{Var}(X)$	variance of X
$\text{Cov}(X, Y)$	covariance of X and Y
$K(x, x')$	transition kernel
$O(n)$	big-O. As $n \to \infty$, $\frac{O(n)}{n} \to$ constant
$o(n)$	small-o. As $n \to \infty$, $\frac{o(n)}{n} \to 0$

Statistics

Y_{com}, Y	complete or augmented data
Y_{obs}	observed data
Y_{mis}, Z	missing data or latent variable
θ, Θ	parameter, parameter space
$L(\theta\|Y_{\text{obs}})$	observed likelihood function of θ for fixed Y_{obs} statistically identical to the joint pdf $f(Y_{\text{obs}}\|\theta)$
$\ell(\theta\|Y_{\text{obs}})$	observed log-likelihood
$\nabla\ell(\theta\|Y_{\text{obs}})$	score vector
$I(\theta\|Y_{\text{obs}})$	observed information, $-\nabla^2\ell(\theta\|Y_{\text{obs}})$
$J(\theta)$	Fisher/expected information, $E\{I(\theta\|Y_{\text{obs}})\|\theta\}$
$\hat{\theta}$	MLE of $\hat{\theta}$
$\text{Se}(\hat{\theta})$	standard error of $\hat{\theta}$
$\text{Cov}(\hat{\theta})$	covariance matrix of $\hat{\theta}$
$\ell(\theta\|Y_{\text{obs}}, Z)$	complete-data log-likelihood
I_{com}	complete information, $I(\theta\|Y_{\text{obs}})\|_{\theta=\hat{\theta}}$
I_{obs}	observed information
I_{mis}	missing information
$\pi(\theta)$	prior distribution/density of θ
$f(\theta\|Y_{\text{obs}}, Z)$	complete-data posterior distribution

$f(Z\|Y_{\text{obs}}, \theta)$	conditional predictive distribution
$f(\theta\|Y_{\text{obs}})$	observed-data posterior distribution
$f(Z\|Y_{\text{obs}})$	marginal predictive distribution
$\{X^{(i)}\}_{i=1}^{m}$	m i.i.d. samples from the distribution of X
$\{X_{(i)}\}_{i=1}^{m}$	order statistics of m i.i.d. samples
$\tilde{\theta}$	mode of $f(\theta\|Y_{\text{obs}})$
$J(y \to x)$	Jacobian determinant from y to x, $\|\partial y/\partial x\|$
$\text{logit}(p)$	logit transformation, $\log(p/(1-p))$

References

Aitchison, J. and Dunsmore, I.R. (1975). *Statistical Prediction Analysis.* Cambridge University Press.

Albert, J.H. (1992). Bayesian estimation of normal ogive item response curves using Gibbs sampling. *J. of Educational Statist.* **17**, 251–269.

Albert, J.H. (1993). Teaching Bayesian statistics using sampling methods and MINITAB. *Am. Statist.* **47**, 182–191.

Albert, J.H. and Chib, S. (1993). Bayesian analysis of binary and polychotomous response data. *J. Am. Statist. Assoc.* **88**, 669–679.

Albert, J.H. and Gupta, A.K. (1983). Estimation in contingency tables using prior information. *J. Roy. Statist. Soc., B* **45**, 60–69.

Albert, J.H. and Gupta, A.K. (1985). Bayesian methods for binomial data with applications to a nonresponse problem. *J. Am. Statist. Assoc.* **80**, 167–174.

Angers, J.F. and Biswas, A. (2003). A Bayesian analysis of zero-inflated generalized Poisson model. *Comput. Statist. Data Anal.* **42**, 37–46.

Arnold, B.C. and Press, S.J. (1989). Compatible conditional distributions. *J. Am. Statist. Assoc.* **84**, 152–156.

Arnold, B.C. and Strauss, D. (1988). Bivariate distributions with exponential conditionals. *J. Am. Statist. Assoc.* **83**, 522–527.

Arnold, B.C., Castillo, E. and Sarabia, J.M. (1999). *Conditional Specification of Statistical Models.* Springer, New York.

Arnold, B.C., Castillo, E. and Sarabia, J.M. (2001). Quantification of incompatibility of conditional and marginal information. *Commun. Statist. — Theory Meth.* **30**, 381–395.

Arnold, B.C., Castillo, E. and Sarabia, J.M. (2002). Exact and near compatibility of discrete conditional distributions. *Comput. Statist. Data Anal.* **40**, 231–252.

Arnold, B.C., Castillo, E. and Sarabia, J.M. (2004). Compatibility of partial or complete conditional probability specifications. *J. of Statist. Planning and Inference* **123**, 133–159.

Arnold, S.F. (1993). Gibbs sampling. In *Handbook of Statistics: Computational Statistics* (C.R. Rao, ed.), Vol.9, 599–625. Elsevier Science Publishers B.V., New York.

Barlow, R.E., Bartholomew, D.J., Bremner, J.M. and Brunk, H.D. (1972). *Statistical Inference Under Order Restrictions.* Wiley, New York.

Bates, D.M. and Watts, D.G. (1988). *Nonlinear Regression Analysis and Its Applications.* Wiley, New York.

Bayes, T. (1763). An essay towards solving a problem in the doctrine of chances. *Philosophical Transactions of the Royal Society,* 330–418. Reprinted with biographical note by G.A. Barnard, in *Biometrika* **45**, 293–315, 1958.

Becker, M.P., Yang, I. and Lange, K. (1997). EM algorithms without missing data. *Statistical Methods in Medical Research* **6**, 38–54.

Berger, J.O. (1980). *Statistical Decision Theory: Foundations, Concepts, and Methods.* Springer, New York.

Besag, J.E. (1974). Spatial interaction and the statistical analysis of lattice systems. *J. Roy. Statist. Soc., B* **36**, 192–236.

Besag, J.E. (1989). A candidate's formula: A curious result in Bayesian prediction. *Biometrika* **76**, 183.

Besag, J.E. and Green, P.J. (1993). Spatial statistics and Bayesian computation (with discussions). *J. Roy. Statist. Soc., B* **55**, 25–37.

Bijleveld, C.C.J.H. and De Leeuw, J. (1991). Fitting longitudinal reduced-rank regression models by alternating least squares. *Psychometrika* **56**, 433–447.

Böhning, D. (1992). Multinomial logistic regression algorithm. *Ann. Institute Statist. Math.* **44**, 197–200.

Böhning, D. (1998). Zero-inflated Poisson models and C.A.MAN: A tutorial collection of evidence. *Biometrical J.* **40**(7), 833–843.

Böhning, D. and Lindsay, B.G. (1988). Monotonicity of quadratic approximation algorithms. *Ann. Institute Statist. Math.* **40**, 641–663.

Bonate, G. (1998). *Analysis of Pretest Posttest Designs.* Chapman & Hall/CRC, Boca Raton.

Booth, J.G. and Hobert, J.P. (1999). Maximizing generalized linear model likelihood with an automated Monte Carlo EM algorithm. *J. Roy. Statist. Soc., B* **61**, 265–285.

Box, G.E.P. and Muller, M.E. (1958). A note on the generation of random normal deviates. *Ann. Math. Statist.* **29**, 610–611.

Box, G.E.P. and Tiao, G.C. (1973). *Bayesian Inference in Statistical Analysis.* Reading, Addison–Wesley, Massachusetts.

Breslow, N.E. and Clayton, D.G. (1993). Approximate inference in generalized linear mixed models. *J. Am. Statist. Assoc.* **88**, 9–25.

Breslow, N.E. and Lin, X.H. (1995). Bias correction in generalized linear mixed models with single component of dispersion. *Biometrika* **82**, 81–91.

Brodsky, B.E. and Darkhovsky, B.S. (1993). *Nonparametric Methods in Change Point Problems.* Series: Mathematics and Its Applications, Vol. 243. Springer, New York.

Broffitt, J.D. (1988). Increasing and increasing convex Bayesian graduation. *Transaction of the Society of Actuaries* **40**, 115–148.

Brooks, S.P. and Roberts, G.O. (1998). Assessing convergence of Markov chain Monte Carlo algorithms. *Statist. and Computing* **8**, 319–335.

Brown, B.W. (1980). Prediction analyses for binary data. In Biostatistics Casebook (R.J. Miller, B. Efron, B.W. Brown and L.E. Moses, eds.). Wiley, New York.

Bulter, J.W. (1958). Machine sampling from given probability distributions. In *Symposium on Monte Carlo Methods* (M.A. Meyer, ed.). Wiley, New York.

Carlin, B.P. and Louis, T.A. (2000). *Bayes and Empirical Bayes Methods for Data Analysis* (2nd Ed.). Chapman & Hall/CRC, Boca Raton.

Carlin, B.P., Gelfand, A.E. & Smith, A.F.M. (1992). Hierarchical Bayesian analysis of changepoint problems. *Appl. Statist.* **41**, 389–405.

Casella, G. (1996). Statistical inference and Monte Carlo algorithms (with discussion). *Test* **5**(2), 249–344.

Casella, G. and George, E.I. (1992). Explaining the Gibbs sampler. *Am. Statist.* **46**, 167–174.

Casella, G. and Robert, C.P. (1998). Post-processing accept-reject samples: Recycling and rescaling. *J. Comput. Graph. Statist.* **7**(2), 139–157.

Casella, G., Lavine, M. and Robert, C.P. (2001). Explaining the perfect sampler. *Am. Statist.* **55**, 299–305.

Castledine, B. (1981). A Bayesian analysis of multiple-recapture sampling for a closed population. *Biometrika* **67**(1), 197 210.

Chao, A. (1998). Capture-recapture. In *Encyclopedia of Biostatistics* (P. Armitage and T. Colton, Editors–in–Chief), 482–486. Wiley, New York.

Chaudhuri, A. and Mukerjee, R. (1988). *Randomized Response: Theory and Techniques.* Marcel Dekker, New York.

Chen, J. and Gupta, A.K. (2000). *Parametric Statistical Change Point Analysis.* Springer, New York.

Chen, M.H. (1994). Importance–weighted marginal Bayesian posterior density estimation. *J. Am. Statist. Assoc.* **89**, 818–824.

Chen, M.H. (2005). Computing marginal likelihoods from a single MCMC output. *Statistica Neerlandica* **59**, 16–29.

Chen, M.H. and Shao, Q.M. (1997). On Monte Carlo methods for estimating ratios of normalizing constants. *Ann. Statist.* **25**, 1563–1594.

Chen, M.H., Shao, Q.M. and Ibrahim, J.G. (2000). *Monte Carlo Methods in Bayesian Computation.* Springer, New York.

Chib, S. (1992). Bayes inference in the Tobit censored regression model. *J. of Econometrics* **51**, 79–99.

Chib, S. (1995). Marginal likelihood from the Gibbs output. *J. Am. Statist. Assoc.* **90**, 1313–1321.

Chib, S. (2000). Bayesian methods for correlated binary data. In *Generalized Linear Models: A Bayesian Perspective* (D.K. Dey, S.K. Ghosh and B.K. Mallick, eds.), 113–131. Marcel Dekker, New York.

Chib, S. and Greenberg, E. (1998). Analysis of multivariate probit models. *Biometrika* **85**, 347–361.

Chiu, H.Y. and Sedransk, J. (1986). A Bayesian procedure for imputing missing values in sample surveys. *J. Am. Statist. Assoc.* **81**, 667–676.

Choi, S.C. and Stablein, D.M. (1982). Practical tests for comparing two proportions with incomplete data. *Appl. Statist.* **31**, 256–262.

Christofides, T.C. (2005). Randomized response technique for two sensitive characteristics at the same time. *Metrika* **62**(1), 53–63.

Collett, D. (1991). *Modeling Binary Data.* Chapman & Hall, London.

Cover, T.M. and Thomas, J.A. (1991). *Elements of Information Theory.* Wiley, New York.

Cowles, M.K. and Carlin, B.P. (1996). Markov chain Monte Carlo convergence diagnostics: A comparative study. *J. Am. Statist. Assoc.* **91**, 883–904.

Cox, D.R. (1972). Regression models and life tables (with discussion). *J. Roy. Statist. Soc., B* **74**, 187–220.

Cox, D.R. and Oakes, D. (1984). *Analysis of Survival Data.* Chapman & Hall, London.

Crowder, M.J., Kimber, A.C., Smith, R.L. and Sweeting, T.J. (1991). *Statistical Analysis of Reliability.* Chapman & Hall, London.

Dalbey, W. and Lock, S. (1982). Inhalation toxicology of diesel fuel obscurant aerosol in Sprague–Dawley rats. *ORNL/TM–8867*, Biology Division, Oak Ridge National Laboratory.

David, H.A. (1981). *Order Statistics* (2nd Ed.). Wiley, New York.

Dawid, A.P. and Skene, A.M. (1979). Maximum likelihood estimation of observer error rates using the EM algorithm, *Appl. Statist.* **28**, 20–28.

De Leeuw, A.R. (1994). Block relaxation algorithms in statistics. In *Information Systems and Data Analysis* (H.H. Bock, W. Lenski and M.M. Richter, eds.), 308–325. Springer, Berlin.

De Leeuw, J. and Heiser, W.J. (1977). Convergence of correction matrix algorithms for multidimensional scaling. In *Geometric Representations of Relational Data* (J. C. Lingoes, E. Roskam and I. Borg, eds.), 735–752. Mathesis Press, Ann Arbor.

Dempster, A.P., Laird, N.M. and Rubin, D.B. (1977). Maximum likelihood from incomplete data via the EM algorithm (with discussion). *J. Roy. Statist. Soc., B* **39**, 1–38.

De Pierro, A.R. (1995). A modified EM algorithm for penalized likelihood estimation in emission tomography. *IEEE Transactions on Medical Imaging* **14**, 132–137.

Devroye, L. (1986). *Non-Uniform Random Variate Generation.* Springer, New York.

Diebolt, J. and Robert, C.P. (1994). Estimation of finite mixture distributions through Bayesian sampling. *J. Roy. Statist. Soc., B* **56**, 363–375.

Elffers, H., Robben, H.S.J. and Hessing, D.J. (1992). On measuring tax evasion. *J. of Economic Psychology* **13**, 545–567.

Escobar, M. and West, M. (1995). Bayesian density estimation and inference using mixtures. *J. Am. Statist. Assoc.* **90**, 577–588.

Evans, M. and Swartz, T. (1995). Methods for approximating integrals in statistics with special emphasis on Bayesian integration problems (with discussions). *Statist. Sci.* **10**, 254–272.

Evans, M. and Swartz, T. (2000). *Approximating Integrals via Monte Carlo and Deterministic Methods.* Oxford University Press, Oxford.

Fang, H.B., Tian, G.L. and Tan, M. (2004). Hierarchical models for tumor xenograft experiments in drug development. *Journal of Biopharmaceutical Statistics* **14**(14), 931–945.

Fang, H.B., Tian, G.L., Xiong, X.P. and Tan, M. (2006). A multivariate random-effects model with restricted parameters: Application to assessing radiation therapy for brain tumors. *Statistics in Medicine* **25**, 1948–1959.

Fang, K.T., Kotz, S. and Ng, K.W. (1990). *Symmetric Multivariate and Related Distributions.* Chapman & Hall, London.

Fox, J. and Tracy, P. (1984). Measuring associations with randomized response. *Soc. Sci. Res.* **13**, 188–197.

Fox, J. and Tracy, P. (1986). *Randomized Response: A Method for Sensitive Surveys.* Sage, Beverly Hills, California.

Gamerman, D. (1997). *Markov Chain Monte Carlo: Stochastic Simulation for Bayesian Inference.* Chapman & Hall, London.

Gasparini, M. and Eisele, J. (2000). A curve-free method for phase I clinical trials. *Biometrics* **56**, 609–615.

Gaver, D.P. and O'Muircheartaigh, I.G. (1987). Robust empirical Bayes analysis of event rates. *Technometrics* **29**, 1–15.

Geisser, S. (1993). *Predictive Inference: An Introduction.* Chapman & Hall, London.

Gelfand, A.E. (1994). Gibbs Sampling. In *Encyclopedia of Statistical Sciences* (S. Kotz, ed.). Wiley, New York.

Gelfand, A.E. (2002). Gibbs sampling. In *Statistics in the 21-st Century* (A.E. Raftery, M.A. Tanner and M.T. Wells, eds.), 341–349. Chapman & Hall/CRC, Boca Raton.

Gelfand, A.E. and Dey, D.K. (1994). Bayesian model choice: Asymptotics and exact calculations. *J. Roy. Statist. Soc., B* **56**, 501–514.

Gelfand, A.E. and Smith, A.F.M. (1990). Sampling-based approaches to calculating marginal densities. *J. Am. Statist. Assoc.* **85**, 398–409.

Gelfand, A.E., Hills, S.E., Racine–Poon, A. and Smith, A.F.M. (1990). Illustration of Bayesian inference in normal data models using Gibbs sampling. *J. Am. Statist. Assoc.* **85**, 972–985.

Gelfand, A.E., Smith, A.F.M. and Lee, T.M. (1992). Bayesian analysis of constrained parameter and truncated data problems using Gibbs sampling. *J. Am. Statist. Assoc.* **87**, 523–532.

Gelman, A. (1996a). Inference and monitoring convergence. In *Markov Chain Monte Carlo in Practice* (W.R. Gilks, S. Richardson and D.J. Spiegelhalter, eds.), 131–143. Chapman & Hall, London.

Gelman, A. (1996b). Bayesian model-building by pure thought: Some principles and examples. *Statistica Sinica* **6**, 215–232.

Gelman, A. and King, G. (1990). Estimating the electoral consequences of legislative redirecting. *J. Am. Statist. Assoc.* **85**, 274–282.

Gelman, A. and Rubin, D.B. (1992). Inference from iterative simulation using multiple sequences (with discussion). *Statist. Sci.* **7**(4), 457–511.

Gelman, A. and Speed, T.P. (1993). Characterizing a joint probability distribution by conditionals. *J. Roy. Statist. Soc., B* **55**, 185–188.

Gelman, A. and Speed, T.P. (1999). Corrigendum: Characterizing a joint probability distribution by conditionals. *J. Roy. Statist. Soc., B* **61**, Part 2, 483.

Gelman, A., Carlin, J.B., Stern, H.S. and Rubin, D.B. (1995). *Bayesian Data Analysis.* Chapman & Hall, London.

Geman, S. and Geman D. (1984). Stochastic relaxation, Gibbs distributions, and the Bayesian restoration of images. *IEEE Transactions on Pattern Analysis and Machine Intelligence* **6**, 721–741.

Geng, Z. and Asano, C. (1989). Bayesian estimation methods for categorical data with misclassification. *Commun. Statist. — Theory Meth.* **18**, 2935–2954.

Geng, Z. and Shi, N.Z. (1990). Isotonic regression for umbrella orderings. *Appl. Statist.* **39**, 397–402.

George, E.I. and Robert, C.P. (1992). Capture-recapture estimation via Gibbs sampling. *Biometrika* **79**, 677–683.

Geweke, J. (1989). Bayesian inference in econometric models using Monte Carlo integration. *Econometrica* **57**, 1317–1340.

Geyer, C.J. (1991). Constrained maximum likelihood exemplified by isotonic convex logistic regression. *J. Am. Statist. Assoc.* **86**, 717–724.

Geyer, C.J. (1992). Practical Markov chain Monte Carlo. *Statist. Sci.* **7**, 473–503.

Ghosh, S.K., Mukhopadhyay, P. and Lu, J.C. (2006). Bayesian analysis of zero-inflated regression models. *J. of Statist. Planning and Inference* **136**, 1360–1375.

Gilks, W.R. and Wild, P. (1992). Adaptive rejection sampling for Gibbs sampling. *Appl. Statist.* **41**, 337–348.

Gilks, W.R., Clayton, D.G., Spiegelhalter, D.J., Best, N.G., McNeil, A.J., Sharples, L.D. and Kirby, A.J. (1993). Modeling complexity: Applications of Gibbs sampling in medicine (with discussion). *J. Roy. Statist. Soc., B* **55**, 39–52.

Gilks, W.R., Richardson, S. and Spiegelhalter, D.J. (1996). *Markov Chain Monte Carlo in Practice.* Chapman & Hall, London.

Givens, G.H. and Raftery, A.E. (1996). Local adaptive importance sampling for multivariate densities with strong nonlinear relationships. *J. Am. Statist. Assoc.* **91**, 132–141.

Gnedenko, B.V. (1962). *The Theory of Probability.* Chelsea, New York.

Greenberg, B.G., Abul–Ela, A.A., Simmons, W.R. & Horvitz, D.G. (1969). The unrelated question randomized response model: Theoretical framework. *J. Am. Statist. Assoc.* **64**, 520–539.

Groer, P.G. and Pereira, C.A.DeB. (1987). Calibration of a radiation detector: Chromosome dosimetry for neutrons. In *Probability and Bayesian Statistics* (R. Viertl, ed.), 225–252. Plenum Press, New York.

Guida, M., Calabria, R. and Pulcini, G. (1989). Bayes inference for a nonhomogeneous Poisson process with power intensity law. *IEEE Transactions on Reliability* **38**, 603–609.

Gumbel, E.J. (1960). Bivariate exponential distributions. *J. Am. Statist. Assoc.* **55**, 698–707.

Gupta, P.L., Gupta, R.C. and Tripathi, R.C. (1996). Analysis of zero-adjusted count data. *Comput. Statist. Data Anal.* **23**, 207–218.

Halpern, A.L. (1999). Minimally selected p and other tests for a single abrupt changepoint in a binary sequence. *Biometrics* **55**, 1044–1050.

Hammersley, J.M. and Clifford, M.S. (1970). Markov fields on finite graphs and lattices. Unpublished.

Hasselblad, V., Stead, A.G. and Crenson, J.P. (1980). Multiple probit analysis with a non-zero background. *Biometrics* **36**, 650–663.

Heilbron, D.C. (1989). Generalized linear models for altered zero probabilities and overdispersion in count data. *Unpublished Technical Report*, Dept of Epidemiology and Biostatistics, U. of California at San Francisco.

Heiser, W.J. (1987). Correspondence analysis with least absolute residuals. *Comput. Statist. and Data Analysis* **5**, 337–356.

Heiser, W.J. (1995). Convergent computing by iterative majorization: Theory and applications in multidimensional data analysis. In *Recent Advances in Descriptive Multi. Analysis* (W.J. Krzanowski, ed.), 157–189. Clarendon Press, Oxford.

Henderson, R. and Matthews, J.N.S. (1993). An investigation of changepoints in the annual number of cases of haemolytic uraemic syndrome. *Appl. Statist.* **42**, 461–471.

Hinde, J. and Demetrio, C.G.B. (1998). Overdispersion: models and estimation. *Comput. Statist. Data Anal.* **27**, 151–170.

Hirotsu, C. (1998). Isotonic inference. In *Encyclopedia of Biostatistics* (P. Armitage and T. Colton, eds.), 2107–2115. Wiley, New York.

Hobert, J.P. and Casella, G. (1996). The effect of improper priors on Gibbs sampling in hierarchical linear models. *J. Am. Statist. Assoc.* **91**, 1461–1473.

Hobert, J.P. and Casella, G. (1998). Functional compatibility, Markov chains, and Gibbs sampling with improper priors. *J. Comp. Graph. Statist.* **7**, 42–60.

Horvitz, D.G., Shah, B.V. and Simmons, W.R. (1967). The unrelated question randomized response model. In *1967 Proceedings of the Social Statistics Section, Am. Statist. Association*, 65–72.

Huber, P.J. (1981). *Robust Statistics.* Wiley, New York.

Hunter, D.R. and Lange, K. (2000). Rejoinder to discussions of "Optimization transfer using surrogate objective functions". *J. Comput. Graph. Statist.* **9**, 52–59.

Hunter, D.R. and Lange, K. (2004). A tutorial on MM algorithms. *Am. Statist.* **58**, 30–37.

Jarrett, R.G. (1979). A note on the intervals between coal-mining disasters. *Biometrika* **66**, 191–193.

Jeffreys, H. (1961). *Theory of Probability* (3rd Ed.). Oxford University Press, Oxford.

Jennrich, R.I. and Schluchter, M.D. (1986). Unbalanced repeated measures models with structured covariance matrices. *Biometrics* **42**, 805–820.

Jiang, J. (1998). Consist estimators in generalized linear mixed models. *J. Am. Statist. Assoc.* **93**, 720–729.

Johnson, M.E. (1987). *Multivariate Statistical Simulation.* Wiley, New York.

Johnson, N.L. and Kotz, S. (1969–1972). *Distributions in Statistics* (4 Vols.). Wiley, New York.

Johnson, N.L., Kotz, S. and Balakrishnan, N. (1994). *Continuous Univariate Distributions, Vol. 1* (2nd Ed.). Wiley, New York.

Johnson, N.L., Kotz, S. and Balakrishnan, N. (1995). *Continuous Univariate Distributions, Vol. 2* (2nd Ed.). Wiley, New York.

Johnson, N.L., Kotz, S. and Kemp, A.W. (1992). *Univariate Discrete Distributions* (2nd Ed.). Wiley, New York.

Johnson, W.O. and Gastwirth, J.L. (1991). Bayesian inference for medical screening tests: Approximations useful for the analysis of a acquired immune deficiency syndrome. *J. Roy. Statist. Soc., B* **53**, 427–439.

Jones, G.L. and Hobert, J.P. (2001). Honest exploration of intractable probability distribution via Markov chain Monte Carlo. *Statist. Sci.* **16**, 312–334.

Joseph, L., Gyorkos, T.W. and Coupal, L. (1995). Bayesian estimation of disease prevalence and the parameters of diagnosis tests in the absence of a gold standard. *Am. J. Epidemiol.* **141**, 263–272.

Kadane, J.B. (1985). Is victimization chronic? A Bayesian analysis of multinomial missing data. *J. of Econometrics* **29**, 47–67.

Kass, R.E. and Raftery, A.E. (1995). Bayes factors. *J. Am. Statist. Assoc.* **90**, 773–795.

Khintchine, A.Y. (1938). On unimodal distributions. *Tomsk. Universitet. Nauchno-issledovatel' skii institut matematiki i mek-haniki IZVESITIIA* **2**, 1–7.

Kiers, H.A.L. and Ten Berge, J.M.F. (1992). Minimization of a class of matrix trace functions by means of refined majorization. *Psychometrika* **57**, 371–382.

Kim, J.M. and Warde, W.D. (2005). Some new results on the multinomial randomized response model. *Commun. Statist. — Theory Meth.* **34**, 847–856.

Kotz, S. and Troutt, M.D. (1996). On vertical density representation and ordering of distributions. *Statistics* **28**, 241–247.

Kotz, S., Fang, K.T. and Liang, J.J. (1997). On multivariate vertical density representation and its application to random number generation. *Statistics* **30**, 163–180.

Kuk, A.Y.C. (1995). Asymptotically unbiased estimation in generalized linear models with random effects. *J. Roy. Statist. Soc., B* **57**, 395–407.

Kuo, L. and Yang, T.Y. (1996). Bayesian computation for nonhomogeneous Poisson process in software reliability. *J. Am. Statist. Assoc.* **91**, 763–773.

Laird, N.M. and Ware, J.H. (1982). Random-effects models for longitudinal data. *Biometrics* **38**, 963–974.

Lakshmi, D.V. and Raghavarao, D. (1992). A test for detecting untruthful answering in randomized response procedures. *J. of Statist. Planning and Inference* **31**(3), 387–390.

Lambert, D. (1992). Zero-inflated Poisson regression, with an application to defects in manufacturing. *Technometrics* **34**, 1–14.

Lange, K. (1999). *Numerical Analysis for Statisticians.* Springer, New York.

Lange, K. (2002). *Mathematical and Statistical Methods for Genetic Analysis* (2nd Ed.). Springer, New York.

Lange, K. and Carson, R. (1984). EM reconstruction for emission and transmission tomography. *J. of Computer Assisted Tomography* **8**, 306–312.

Lange, K. and Fessler, J.A. (1995). Globally convergent algorithms for maximum a posteriori transmission tomography. *IEEE Transactions on Image Processing* **4**, 1430–1438.

Lange, K., Hunter, D.R. and Yang, I. (2000). Optimization transfer using surrogate objective functions (with discussion). *J. Comput. Graph. Statist.* **9**, 1–20.

Larsen, R.I., Gardner, D.E. and Coffin, D.L. (1979). An air quality data analysis system for interrelating effects, standards and needed sourced reductions. Part 5: No. 2, Mortality of mice. *J. Air. Pollut. Control Assoc.* **39**, 113–117.

Lee, A.H., Xiang, L. and Fung, W.K. (2004). Sensitivity of score tests for zero-inflation in count data. *Statist. in Medicine* **23**, 2757–2769.

Lee, D. (1997). Selecting sample sizes for the sampling/importance resampling filter. *Proceedings of the Section on Bayesian Statistical Science*, ASA, 72–77.

Lee, E.T. (1974). A computer program for linear logistic regression analysis. *Computer Program in Biomedicine* **4**, 80–92.

Lee, R.M. (1993). *Doing Research on Sensitive Topics.* Sage, Newbury Park, CA.

Lehmann, E.L. (1983). *Theory of Point Estimation.* Wiley, New York.

Leonard, T. (2000). *A Course in Categorical Data Analysis.* Chapman & Hall/CRC, Boca Raton.

Li, K.H. (2004). The sampling/importance resampling algorithm. In *Applied Bayesian Modeling and Causal Inference from Incomplete Data Perspectives* (A. Gelman and X.L. Meng, eds.), 265–276. Wiley, New York.

Li, K.H. (2007). Pool size selection for the sampling/importance resampling algorithm. *Statistica Sinica* **17**(3), 895–907.

Lin, X.H. and Breslow, N.E. (1996). Bias correction in generalized linear mixed models with multiple components of dispersion. *J. Am. Statist. Assoc.* **91**, 1007–1016.

Lindley, D. (1995). Simplicity. *RSS News* **22**, 1–3.

Little, R.J.A. and Rubin, D.B. (2002). *Statistical Analysis with Missing Data* (2nd Ed.). Wiley, New York.

Liu, C.H. (1999). Efficient ML estimation of the multivariate normal distribution from incomplete data. *J. Multi. Anal.* **69**, 206–217.

Liu, C.H. (2000). Estimation of discrete distributions with a class of simplex constraints. *J. Am. Statist. Assoc.* **95**, 109–120.

Liu, C.H. and Rubin, D.B. (1994). The ECME algorithm: A simple extension of EM and ECM with faster monotone convergence. *Biometrika* **81**, 633–648.

Liu, C.H., Rubin, D.B. and Wu, Y.N. (1998). Parameter expansion to accelerate EM: The PX-EM algorithm. *Biometrika* **85**, 755–770.

Liu, J.S. (2001). *Monte Carlo Strategies in Scientific Computing.* Springer, New York.

Liu, J.S. (1994). The collapsed Gibbs sampler in Bayesian computation with application to a gene-regulation problem. *J. Am. Statist. Assoc.* **89**(427), 958–966.

Liu, J.S., Wong, W.H. and Kong, A. (1994). Covariance structure of the Gibbs sampler with applications to the comparisons of estimators and augmentation schemes. *Biometrika* **81**, 27–40.

Liu, J.S., Wong, W.H. and Kong, A. (1995). Covariance structure and convergence rate of the Gibbs sampler with various scans. *J. Roy. Statist. Soc., B* **57**, 157–169.

Louis, T.A. (1982). Finding the observed information matrix when using the EM algorithm. *J. Roy. Statist. Soc., B* **44**, 226–233.

Lyles, R., Taylor, D.J., Hanfelt, J.J. and Kupper, L.L. (2001). An alternative parametric approach for discrete missing data problems. *Commun. Statist. — Theory Meth.* **30**, 1969–1988.

Maas, B., Garnett, W.R., Pollock, I.M. and Carnstock, T.J. (1987). A comparative bioavailability study of Carbamazepine tablets and the chewable formulation. *Therapeutic Drug Monitoring* **9**, 28–33.

Maguire, B.A., Pearson, E.S. and Wynn, A.H.A. (1952). The time intervals between industrial accidents. *Biometrika* **38**, 168–180.

Marshall, A. (1956). The use of multi-stage sampling schemes in Monte Carlo computations. In *Symposium on Monte Carlo Methods* (M. Mayer, ed.), 123–140. Wiley, New York.

Marshall, A.W. and Olkin, I. (1979). *Inequality: Theory of Majorization and Its Applications.* Academic, San Diego.

Marske, D. (1967). Biochemical oxygen demand data interpretation using sums of squares surface. M.Sc. Thesis, University of Wisconsin.

McAllister, M.K. and Ianelli, J.N. (1997). Bayesian stock assessment using catch-age data and the sampling/importance resampling algorithm. *Canad. J. Fisheries and Aquatic Sci.* **54**, 284–300.

McAllister, M.K., Pikitch, E.K., Punt, A.E. and Hilborn, R. (1994). A Bayesian approach to stock assessment and harvest decisions using the sampling/importance resampling algorithm. *Canad. J. Fisheries and Aquatic Sci.* **51**, 2673–2687.

McCullagh, P. and Nelder, J.A. (1989). *Generalized Linear Models* (2nd Ed.). Chapman & Hall/CRC, Boca Raton.

McCulloch, C.E. (1994). Maximum likelihood variance components estimation for binary data. *J. Am. Statist. Assoc.* **89**, 330–335.

McCulloch, C.E. (1997). Maximum likelihood algorithms for generalized linear mixed models. *J. Am. Statist. Assoc.* **92**, 162–170.

McLachlan, G.J. (1997). *Recent Advances in Finite Mixture Models.* Wiley, New York.

McLachlan, G.J. and Krishnan, T. (1997). *The EM Algorithm and Extensions.* Wiley, New York.

Meng, X.L. (1996). Comments on "Statistical inference and Monte Carlo algorithms," by G. Casella. *Test* **5**(2), 310–318.

Meng, X.L. and Rubin, D.B. (1991). Using EM to obtain asymptotic variance–covariance matrices: The SEM algorithm. *J. Am. Statist. Assoc.* **86**, 899–909.

Meng, X.L. and Rubin, D.B. (1993). Maximum likelihood estimation via the ECM algorithm: A general framework. *Biometrika* **80**, 267–278.

Meng, X.L. and van Dyk, D. (1997). The EM algorithm — an old folk-song sung to a fast new tune (with discussion). *J. Roy. Statist. Soc., B* **59**, 511–567.

Meng, X.L. and van Dyk, D. (1998). Fast EM-type implementations for mixed effects models. *J. Roy. Statist. Soc., B* **60**, 559–578.

Mengersen, K.L., Robert, C.P. and Guihenneuc–Jouyaux, C. (1999). MCMC convergence diagnostics: A review. In *Bayesian Statistics, 6* (J.M. Bernardo, J.O. Berger, A.P. Dawid and A.F.M. Smith, eds.), 415–440. Oxford University Press, Oxford.

Metropolis, N. and Ulam, S. (1949). The Monte Carlo method. *J. Am. Statist. Assoc.* **44**, 335–341.

Michael, J.R., Schucany, W.R. and Hass, R.W. (1976). Generating random variates using transformations with multiple roots. *Am. Statist.* **30**, 88–90.

Milford, D.V., Taylor, C.M., Gutteridge, B., Hall, S.M., Rowe, B. and Kleanthous, H. (1990). Haemolytic uraemic syndromes in the British Isles 1985–8: association with verocytotoxin producing Escherichia coli. Part 1: Clinical and epidemiological aspects. *Arch. Dis. Child.* **65**(7), 716–721.

Mudholkar, G.S. and George, G.O. (1978). A remark on the shape of the logistic distribution. *Biometrika* **65**, 667–668.

Murray, G.D. (1977). Contribution to the discussion of paper by A.P. Dempster, N.M. Laird and D.B. Rubin. *J. Roy. Statist. Soc., B* **39**, 27–28.

Newton, M.A. and Raftery, A.E. (1994). Approximate Bayesian inference with the weighted likelihood bootstrap (with discussion). *J. Roy. Statist. Soc., B* **56**, 3–48.

Ng, K.W. (1969). Generalizations of Some Fixed Point Theorems In Metric Spaces. M.Sc. Thesis in the University of Alberta, Canada.

Ng, K.W. (1970). A Remark on Contractive Mappings. *Canadian Mathematical Bulletin* **13**, 111–113.

Ng, K.W. (1995a). Explicit formulas for unconditional pdf. Research Report No. 82 (March 1995), Department of Statistics, the University of Hong Kong, Hong Kong.

Ng, K.W. (1995b). On the inversion of Bayes theorem. Presentation in *The 3rd ICSA Statistical Conference*, August 17–20, Beijing, P.R. China.

Ng, K.W. (1996). Inversion of Bayes formula without positivity assumption. Presentation in *Sydney International Statistical Congress 1996*, ASC Contributed Session: Topics in Statistical Inference III, July 12, 8:30–10:20 am, Sydney, Australia. Abstract #438 in Final Programme.

Ng, K.W. (1997a). Inversion of Bayes formula: Explicit formulas for unconditional pdf. In *Advances in the Theory and Practice in Statistics — A Volume in Honor of Samuel Kotz* (N.L. Johnson and N. Balakrishnan, eds.), 571–584. Wiley, New York.

Ng, K.W. (1997b). Applications of inverse Bayes formula. Presentation in *The 1997 International Symposium on Contemporary Multivariate Analysis and Its Applications*, under the I. Theme: *Bayesian Computation* organized by A. Lo and W.H. Wong, Preprint p. I.1–10, May 19–22, 1997, Hong Kong.

Ng, K.W., Tang, M.L., Tan, M. and Tian, G.L. (2008). Grouped Dirichlet distribution: A new tool for incomplete categorical data analysis. *J. Multi. Anal.* **99**(3), 490–509.

Ng, K.W., Tang, M.L., Tian, G.L. and Tan, M. (2009). The nested Dirichlet distribution and incomplete categorical data analysis. *Statistica Sinica* **19**(1), 251–271.

Nordheim, E.V. (1984). Inference from nonrandomly missing categorical data: An example from a genetic study on Turner's syndrome. *J. Am. Statist. Assoc.* **79**, 772–780.

Nyquist, H., Rice, S.O. and Riordan, J. (1954). The distribution of random determinants. *Quarterly of Appl. Math.* **42**, 97–104.

Odell, P.L. and Feiveson, A.H. (1966). A numerical procedure to generate a sample covariance matrix. *J. Am. Statist. Assoc.* **61**, 199–203.

Ortega, J.M. and Rheinboldt, W.C. (1970). *Iterative Solutions of Nonlinear Equations in Several Variables.* Academic, New York.

Papageorgiou, H. (1983). On characterizing some bivariate discrete distributions. *Australian J. of Statist.* **25**, 136–144.

Patil, G.P. (1965). On a characterization of multivariate distribution by a set of its conditional distributions. In *Handbook of the 35th International Statistical Institute Conference in Belgrade.* International Statistical Institute.

Paulino, C.D.M. and Pereira, C.A.B. (1995). Bayesian methods for categorical data under informative general censoring. *Biometrika* **82**, 439–446.

Philippe, A. (1997a). Simulation output by Riemann sums. *J. Statist. Comput. Simul.* **59**(4), 295–314.

Philippe, A. (1997b). Importance sampling and Riemann sums. *Prepub. IRMA* **43**, VI, Université de Lille.

Pievatolo, A. and Rotondi, R. (2000). Analyzing the interevent time distribution to identify seismicity phases: a Bayesian nonparametric approach to the multiple-changepoint problem. *Appl. Statist.* **49**, 543–562.

Pothoff, R.F. and Roy, S.N. (1964). A generalized multivariate analysis of variance model useful especially for growth curve problems. *Biometrika* **51**, 313–326.

Press, S.J. (1989). *Bayesian Statistics: Principles, Models and Applications.* Wiley, New York.

Qiu, Z., Song, P. and Tan, M. (2002). Bayesian hierarchical models for multi-level ordinal data using WinBUGS. *Journal of Biopharmaceutical Statistics* **12**, 121–135.

Qu, Y., Tan, M. and Kutner, M.H. (1996). Random-effects models in latent class analysis for evaluating accuracy of diagnostic tests. *Biometrics* **52**, 797–810.

Raftery, A.E. and Akman, V.E. (1986). Bayesian analysis of a Poisson process with a change-point. *Biometrika* **73**, 85–89.

Raftery, A.E., Givens, G.H. and Zeh, J.E. (1995). Inference from a deterministic population dynamics model for bowhead whales. *J. Am. Statist. Assoc.* **90**, 402–416.

Ramgopal, P., Laud, P.W. and Smith, A.F.M. (1993). Nonparametric Bayesian bioassay with prior constraints on the shape of the potency curve. *Biometrika* **80**, 489–498.

Rao, C.R. (1973). *Linear Statistical Inferences and Its Applications* (2nd Ed.). Wiley, New York.

Raudenbush, S.W., Yang, M.L. and Yosef, M. (2000). Maximum likelihood for generalized linear models with nested random effects via high-order, multivariate Laplace approximation. *J. Comput. Graph. Statist.* **9**, 141–157.

Ridout, M.S., Demetrio, C.G.B. and Hinde, J.P. (1998). Models for count data with many zeros. *Proceedings of the XIXth International Biometrics Conference*, Cape Town, 179–192.

Ritter, C. and Tanner, M.A. (1992). Facilitating the Gibbs sampler: The Gibbs stopper and the griddy-Gibbs sampler. *J. Am. Statist. Assoc.* **87**, 861–868.

Robert, C.P. (1995). Simulation of truncated normal variables. *Statist. Comput.* **5**, 121–125.

Robert, C.P. (1996). Mixtures of distributions: inference and estimation. In *Markov Chain Monte Carlo in Practice* (W.R. Gilks, S. Richardson and D.J. Spiegelhalter, eds.), 441–464. Chapman & Hall, London.

Robert, C.P. (1998). *Discretization and MCMC Convergence Assessment.* Lecture Notes in Statistics, Vol. 135. Springer, New York.

Robert, C.P. and Casella, G. (1999). *Monte Carlo Statistical Methods.* Springer, New York.

Roberts, G.O. and Polson, N.G. (1994). On the geometric convergence of the Gibbs sampler. *J. Roy. Statist. Soc., B* **56**, 377–384.

Robertson, T., Wright, F.T. and Dykstra, R.L. (1988). *Order Restricted Statistical Inference.* Wiley, New York.

Rodrigues, J. (2003). Bayesian analysis of zero-inflated distributions. *Commun. Statist. — Theory Meth.* **32**(2), 281–289.

Rosenblatt, M. (1952). Remarks on a multivariate transformation. *Ann. Math. Statist.* **23**, 470–472.

Ross, S.M. (1983). *Stochastic Processes.* Wiley, New York.

Ross, S.M. (1991). *A Course in Simulation.* Macmillan Publishing Company, New York.

Rubin, D.B. (1976). Inference and missing data. *Biometrika* **63**, 581–592.

Rubin, D.B. (1987a). *Multiple Imputation for Nonresponse in Surveys.* Wiley, New York.

Rubin, D.B. (1987b). Comments on "The calculation of posterior distributions by data augmentation," by M.A. Tanner and W.H. Wong. *J. Am. Statist. Assoc.* **82**, 543–546.

Rubin, D.B. (1988). Using the SIR algorithm to simulate posterior distributions (with discussions). In *Bayesian Statistics*, Vol.3 (J.M. Bernardo, M.H. DeGroot, D.V. Lindley and A.F.M. Smith, eds.), 395–402. Oxford University Press, Oxford.

Rubin, D.B. and Thayer, T.T. (1982). EM algorithm for ML factor analysis. *Psychometrika* **47**, 69 76.

Rubinstein, R.Y. (1997). Optimization of computer simulation models with rare events. *European J. of Operational Research* **99**, 89–112.

Rubinstein, R.Y. and Kroese, D.P. (2004). *The Cross-Entropy Method.* Springer, New York.

Schafer, J.L. (1997). *Analysis of Incomplete Multivariate Data.* Chapman & Hall, London.

Schervish, M.J. and Carlin, B.P. (1992). On the convergence of successive substitution sampling. *J. Comput. Graph. Statist.* **1**, 111–127.

Schmee, J. and Hahn, G.J. (1979). A simple method for regression analysis with censored data. *Technometrics* **21**, 417–434.

Schmoyer, R.L. (1984). Sigmoidally constrained maximum likelihood estimation in quantal bioassay. *J. Am. Statist. Assoc.* **79**, 448–453.

Schoenfeld, D.A. (1986). Confidence bounds for normal means under order restrictions with application to dose-response curves, toxicology experiments and low-dose extrapolation. *J. Amer. Statist. Assoc.* **81**, 186–195.

Schukken, Y.H., Casella, G. and van den Broek, J. (1991). Overdispersion in clinical mastitis data from dairy herds: A negative binomial approach. *Preventive Veterinary Medicine* **10**, 239–245.

Seshadri, V. and Patil, G.P. (1964). A characterization of a bivariate distribution by the marginal and the conditional distributions of the same component. *Ann. Institute Statist. Math.* **15**, 215–221.

Shepp, L.A. and Vardi, Y. (1982). Maximum likelihood reconstruction for emission tomography. *IEEE Transactions on Image Processing* **2**, 113–122.

Shi, N.Z. (1988). A test of homogeneity for umbrella alternatives and tables of the level probabilities. *Commun. Statist. — Theory Meth.* **17**, 657–670.

Shuster, J. (1968). On the inverse Gaussian distribution function. *J. Am. Statist. Assoc.* **63**, 1514–1516.

Siegmund, D. (1988). Confidence sets in change point problems. *Int. Statist. Rev.* **56**, 31–48.

Silvapulle, M.J. and Sen, P.K. (2005). *Constrained Statistical Inference: Inequality, Order, and Shape Restrictions.* Wiley, New York.

Singhal, A., Davies, P., Sahota, A., Thomas, P.W. and Serjeant, G.R. (1993). Resting metabolic rate in homozygous sickle cell disease. *American J. of Clinical Nutrition* **57**, 32–34.

Skare, Ø., Bølviken, E. and Holden, L. (2003). Improved sampling importance resampling and reduced bias importance sampling. *Scand. J. Statist.* **30**, 719–737.

Smith, A.F.M. (1975). A Bayesian approach to inference about a change-point in a sequence of random variables. *Biometrika* **62**, 407–416.

Smith, A.F.M. (1980). Changepoint problems: Approaches and applications. In *Bayesian Statistics*, Vol. 1 (J.M. Bernardo, M.H. DeGroot, D. V. Lindley and A.F.M. Smith, eds.), 83–89. Valencia University Press, Valencia.

Smith, A.F.M. and Cook, D.G. (1980). Straight lines with a change-point: A Bayesian analysis of some renal transplant data. *Appl. Statist.* **29**, 180–189.

Smith, A.F.M. and Gelfand, A.E. (1992). Bayesian statistics without tears: A sampling–resampling perspective. *Am. Statist.* **46**, 84–88.

Smith, A.F.M. and Roberts, G.O. (1993). Bayesian computation via the Gibbs sampler and related Markov chain Monte Carlo methods (with discussion). *J. Roy. Statist. Soc., B* **55**, 3–23.

Song, C.C., Li, L.A., Chen, C.H., Jiang, T.J. and Kuo, K.L. (2006). Revisiting the compatible conditional distributions. Technical Report of Department of Mathematical Sciences, National Chengchi University, Taiwan.

Stephens, D.A. (1994). Bayesian retrospective multiple-changepoint identification. *Appl. Statist.* **43**, 159–178.

Stigler, S.M. (1983). Who discovered Bayes's theorem? *Am. Statist.* **37**, 290–296.

Strauss, S.M., Rindskopf, D.M., and Falkin, G.P. (2001). Modeling relationships between two categorical variables when data are missing: Examining consequences of the missing data mechanism in an HIV data set. *Multi. Behavioral Research* **36**(4), 471–500.

Tan, M., Fang, H.B. and Tian, G.L. (2005). Statistical analysis for tumor xenograft experiments in drug development. In *Contemporary Multivariate Analysis and Experimental Designs — In Celebration of Professor Kai–Tai Fang's 65th Birthday* (J. Fan and G. Li, eds.), 351–368. World Scientific Publishing Co. Ltd., New Jersey.

Tan, M., Tian, G.L. and Fang, H.B. (2003). Estimating restricted normal means using the EM-type algorithms and IBF sampling, In *Development of Modern Statistics and Related Topics — In Celebration of Professor Yaoting Zhang's 70th Birthday* (J. Huang and H. Zhang, eds.), 53–73. World Scientific Publishing Co. Ltd., New Jersey.

Tan, M., Tian, G.L. and Fang, H.B. (2007). An efficient MCEM algorithm for fitting generalized linear mixed models for correlated binary data. *J. Statist. Comput. Simul.* **77**(11), 929–943.

Tan, M., Tian, G.L. and Ng, K.W. (2003). A noniterative sampling method for computing posteriors in the structure of EM-type algorithms. *Statistica Sinica* **13**(3), 625–639.

Tan, M., Tian, G.L. and Ng, K.W. (2006). Hierarchical models for repeated binary data using the IBF sampler. *Comput. Statist. Data Anal.* **50**(5), 1272–1286.

Tan, M., Tian, G.L. and Tang, M.L. (2009). Sample surveys with sensitive questions: A non-randomized response approach. *The American Statistician* **63**(1), 9–16.

Tan, M., Tian, G.L. and Xiong, X.P. (2001). Explicit Bayesian solution for incomplete pre-post test problems using inverse Bayes formulae. *Commun. Statist. — Theory Meth.* **30**(6), 1111–1129.

Tan, M., Fang, H.B., Tian, G.L. and Houghton, P.J. (2002). Small-sample inference for incomplete longitudinal data with truncation and censoring in tumor xenograft models. *Biometrics* **58**(3), 612–620.

Tan, M., Fang, H.B., Tian, G.L. and Houghton, P.J. (2005). Repeated–measures models with constrained parameters for incomplete data in tumor xenograft experiments. *Statistics in Medicine* **24**, 109–119.

Tan, M., Fang, H.B., Tian, G.L. and Wei, G. (2005). Testing multivariate normality in incomplete data of small sample size. *J. Multi. Anal.* **93**, 164–179.

Tan, M., Qu, Y., Mascha, E. and Schubert, A. (1999). A Bayesian hierarchical model for multi-level repeated ordinal data: Analysis of oral practice examinations in a large anesthesiology training program. *Statistic in Medicine* **18**, 1983–1992.

Tan, M., Tian, G.L., Fang, H.B. and Ng, K.W. (2007). A fast EM algorithm for quadratic optimization subject to convex constraints. *Statistica Sinica* **17**(3), 945–964.

Tang, M.L., Ng, K.W., Tian, G.L. and Tan, M. (2007). On improved EM algorithm and confidence interval construction for incomplete $r \times c$ tables. *Comput. Statist. Data Anal.* **51**(6), 2919–2933.

Tanner, M.A. (1993). *Tools for Statistical Inference: Observed Data and Data Augmentation Methods* (3rd Printing). Springer–Verlag, New York.

Tanner, M.A. (1996). *Tools for Statistical Inference: Methods for the Exploration of Posterior Distributions and Likelihood Functions* (3rd Ed.). Springer–Verlag, New York.

Tanner, M.A. and Wong, W.H. (1987). The calculation of posterior distributions by data augmentation (with discussion). *J. Am. Statist. Assoc.* **82**, 528–550.

Tarr, P.I., Neill, M.A., Allen, J., Siccardi, C.J., Watkins, S.L. and Hickman, R.O. (1989). The increasing incidence of the hemolytic–uremic syndrome in King County, Washington: Lack of evidence for ascertainment bias. *Am. J. Epidemiol.* **129**(3), 582–586.

Tian, G.L. (2000). *Bayesian Analysis for Incomplete Data and Survey Techniques for Sensitivity Questions.* Postdoctoral Research Report, *Department of Probability and Statistics, Peking University*, Beijing, P.R. China.

Tian, G.L. and Tan, M. (2003). Exact statistical solutions using the inverse Bayes formulae. *Statist. & Prob. Letters* **62**(3), 305–315.

Tian, G.L., Ng, K.W. and Geng, Z. (2003). Bayesian computation for contingency tables with incomplete cell-counts. *Statistica Sinica* **13**(1), 189–206.

Tian, G.L., Ng, K.W. and Tan, M. (2008). EM-type algorithms for computing restricted MLEs in multivariate normal distributions and multivariate t-distributions. *Comput. Statist. Data Anal.* **52**(10), 4768–4778.

Tian, G.L., Tan, M. and Ng, K.W. (2007). An exact noniterative sampling procedure for discrete missing data problems. *Statistica Neerlandica* **61**(2), 232–242.

Tian, G.L., Tang, M.L. and Ng, K.W. (2009). A review on the development of compatibility and uniqueness of two conditional distributions. *International Statistical Review*, in press.

Tian, G.L., Ng, K.W., Li, K.C. and Tan, M. (2009). Noniterative sampling–based Bayesian methods for identifying changepoints in the sequence of cases of hemolytic uremic syndrome. *Comput. Statist. Data Anal.* **53**(9), 3314-3323.

Tian, G.L., Tan, M., Ng, K.W. and Tang, M.L. (2009). A unified method for checking compatibility and uniqueness for finite discrete conditional distributions. *Commun. Statist. — Theory Meth.* **38**, 115–129.

Tian, G.L., Tang, M.L., Yuen, K.C. and Ng, K.W. (2009). Further properties and new applications for the nested Dirichlet distribution. *Comput. Statist. Data Anal.*, in press.

Tian, G.L., Yu, J.W., Tang, M.L. and Geng, Z. (2007). A new nonrandomized model for analyzing sensitive questions with binary outcomes. *Statist. in Medicine* **26**(23), 4238–4252.

Tian, G.L., Yuen, K.C., Tang, M.L. and Tan, M. (2009). Bayesian nonrandomized response models for surveys with sensitive questions. *Statistics and Its Interface* **2**, 13–25.

Tierney, L. and Kadane, J.B. (1986). Accurate approximations for posterior moments and marginal densities. *J. Am. Statist. Assoc.* **81**, 82–86.

Troutt, M.D. (1991). A theorem on the density of the density ordinate and an alternative interpretation of the Box–Muller method. *Statistics* **22**(3), 463–466.

Troutt, M.D. (1993). Vertical density representation and a further remark on the Box–Muller method. *Statistics* **24**, 81–83.

Vardi, Y. and Lee, D. (1993). From image deblurring to optimal investments: Maximum likelihood solutions for positive linear inverse problems (with discussion). *J. Roy. Statist. Soc., B* **55**, 569–612.

Verbeke, G. and Molenberghs, G. (2000). *Linear Mixed Models for Longitudinal Data.* Springer, New York.

von Neumann, J. (1951). Various techniques used in connection with random digits. *National Bureau of Standards Appl. Math. Series* **12**, 36–38.

Warner, S.L. (1965). Randomized response: A survey technique for eliminating evasive answer bias. *J. Am. Statist. Assoc.* **60**, 63–69.

Wei, G.C.G. and Tanner, M.A. (1990). Posterior computations for censored regression data. *J. Am. Statist. Assoc.* **85**, 829–839.

Wesolowski, J. (1995a). Bivariate discrete measures via a power series conditional distribution and a regression function. *J. of Multivariate Analysis* **55**, 219–229.

Wesolowski, J. (1995b). Bivariate distributions via a Pareto conditional distribution and a regression function. *Ann. Institute Statist. Math.* **47**, 177–183.

West, M. and Harrison, J. (1989). *Bayesian Forecasting and Dynamic Models.* Springer, New York.

Wilks, S.S. (1932). Moments and distributions of estimates of population parameters from fragmentary samples. *Ann. Math. Statist.* **2**, 163–195.

Williams, R., Mackert, P., Fletcher, L., Olivi, S., Tian, G.L. and Wang, W. (2002). Comparison of energy prediction equations with measured resting energy expenditure in children with sickle cell anemia. *J. Am. Dietetic Assoc.* **102**(7), 956–961.

Worsley, K.J. (1986). Confidence regions and tests for a changepoint in a sequence of exponential family random variables. *Biometrika* **73**, 91–104.

Wu, Y.H. (2005). *Inference for Change Point and Post Change Means After a CUSUM Test.* Lecture Notes in Statistics, Vol. 180. Springer, New York.

Yakowitz, S., Krimmel, J.E. and Szidarovszky, F. (1978). Weighted Monte Carlo integration. *SIAM J. Numer. Anal.* **15**(6), 1289–1300.

Yip, P. (1988). Inference about the mean of a Poisson distribution in the presence of a nuisance parameter. *Australian J. Statist.* **30**, 299–306.

Yu, J.W., Tian, G.L. and Tang, M.L. (2008a). Statistical inference and prediction for the Weibull process with incomplete observations. *Comput. Statist. Data Anal.* **52**, 1587–1603.

Yu, J.W., Tian, G.L. and Tang, M.L. (2008b). Two new models for survey sampling with sensitive characteristic: Design and analysis. *Metrika* **67**(3), 251–263.

Zeger, S.L. and Karim, M.R. (1991). Generalized linear models with random effects: A Gibbs sampling approach. *J. Am. Statist. Assoc.* **86**, 79–86.

Zellner, A. and Min, C.K. (1995). Gibbs sampler convergence criteria. *J. Am. Statist. Assoc.* **90**, 921–927.

Zhou, X.H., Obuchowski, N.A. and McClish, D.K. (2002). *Statistical Methods in Diagnostic Medicine.* Wiley, New York.

Zhou, Y.Q. and Weng, Z.X. (1992). *Reliability Growth.* Science Press, Beijing, P.R. China.

Author Index

Subject Index